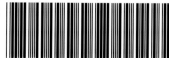

MANUAL OF PERIPHERAL VASCULAR INTERVENTION

MANUAL OF PERIPHERAL VASCULAR INTERVENTION

Editors

Ivan P. Casserly, MB, BCh

Department of Cardiology
Denver Veteran Affairs Medical Center
Denver, Colorado

Ravish Sachar, MD

Department of Cardiovascular Medicine
Wake Heart and Vascular Associates
Raleigh, North Carolina

Jay S. Yadav, MD

Department of Cardiovascular Medicine
Cleveland Clinic Foundation
Cleveland, Ohio

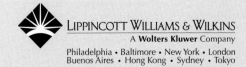

LIPPINCOTT WILLIAMS & WILKINS
A **Wolters Kluwer** Company
Philadelphia • Baltimore • New York • London
Buenos Aires • Hong Kong • Sydney • Tokyo

Acquisitions Editor: Frances R. DeStefano
Managing Editor: Joanne P. Bersin
Production Editor: Dave Murphy
Manufacturing Manager: Ben Rivera
Marketing Manager: Kathy Neely
Creative Director: Doug Smock
Design: Joseph DePinho
Compositor: TechBooks
Printer: Edwards Brothers

© 2005 by LIPPINCOTT WILLIAMS & WILKINS
530 Walnut Street
Philadelphia, PA 19106 USA
LWW.com

Printed in the USA

Library of Congress Cataloging-in-Publication Data

Manual of peripheral vascular intervention / editors, Ivan P. Casserly, Ravish Sachar, Jay S. Yadav.
  p. ; cm.
Includes bibliographical references and index.
ISBN 0-7817-5238-8 (alk. paper)
  1. Peripheral vascular diseases—Handbooks, manuals, etc.   2. Peripheral vascular diseases—Surgery—Handbooks, manuals, etc.   I. Casserly, Ivan P.   II. Sachar Ravish.
III. Yadav, Jay S.
  [DNLM: 1. Peripheral Vascular Diseases—surgery.   2. Vascular Surgical Procedures. WG 500 M2937 2005]
  RC694.M365 2005 616.1′31—dc22

                                                                                           2005007884

Care has been taken to confirm the accuracy of the information presented and to describe generally accepted practices. However, the authors, editors, and publisher are not responsible for errors or omissions or for any consequences from application of the information in this book and make no warranty, expressed or implied, with respect to the currency, completeness, or accuracy of the contents of the publication. Application of this information in a particular situation remains the professional responsibility of the practitioner.

The authors, editors, and publisher have exerted every effort to ensure that drug selection and dosage set forth in this text are in accordance with current recommendations and practice at the time of publication. However, in view of ongoing research, changes in government regulations, and the constant flow of information relating to drug therapy and drug reactions, the reader is urged to check the package insert for each drug for any change in indications and dosage and for added warnings and precautions. This is particularly important when the recommended agent is a new or infrequently employed drug.

Some drugs and medical devices presented in this publication have Food and Drug Administration (FDA) clearance for limited use in restricted research settings. It is the responsibility of the health care provider to ascertain the FDA status of each drug or device planned for use in their clinical practice.

10 9 8 7 6 5 4 3 2 1

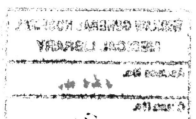

To the many gifted invasive cardiologists with whom I have trained (especially Drs. Franco, Taniuchi, Tuzcu, Whitlow and Yadav), for taking the time and having the patience to impart their knowledge, and to my parents for their selflessness and unwavering support.

Ivan P. Casserly

To my family: my parents, who have made everything possible; and my wife, Jignasa, and my children, Nikhil and Natasha, who make it all worthwhile. And to Jay, a mentor and a friend whose vision is a constant guide.

Ravish Sachar

To my wife (Marshalla) and my children (Nevin, Chethan, Priya and Daven) for making every day a pleasure and the remarkably talented interventional cardiology fellows at the Cleveland Clinic who make teaching a joy and a privilege.

Jay S. Yadav

Contents

Preface

The endovascular treatment of peripheral vascular disease has emerged as a viable alternative for patients, over conventional surgery. Improvements in catheter, balloon, and stent design, as well as the advent of distal emboli protection, have collectively enabled the safe, efficacious, and durable treatment of obstructive and aneurysmal vascular disease. These advances reflect the collective efforts of specialists from the fields of interventional cardiology, vascular surgery, and interventional radiology.

One of the major challenges in a burgeoning field such as peripheral vascular intervention, is that there are insufficient numbers of accredited fellowship positions dedicated solely to percutaneous peripheral vascular intervention. As a result, operators often finish fellowships with minimal specific training in peripheral vascular disease, and have to continue the learning process "on the job." Furthermore, for those already in practice, retraining in peripheral vascular intervention is often a difficult, and haphazard process, consisting of didactic and "hands-on" training through short courses offered in various institutions. For those who are already trained, this rapidly evolving field mandates that physicians constantly keep abreast of newer developments.

This book seeks to address some of the above challenges. First and foremost, this is a *manual* of peripheral vascular intervention, with a firm emphasis on *how to perform* peripheral vascular interventions. For this reason, we purposefully invited authors with the greatest hands-on experience to write the chapters and provide their insights. Every effort has been made to graphically illustrate the techniques and provide real-life examples of these procedures. There is also an obligation for operators to have a sound understanding of the clinical and non-invasive evaluation of patients with peripheral vascular disease, and a working knowledge of the anatomy and biology of the vascular bed in which they intend to intervene. We have therefore provided this information in as succinct a manner as possible, for each vascular bed.

We have tried to address intervention in all of the vascular territories. Some of the chapters, such as intracranial stenting, detail procedures that in many cases, are still experimental, and should be performed only by physicians with a firm grasp of intracerebral intervention. Carotid angioplasty and stenting has recently been approved by the FDA as an alternative to surgery, for patients with high-risk clinical and anatomic features. As such, we hope that the chapter on carotid intervention is especially useful. Other chapters, such as those on subclavian, iliofemoral, and infrapopliteal interventions, offer insights we hope will help even experienced operators.

Peripheral vascular intervention is an exciting and challenging field. While this book is not meant to serve as a replacement for essential didactic and hands-on training, our hope is that both trainees and experienced operators in each of the disciplines involved in performing peripheral vascular intervention will find this a useful and practical manual.

Ivan P. Casserly MB, BCh
Ravish Sachar MD
Jay S. Yadav MD

Contributor List

Alex Abou-Chebl, MD
Interventional Neurology
Section of Stroke & Neurologic Intensive Care
Department of Neurology
The Cleveland Clinic Foundation
Cleveland, Ohio

Gary M. Ansel, MD
Clinical Director of Peripheral Vascular Intervention
Mid-Ohio Cardiology and Vascular Consultants
Columbus, Ohio

Herbert D. Aronow, MD, MPH
Assistant Professor of Medicine
Director, Cardiac Catheterization Laboratory
Philadelphia Veteran's Affairs Medical Center
Director, Peripheral Intervention
Hospital of the University of Pennsylvania
Philadelphia, Pennsylvania

Christopher T. Bajzer, MD
Associate Director, Carotid & Peripheral
    Intervention
Sections of Vascular Medicine & Interventional
    Cardiology
Department of Cardiovascular Medicine
The Cleveland Clinic Foundation
Cleveland, Ohio

Giancarlo Biamino, MD
Professor of Medicine
Center for Cardiology, Angiology & Vascular
    Intervention
Director, Clinical and Interventional Angiology
Dept. for Clinical Angiology
Heart Center
University Leipzig
Leipzig, Germany

Ivan P. Casserly, MB, BCh
Assistant Professor of Medicine
Director of Interventional Cardiology
Denver Veterans Affairs Medical Center
Denver, CO

Albert W. Chan, MD, MSc, FRCP(C), FACC
Associate Director
Catheterization Laboratory
Ochsner Clinic Foundation
New Orleans, Louisiana

Leslie Cho, MD
Assistant Professor of Medicine
Director of Carotid Intervention
Loyola University Medical Center
    Stritch School of Medicine
Chicago, Illinois

Christopher J. Cooper, MD
Associate Professor & Director of Cardiovascular
    Research
Department of Medicine
Chief, Division of Cardiology
Medical College of Ohio
Toledo, Ohio

Kent W. Dauterman, MD, FACC
Director of Cardiology
Rogue Valley Medical Center
Medford, Oregon

Jeffrey Goldstein, MD
Interventional Cardiologist
Prairie Cardiovascular Consultants
Springfield, Illinois

Samir R. Kapadia, MD
Interventional Cardiologist
Department of Cardiovascular
    Medicine
The Cleveland Clinic Foundation
Cleveland, Ohio

Mahmoud B. Malas, MD
Division of Vascular Surgery, Department
    of Surgery
Montefiore Medical Center
Albert Einstein College of Medicine
Bronx, New York

Fred Moeslein, MD, PhD
Division of Radiology
Cleveland Clinic Foundation
Cleveland, Ohio

Debabrata Mukherjee, MD, MS, FACC
Associate Professor of Medicine
Division of Cardiovascular Medicine
University of Kentucky
Lexington, KY

Takao Ohki, MD
Chief of Vascular and Endovascular Surgery
Montefiore Medical Center
Albert Einstein College of Medicine
Bronx, New York

Jeffrey W. Olin, DO
Zena & Michael A. Wiener Cardiovascular
   Institute
Mt. Sinai School of Medicine
New York, New York

Kenneth Ouriel, MD
Chairman
Division of Surgery
The Cleveland Clinic Foundation
Cleveland, Ohio

Darren Postoak, MD
Assistant Professor
Cardiovascular and Interventional Radiology
University of Texas Health Science Center at
   San Antonio
San Antonio, Texas

Stephen Ramee MD, FACC
Section Head, Interventional Cardiology
Director, Cardiac Catheterization Laboratory
Ochsner Heart and Vascular Institute
New Orleans, Louisiana

Joel P. Reginelli, MD
Interventional Cardiologist
The Cardiology Center of Cincinnati
Cincinnati, Ohio

Krishna Rocha-Singh, MD
Assistant Professor of Medicine
Southern Illinois University School of Medicine
Prairie Cardiovascular Consultants
Springfield, Illinois

Marco Roffi, MD
Andreas Grüntzig Cardiovascular Catheterization
   Laboratories

University Hospital
Zurich, Switzerland

Ken Rosenfeld, MD
Director, Cardiac and Vascular Invasive Service
Massachusetts General Hospital
Boston, Massachusetts

Mark J. Sands, MD
Section Head Vascular and Interventional
   Radiology
The Cleveland Clinic Foundation
Cleveland, Ohio

Mitchell J. Silver, MD
Department of Cardiology and Vascular Medicine
Mid-Ohio Cardiology and Vascular Consultants
Columbus, Ohio

E. Murat Tuzcu, MD
Professor of Medicine
Cleveland Clinic Lerner College of Medicine
Case Western Reserve University
Cleveland, Ohio

Christopher J. White, MD, FACC
Chairman, Department of Cardiology
Director, Ochsner Heart & Vascular Institute
New Orleans, Louisiana

Mark H. Wholey, MD
Chairman, Pittsburgh Vascular Institute
University of Pittsburgh Medical Center
   Shadyside
5230 Centre Ave
Pittsburg, Pennsylvania

Michael Wholey, MD, MBA
Associate Professor and Chief
   Cardiovascular and Interventional Radiology
University of Texas
Health Science Center at San Antonio
San Antonio, Texas

Jay S. Yadav, MD
Director Peripheral Vascular Intervention
Department of Cardiovascular Medicine
The Cleveland Clinic Foundation
Cleveland, OH

Khaled M. Ziada, MD
Assistant Professor of Medicine
Gill Heart Institute
Division of Cardiovascular Medicine
University of Kentucky

Acknowledgements

Firstly, we would like to thank all of the contributing authors who took time from their busy clinical schedules to write their respective chapters. We owe a tremendous debt of gratitude to Marion Tomasko in the graphics department at the Cleveland Clinic who worked tirelessly in putting together many of the wonderful graphical illustrations in this book from our feeble sketches. We couldn't have completed this book without her help. Finally we thank the many people at Lippincott, Williams & Wilkins who have helped make this book a reality. Special thanks to Erin McMullan, Joanne Bersin and Ruth Weinberg.

Ivan P. Casserly
Ravish Sachar
Jay S. Yadav

CHAPTER 1

Guidelines for Training and Credentialing in Peripheral Vascular Intervention

Christopher J. White

BACKGROUND

There are compelling reasons for interventional cardiologists to undertake percutaneous treatment of noncoronary vascular diseases with a total body approach to patients with atherosclerotic diseases (1). Atherosclerosis is a systemic disease that often involves several vascular beds resulting in the common occurrence of both cardiac and noncardiac vascular problems (2,3). There is general agreement that a shortage of trained providers necessary to meet the rapidly increasing demand for percutaneous revascularization exists. Interventional cardiologists possess the technical skills necessary to perform peripheral vascular intervention but in general, have an inadequate knowledge base for vascular medicine, which is necessary. In recognition of the need for adult cardiovascular-medicine trainees to gain broader expertise in vascular medicine and vascular intervention, a Core Cardiology Training Symposium (COCATS-11) was developed (4).

Noncoronary vascular disease is frequently an important aspect of the management of patients with heart disease. Renovascular hypertension is the most common cause of secondary hypertension in patients with atherosclerosis. Renovascular hypertension causes resistant hypertension, which negatively impacts the medical management of angina pectoris and congestive heart failure. Peripheral-vascular symptoms, such as claudication, impair the effectiveness of cardiovascular rehabilitation programs. Coronary-artery atherosclerosis is the most common cause of morbidity and mortality in patients with atherosclerotic peripheral vascular disease.

FEASIBILITY OF CARDIOLOGISTS PERFORMING PERIPHERAL VASCULAR INTERVENTION

As experienced coronary interventionalists, the author and colleagues reported our initial experience in peripheral angioplasty in 164 consecutive patients over a 20-month period (5). Prior to performing angioplasty, the aforementioned providers observed the performance of peripheral angioplasty in several angiographic laboratories with high-volume case loads. The providers were proctored for initial cases by a qualified outside operator, and the initial cases were reviewed and discussed with an experienced vascular surgeon.

Lower extremity percutaneous transluminal angioplasty (PTA) was performed in 116 patients, upper extremity PTA in 30 patients, and renal artery PTA in 18 patients (Table 1-1).

Successful results were obtained in 92% (191/208) of the lesions attempted, with a successful PTA in 99% (155/157) of stenoses versus 71% (36/51) of occlusions ($p < 0.01$) (Figs. 1-1 and 1-2).

In no patient did a failed attempt result in worsening of the patient's clinical condition or

TABLE 1-1

Demographic of Initial Experience PTA Patients

- Patients   = 164
  Lower extremity = 116
  Upper extremity = 30
  Renal artery   = 18
- Vessels   = 208
- Lesion length   = 5.8 ± 8.0 cm
- Occlusions   = 25%

Adapted from White et al. Initial results of peripheral vascular angioplasty performed by experienced interventional cardiologists. *Am J Cardiol.* 1992; 69:1249–1250.

the need for emergency surgery. The overall major complication rate of 4.3% (7/164) was similar to other studies published in the literature.

Our experience supported the hypothesis that experienced interventional cardiologists, working in partnership with vascular surgeons, possessed the necessary technical skills to perform peripheral vascular angioplasty in a safe and effective manner. Our vascular surgery colleagues provided guidance in patient and lesion selection, which compensated for our limited fund of knowledge regarding vascular medicine. Our results did not demonstrate a learning curve. The percentage of patients with totally occluded vessels (25%) and the average lesion length (5.8 ± 8.0 cm) attests to the relatively difficult lesions routinely accepted for treatment.

Achieving a success rate of 92% for all lesions and a 99% success rate for stenoses suggested that coronary angioplasty skills are transferable to the treatment of noncoronary vascular lesions, and quite effectively. Our results of success rates

that were higher for nontotal occlusions and lesions of shorter length were consistent with the reported outcomes for vascular intervention in the literature.

FELLOWSHIP TRAINING IN NONCORONARY DIAGNOSTIC ANGIOGRAPHY

Cardiology fellows currently receive training in invasive cardiac and noncardiac angiography. An example of this training would be performing ascending and descending aortography in patients with suspected aortic dissection. These angiographic studies may include selective angiography of the aortic arch vessels, mesenteric vessels, renal arteries, and iliofemoral arteries. Another example is the routine performance of selective angiography of the subclavian, internal mammary, and gastroepiploic arteries, to determine patency of coronary bypass grafts. Screening renal angiography is frequently done in patients who are at increased risk for renal artery stenosis. Finally, routine imaging of the iliac and femoral arteries is commonly performed prior to placement of vascular closure devices.

Cardiologists performing noncardiac angiography are responsible for the accurate interpretation of the images they obtain. They must accept the liability for errors or omissions in their interpretation of noncoronary angiography, just as they do for coronary angiography. Physicians who feel insecure in their ability to interpret these films may ask for assistance or over-reading of the films by another qualified physician. Peer review of angiographic studies, in a non-threatening environment, leads to improved quality of peripheral angiographic studies and

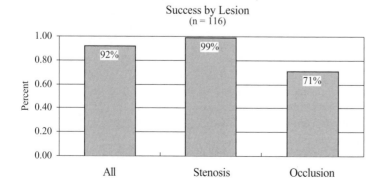

FIGURE 1-1 ● Success by lesion type. Adapted from White et al. Initial results of peripheral vascular angioplasty performed by experienced interventional cardiologists. *Am J Cardiol.* 1992; 69:1249–1250.

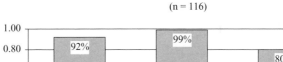

Success by Lesion Length
(n = 116)

FIGURE 1-2 ● Success by lesion length. Adapted from White et al.[5] Initial results of peripheral vascular angioplasty performed by experienced interventional cardiologists. *Am J Cardiol.* 1992; 69:1249–1250.

provides opportunities for less experienced angiographers to enhance their understanding of peripheral vascular anatomy, collateral circulations, and anatomic variations.

FELLOWSHIP TRAINING REQUIREMENTS FOR PERIPHERAL VASCULAR INTERVENTION

The American College of Cardiology Core Cardiology Training Symposium document provides guidelines for training in catheter based, peripheral vascular interventions (4). For the cardiovascular trainee wishing to acquire competence as a peripheral vascular interventionalist, a minimum of 12 months of training is recommended (Table 1-2). This period is in addition to the

TABLE 1-2

Recommended Fellowship Training Requirements for Cardiovascular Physicians

- Duration of training[1]—12 months
- Diagnostic coronary angiograms[2]—300 cases (200 as the primary operator)
- Diagnostic peripheral angiograms—100 cases (50 as primary operator)
- Peripheral interventional cases[3]—50 cases (25 as primary operator)

---

[1] After completing core cardiovascular training with at least eight months of cardiac catheterization.
[2] Coronary catheterization procedures should be completed prior to beginning interventional training.
[3] The case mix should be evenly distributed among the different vascular beds. Supervised cases of thrombus management for limb ischemia and venous thrombosis, utilizing percutaneous thrombolysis or thrombectomy, should be included.

required core cardiology training, and a minimum of 8 months in diagnostic cardiac catheterization in an ACGME-accredited fellowship program.

It is recommended that a cardiology fellow perform 300 coronary diagnostic procedures, including 200 with supervised primary responsibility, prior to beginning interventional training. The trainee in an ACGME-accredited program should participate in a minimum of 100 diagnostic peripheral angiograms and 50 noncardiac peripheral vascular interventional cases during the interventional training period. The case mix should be evenly distributed among the different vascular beds. Cases of thrombus management for limb ischemia or venous thrombosis, utilizing percutaneous thrombolysis or thrombectomy, should be included.

Advanced training in peripheral vascular intervention may be undertaken concurrently with a fourth year of training for coronary interventions. Peripheral vascular interventional training should include experience on an inpatient vascular medicine consultation service, in a noninvasive vascular-diagnostic laboratory, and include experience in longitudinal care of outpatients with vascular disease. Comprehensive training in vascular medicine, as discussed previously in this document, is not a prerequisite for noncoronary interventional training.

ALTERNATIVE TRAINING PATHWAYS FOR PERIPHERAL VASCULAR DISEASE (PVD) INTERVENTION

Many physicians with specialty training and board certification in interventional cardiology are currently performing peripheral vascular interventional procedures. These physicians have received either formal training in accredited programs or on-the-job training. Unfortunately, there currently exists little or no cooperation among the specialty training programs, with regard to peripheral vascular interventional training. There has been no uniform standard by which physicians with an interest in performing peripheral vascular interventional procedures may be measured.

An on-going turf war between competing subspecialties in many hospitals, over the provision of these services, is clearly not in the best interests of patients. Several professional societies including the American College of Cardiology, the American Heart Association, the American Society of Cardiovascular Interventionists, the Society of Cardiovascular Interventional Radiologists, the Society of Vascular Surgery, and the Society for Cardiovascular Angiography and Interventions have published disparate guidelines for the performance of peripheral angioplasty (6–11).

The realization that there is a need for cardiologists to provide noncoronary vascular care to patients with concomitant PVD has prompted revision of prior guidelines that were not cardiology specific (12). This was done in order to provide a more focused view of the role of the cardiologist, specifically the interventional cardiologist, in the management of these patients. Peripheral vascular intervention is currently being performed by cardiologists with widely varying backgrounds and clinical experience. Competency to perform peripheral vascular percutaneous interventions may be broken down into three categories or skill sets (Table 1-3).

Unrestricted Certification

Completion of at least 100 diagnostic peripheral angiograms, with a minimum of 50 peripheral interventional procedures, has been recommended for unrestricted certification (Table 1-4).

The physician should have been the supervised primary operator for one-half of the procedures. These procedures should be performed under the guidance of a credentialed peripheral-vascular interventionalist.

TABLE 1-3

Skills for Optimal Endovascular Intervention

- **Cognitive:** The fund of knowledge required is derived from the specialties of vascular medicine and angiology. It includes the knowledge of the natural history of the disease, the anatomy and physiology of the affected organ systems, interpretation of noninvasive tests, and an understanding of the indications for treatment and expected outcomes (risks and benefits) of the treatment options.
- **Procedural:** These skills involve the full range of invasive percutaneous cardiovascular techniques including gaining vascular access, performing diagnostic angiography, performing angioplasty and intervention, administering thrombolytic agents, and recognizing and managing complications of these procedures.
- **Clinical:** This category encompasses the skills necessary to manage inpatients and outpatients with noncardiac vascular diseases. It includes the ability to admit patients to the hospital and provide daily care. The ability to perform a complete history and physical examination, and to integrate the patient's history, physical examination and noninvasive laboratory data to make accurate diagnoses is required. Finally, it requires establishing a doctor-patient relationship and continuity of care in order provide long-term care for this chronic disease.

The case mix should be evenly distributed, so as to ensure exposure to diagnosis and intervention in a variety of different vascular beds. Experience that is heavily weighted toward treatment of one specific site (e.g., renal) to the exclusion of other vascular distributions (e.g., infrainguinal) may not provide adequate expertise for the latter. To achieve the balanced experience required for unrestricted competence, the following three broadly defined vascular territories should be evenly represented: 1) aortoiliac and brachiocephalic arteries (i.e., subclavian and axillary); 2) abdominal visceral arteries (i.e., renal and mesenteric arteries); and 3) infrainguinal arteries (i.e., femoral, popliteal, tibial, and peroneal arteries). In addition, unrestricted competence requires separate, supervised cases of thrombus management for limb ischemia or venous thrombosis, utilizing catheter-based thrombolysis or

TABLE 1-4

Suggested Alternative Pathways for Achieving Competency in Peripheral Vascular Intervention

Unrestricted Certification
- Diagnostic angiograms—100 cases (50 as primary operator)
- Peripheral interventions—50 cases (25 as primary operator)
  —aortoiliac, brachiocephalic arteries and extracranial carotid arteries
  —abdominal and visceral (renal and mesenteric) arteries
  —infrainguinal arteries
  —thrombolysis/thrombectomy

Restricted Certification
- Diagnostic angiograms—30 cases per specific vascular territory (15 as primary operator)
- Peripheral interventions
  —aortoiliac and brachiocephalic—15 cases (8 as primary operator)
  —abdominal and visceral (mesenteric and renal)—15 cases (8 as primary operator)
  —infrainguinal—15 cases (8 as primary operator)

thrombectomy, in a nonspecified vascular bed. Familiarity with thrombolytic agents and their uses is also required. Facility with other devices and technologies (e.g., mechanical) available for thrombus management is also desirable.

Obtaining competence in the performance of procedures and interventions in the extracranial cerebral vessels (i.e., carotid and vertebral arteries) is considered by many to be a unique category. There are unique challenges associated with gaining vascular access to the carotid and vertebral arteries, and in performing interventions in these circulatory beds. Secondly, there are obvious special issues related to the distribution and target organ of these vessels, which only allow very narrow safety margins. For those performing carotid or vertebral procedures, suggested requirements for achievement of competence include mastery of the cognitive and clinical skills pertaining specifically to this vascular bed and these procedures. This includes, as with other sites, a complete understanding of the anatomic and pathologic characteristics unique to this vascular bed and the abil-

ity to interpret relevant angiographic images. To achieve competence, additional diagnostic cerebrovascular angiograms and interventions should be performed, with appropriate documentation, follow-up monitoring, and outcomes assessment. As with procedures in other regional vascular venues, it is anticipated that for some physicians to achieve competence, supervising faculty will recommend additional cases beyond the minimum number.

Restricted Certification

Achieving competence in performing peripheral-vascular intervention need not be an all-or-nothing phenomenon. Rather, levels of competence in specific procedures or regional vascular territories may be achieved, particularly for those established physicians who have already completed formal training in coronary intervention or vascular surgery. A physician might become competent to perform interventions only in some regional circulations, but not in others. This is termed restricted certification. For example, one might acquire the skills to perform percutaneous renal, iliac, and subclavian intervention, yet not have adequate background or expertise to perform infrapopliteal or carotid intervention.

Competence in one area may be partly or wholly transferable to another, depending upon the degree of overlap or similarity between the vascular beds, the disease states, and the knowledge and skill sets involved. For example, the technical skills required to perform iliac artery intervention are partly transferable to subclavian-artery intervention, since the size of these vessels is comparable, and the therapeutic procedures are similar. In contrast, expertise in iliac artery revascularization does not confer comparable ability to perform carotid stenting, tibioperoneal angioplasty, or catheter-based thrombolysis, because of the dissimilarity of these interventions and their associated vascular territories.

Restricted certification may be achieved for each of the three major vascular territories defined previously (e.g., aortoiliac and brachiocephalic vessels; abdominal visceral arteries; and infrainguinal arteries) in which competence is sought; supervised performance of a minimum of diagnostic angiograms and interventions is required (Table 1-4). One-half of the diagnostic angiograms and one-half of the interventions in the specific territory must have been performed as the supervised primary operator. The cognitive and clinical skills pertaining to the particular territory should also have been mastered. Utilizing a restricted certification approach, a practicing physician possessing the requisite catheter skills may initially achieve competence in one, or more, selected territories and subsequently, may elect to progress in a step-wise fashion to gain unrestricted certification.

MAINTAINING CLINICAL COMPETENCY

Maintaining skill levels in catheter-based, peripheral vascular (noncoronary) interventions is an ongoing and continuing process. The physician's cognitive-knowledge base in PVD management and techniques must remain up to date. The physician must commit to ongoing education and life-long learning, through documented attendance at continuing medical education (CME) seminars in the field of expertise. Technical skills should be maintained via performance of a minimum of 25 peripheral vascular intervention cases annually, and with documentation of success and complication rates. Continuing appropriate board certification in his/her specific medical specialty or subspecialty, as well as appropriate recertification, is required.

CONCLUSION

There is evidence that the technical skills necessary to perform coronary intervention are transferable to the peripheral vasculature. However, an understanding of the natural history of peripheral disease, patient- and lesion-selection criteria, and the knowledge of treatment alternatives, are essential elements required to perform these procedures safely and effectively. For interventional cardiologists who are inexperienced in the treatment of PVD, appropriate preparation and training, including a team approach that involves an experienced vascular surgeon, are both de-sirable and necessary before attempting percutaneous peripheral angioplasty.

Clearly, patients with PVD are being under diagnosed and under treated. Patient care will benefit by increasing the number of physicians who may provide this needed care with either a restricted or unrestricted certification. Criticisms that the standards are being lowered may be countered by the implementation of on-going quality assurance programs.

There are inherent advantages for patients when the interventionalist performing the procedure is also the clinician responsible for the pre- and postprocedure care, analogous to the vascular surgeon who cares for patients before and after surgical procedures. Judgments regarding the indications, timing, and risk-to-benefit ratio of procedures, are enhanced by a long-term relationship between physician and patient. Finally, in view of the increased incidence of coronary artery disease in patients with atherosclerotic PVD, the participation of a cardiologist is appropriate.

REFERENCES

1. Isner JM, Rosenfield K. Redefining the treatment of peripheral artery disease. Role of percutaneous revascularization. *Circulation*. 1993;88:1534–1537.
2. Criqui MH. Peripheral arterial disease and subsequent cardiovascular mortality: a strong and consistent association. *Circulation*. 1990;82:2246–2247.
3. Hertzer NR. The natural history of peripheral vascular disease: Implications for its management. *Circulation*. 1991;83(2 Suppl):I12–I19.
4. Beller GA, Bonow RO, Fuster V, et al. ACC Revised Recommendations for Training in Adult Cardiovascular Medicine Core Cardiology Training II (COCATS 2) (Revision of the 1995 COCATS Training Statement). American College of Cardiology, March 8, 2002. Accessed 12-15-04, available at http://www.acc.org/clinical/training/COCATS2.pdf
5. White CJ, Ramee SR, Collins TJ, et al. Initial results of peripheral vascular angioplasty performed by experienced interventional cardiologists. *Am J Cardiol*. 1992;69:1249–1250.
6. Wexler L, Levin DC, Dorros G, et al. Training standards for physicians performing peripheral angioplasty: New developments. *Radiology*. 1991;178:19–21.
7. Guidelines for Percutaneous Transluminal Angioplasty. Standards of Practice Committee of the Society of Cardiovascular and Interventional Radiology. *Radiology*. 1990;177:619–626.
8. Guidelines for Performance of Peripheral Percutaneous Transluminal Angioplasty. The Society for Cardiac Angiography and Interventions Interventional Cardiology

Committee Subcommittee on Peripheral Interventions. *Cathet Cardiovasc Diagn.* 1988;21:128–129.

9. Pentecost MJ, Criqui MH, Dorros G, et al. Guidelines for peripheral percutaneous transluminal angioplasty of the abdominal aorta and lower extremity vessels. *Circulation.* 1994;84:511–531.

10. Spittell JA Jr, Nanda NC, Creager MA, et al. Recommendations for peripheral transluminal angioplasty: training and facilities. American College of Cardiology Peripheral Vascular Disease Committee. *J Am Coll Cardiol.* 1993;21:546–548.

11. Levin DC, Becker GJ, Dorros G, et al. Training standards for physicians performing peripheral angioplasty and other percutaneous peripheral vascular interventions. *J Vasc Intervent Radiol.* 2003;9 (Pt2):S359–S361.

12. Babb JD, Collins TJ, Cowley MJ, et al. Revised guidelines for the performance of peripheral vascular intervention. *Cathet Cardiovasc Intervent.* 1999;46:21–23.

CHAPTER 2

Noninvasive Evaluation of Arterial Disease

Khaled M. Ziada and Jeffrey W. Olin

Although an accurate medical history and physical examination remain the cornerstones of diagnosing arterial disease, clinicians should be aware of the limitations of clinical evaluation. For example, while 10% to 30% of patients with peripheral arterial disease (PAD) have typical claudication, and 20% to 40% have atypical leg symptoms, nearly 50% are totally asymptomatic (1,2). Moreover, early symptoms may be subtle or vague, with patients often not seeking medical attention until the advanced stages of the disease. This highlights the need for objective noninvasive methods to diagnose PAD. In addition, these methods are also essential in evaluating the location and severity of known disease, and assessing the success or failure of various therapies for PAD. The accuracy of noninvasive tests in the diagnosis, evaluation, and follow-up monitoring of PAD have resulted in a significant reduction in the need for invasive angiographic studies, which provides considerable savings for the health-care system without compromising quality of care. The purpose of this chapter is to outline the array of noninvasive tests that may be used to objectively assess peripheral vascular diseases.

LOWER LIMB ISCHEMIA

Limb Blood Pressure

Several physiologic facts about arterial pressure are important in interpreting limb pressure studies in patients with obstructive arterial disease of the extremities. First, systolic blood pressure measured distal to a hemodynamically significant obstructive lesion is *lower* than that measured proximally. The degree of 'regional hypotension' is directly related to the severity of the obstruction (3,4). Second, systolic pressure in the arterial system normally *increases* from the central aorta to the peripheral arteries. This is caused by reflection waves from the arterioles, bifurcation points and branches, which amplify the systolic pressure wave in the peripheral artery (5). In addition, the distensibility of the central aorta tends to dampen the peak of the systolic wave centrally, contributing to the same effect. Third, conditions that increase stiffness in the peripheral arteries, most commonly calcification, will result in an exaggerated increase in the difference between peripheral and central systolic pressures.

When evaluating limb pressures in the extremity, the following practice is used: a continuous wave Doppler device is used to detect flow in the artery of interest distal to a pneumatic cuff. The cuff is inflated to occlusive pressure and then gradually deflated. The systolic pressure is the point at which the flow signal is restored. Obviously, the cuff width should be proportional to the circumference of the limb segment under investigation; otherwise spuriously elevated (cuff too small) or reduced (cuff too large) values may be obtained.

The Ankle-Brachial Index

The Ankle-Brachial Index (ABI) is defined as the ratio between the systolic pressure measured over the posterior tibial or dorsalis pedis arteries (generally using the highest value), and the higher of the systolic pressures measured in both arms. A normal ABI is 0.9–1.30. A value over 1.30 indicates that the blood vessels are calcified, and not compressible, which typically occurs in patients with diabetes or end-stage renal disease. Under these circumstances, the ABI is artifactually increased and may be falsely read as normal (6,7). When this situation is suspected, the toe-brachial index (TBI), the ratio of the systolic pressure of the toe to that of the arm, should be used. A normal TBI is greater than 0.6. Greater weight should also be given to the pulse volume recordings (see below) in this setting.

A reduction in the ABI value indicates reduced arterial flow to the lower extremity (3,4,8). The degree of reduction correlates with severity of disease, but *does not* define the disease location. Values between 0.7–0.89 and 0.4–0.69 reflect mild and moderate disease, respectively, and are consistent with patients experiencing claudication. An ABI of less than or equal to 0.4 denotes severe disease and is consistent with short distance claudication or rest pain (9). Patients exhibiting critical limb ischemia almost always have an ABI of less than 0.40 and multi-level disease. The ABI is the method most commonly used to define lower extremity PAD in large population-based studies (10–12). Moreover, it has been correlated with clinical outcomes of different patient populations with vascular risk factors and coronary artery disease (13–16).

It should be noted that the ABI could be normal in the face of a hemodynamically significant stenosis. This most commonly occurs with disease in the aortoiliac segment. If the patient has a normal ABI but gives a convincing history of claudication, they should undergo a treadmill test to reproduce their symptoms and measure the ankle pressures after exercise. A decrease in ankle pressure (and ABI) due to a fixed amount of blood being delivered to the dilated vascular bed distally strongly supports the diagnosis of PAD.

Segmental Limb Pressures

The ABI serves as a useful screen to detect the presence of disease at some point along the length of the lower extremity (to the level of the ankle). Segmental limb pressures assess the systolic pressures at the upper and lower thigh, calf, and ankle, which helps define the segmental location of disease and the severity of disease in an arterial segment (Figs. 2-1, 2-2, 2-3).

After the ABI is calculated, the upper thigh cuff is inflated to occlusive pressure, and with a Doppler device placed over the dorsalis pedis artery, the cuff is deflated and the systolic pressure is recorded. This process is repeated with the cuff inflated at the lower thigh, upper calf, and ankle. Normally, the difference between systolic pressure at two consecutive levels should be less than 20 mmHg. A larger difference indicates obstructive disease in the arterial segment proximal to the cuff. The difference between the two limbs at the same level should also be less than 20 mmHg. A larger difference indicates obstructive disease proximal to the cuff on the side with the lower pressure (17). In addition to comparing pressures at different levels and between limbs, the absolute levels of pressure may be of value: an ankle pressure less than 50 mmHg is considered to be a sign of very poor perfusion and an unfavorable predictor of ulcer healing (18).

It is important to understand that pressures measured using this technique may be artifactually high. Using cuff measurements, the proximal thigh pressure is expected to be 20 mmHg to 30 mmHg higher than the brachial pressure. In addition to the increasing systolic pressure in the peripheral arteries, it is also possible that the pressure inside the cuff may not be fully transmitted to the artery embedded deep in the thigh. This may result in overestimation of the systolic pressure in the proximal thigh and underestimation of an aortoiliac obstruction. Therefore, if the systolic pressure in the thigh is equal to the brachial pressure, this should raise the possibility of aortoiliac disease (19). For that reason, we routinely measure a Doppler waveform at the common femoral artery. If it is normal (i.e., triphasic, see below), it is very unlikely that the patient has iliac disease.

Doppler Velocity Patterns

One of the valuable diagnostic clues that may be provided by a vascular laboratory is an analysis

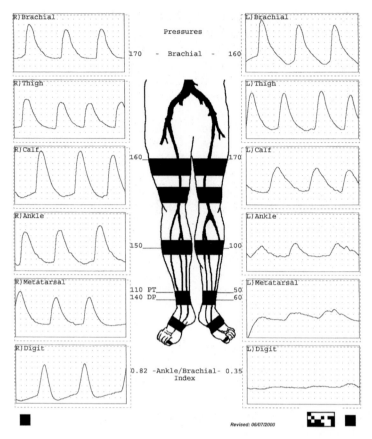

FIGURE 2-1 ● **Non-invasive assessment (ankle-brachial index [ABI], segmental limb pressures, and pulse volume recordings [PVR]) of lower extremity arterial circulation, in 73 year-old male with known peripheral vascular disease.** ABI - Right ABI is mildly reduced at 0.82 (140/170), left ABI is severely reduced at 0.35 (60/170). Segmental Limb Pressures and PVRs - Right-sided segmental-limb pressures show a 10-mmHg drop in gradient between the upper thigh, upper calf, and ankle. There is no segmental drop >20 mmHg, so one is unable to determine the level of disease causing the mild decrease in ABI. Note that the upper thigh pressure is less than the brachial pressure, raising a suspicion for aortoiliac disease. However, the PVR at this site appears normal suggesting that there is no significant aortoiliac disease. The remaining PVRs on the right side also appear normal.

Left-sided segmental limb pressures show significant (i.e., >20mmHg) drops in pressure between the upper thigh and the upper calf, and between the calf and the ankle, suggesting the presence of significant, left-sided, superficial femoral and popliteal artery disease, and below-knee disease. The metatarsal PVR tracings show marked diminution in amplitude, and the digit PVR tracing is flat, suggesting severe small-vessel disease in the left foot.

of the velocity waveforms of arterial flow. These waveforms are obtained using a Doppler device placed over the different segments of the arterial tree. The changes in the direction and velocity of arterial flow may be displayed on a screen and printed for documentation.

The normal Doppler tracing in the lower extremity vessels is described as triphasic: a main forward-flow systolic phase, a reverse-flow phase coinciding with late systole, and a secondary smaller forward-flow phase seen in diastole (Fig. 2-4A) (20). The presence of a normal tracing virtually excludes the presence of a proximal lesion

producing more than 50% stenosis. With early disease, the reverse-flow phase is lost leading to a biphasic wave. With more advanced disease, the amplitude of the forward systolic wave diminishes, and the wave becomes monophasic (Fig. 2-4B) (17). By obtaining waveforms at different levels, the location of the obstructive lesion may be identified.

Pulse Volume Recordings (PVR)

During the cardiac cycle, there are pulsatile volume changes in the limb. Since the volume of

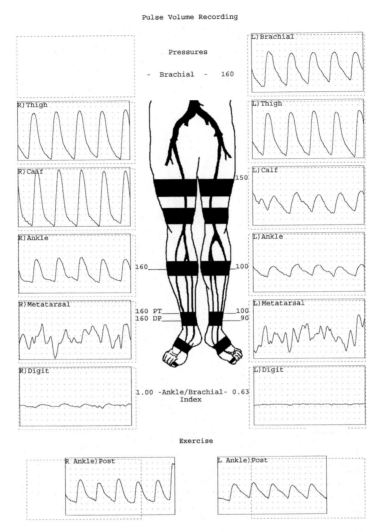

FIGURE 2-2 ● **Noninvasive evaluation (ankle-brachial index (ABI), segmental limb pressures, pulse volume recordings (PVR, and exercise study) of lower extremities in 65-year-old female with left leg claudication.** Brachial Pressures - The patient had a known right subclavian artery stenosis, making use of the left brachial artery pressure mandatory.

ABI - Right ABI is normal at 1.0 (160/160). Left ABI is moderately reduced at 0.63 (100/160). Segmental Limb Pressures and PVRs - Right-sided segmental limb pressures are identical from the upper thigh to the ankle, suggesting no significant disease in the superficial femoral artery, popliteal artery, or large below-knee arteries. The associated PVRs at these locations are normal. Note that the calf PVR is of greater amplitude than the thigh PVR, which is a normal finding. There is artifact in the PVR tracing from the metatarsal region, making interpretation difficult. The flat PVR from the digits suggests severe, small-vessel disease in the right foot.

Left-sided segmental limb pressures show a significant drop (>20 mmHg) in pressure between the thigh and upper calf. The PVR at the calf is of smaller amplitude than at the thigh, which is markedly abnormal. The PVR at the ankle is further diminished in amplitude, compared to the calf. These findings are consistent with femeropopliteal and intrapopliteal artery disease. The flat PVR tracing in the digits is consistent with severe, small-vessel disease in the left foot.

Exercise test - Following exercise, the left brachial pressure was 150 mmHg, the right ankle pressure was 140 mmHg, and the left ankle pressure was 80 mmHg. This response is within the normal range, in that there was a <20-mmHg drop in ankle pressures following exercise. Consistent with this conclusion is the fact that the PVR tracings from the ankles did not change with exercise.

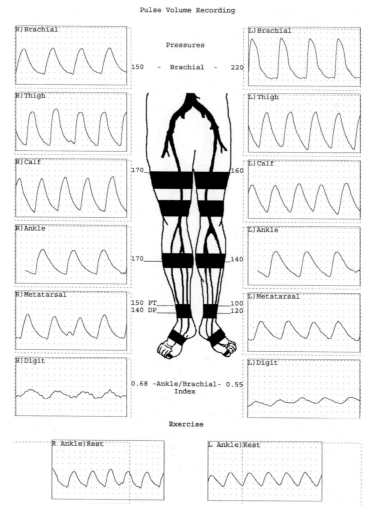

Pulse Volume Recording

FIGURE 2-3 ● **Noninvasive evaluation (ankle-brachial index (ABI), segmental limb pressures, pulse volume recordings (PVR), and exercise study) of lower extremities, in 78-year-old female with bilateral lower extremity claudication.** Brachial Pressure - Note the 70-mmHg pressure difference between the right and left brachial artery measurements, suggesting right-sided disease involving the innominate or subclavian artery. The right brachial PVR is decreased in amplitude and consistent with this diagnosis. The left brachial pressure must be used for ABI measurements in this patient. ABI – The ABI is moderately reduced in both limbs (Right 0.68, 150/220) (Left 0.55, 120/220). Segmental Limb Pressures and PVRs – There is a 50-mmHg drop in pressure between the left brachial pressure and the right upper thigh pressure, consistent with right-sided aortoiliac, common femoral, or profunda femoral disease. Although, there is no pressure drop between the right upper thigh and right calf pressure, the PVR tracing at the calf is lower in amplitude than at the thigh, which is abnormal, and suggestive of right-sided, superficial femoral and popliteal artery disease. There is a further 20-mmHg drop in pressure between the right upper calf and ankle, consistent with below-knee disease. The PVR in the right digit is severely blunted, suggesting severe, small-vessel disease in the right foot.

There is a 60-mmHg drop in pressure between the left brachial pressure and left upper thigh pressure, consistent with left-sided aortoiliac, left common femoral, or profunda femoral disease. There are further significant pressure drops (20 mmHg) between the left upper thigh and calf, and the left calf and ankle, consistent with left-sided superficial femoral and popliteal artery disease, and left-sided below-knee disease. The gradual drop in amplitude of the PVR waveforms at these levels is consistent with this conclusion. The severely blunted PVR waveform from the digits suggests severe, small-vessel disease in the left foot. Exercise test – Following exercise, the left brachial pressure was 220 mmHg, the right ankle pressure was 130 mmHg, and the left ankle was 90 mmHg. This represents a drop of 20 mmHg and 30 mmHg in the right and left ankle pressures, respectively, which is abnormal. Qualitatively, there is a drop in the amplitude of the ankle PVRs, consistent with an abnormal response to exercise.

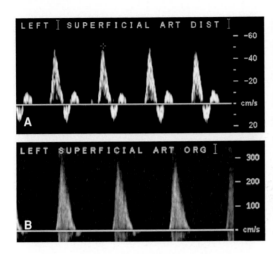

FIGURE 2-4 ● **Doppler-velocity patterns in lower extremity. A:** Normal triphasic waveform. **B:** Monophasic waveform indicative of significant proximal stenosis.

tissue and venous blood is relatively constant, the change in volume is directly related to the arterial flow. Using the same pneumatic cuffs that were utilized to measure segmental blood pressures, these volume changes may be measured using a pulse volume recorder. The cuff is inflated to a set pressure approximately 60 mmHg (in the presence of severe ischemia, especially in the foot and toe, the pressure in the cuff should be reduced). With each heartbeat, the limb expands leading to a change in the cuff pressure. That change may be presented on a spectral display and printed on a graduated chart, producing a plethysmographic tracing. Generally, every 1-mmHg change in the cuff pressure produces 20 mm of deflection on the spectral display. The PVR tracings are similar to arterial pulse wave tracings: rapid systolic upstroke followed by a rapid down stroke, interrupted by a prominent dicrotic notch (Figs. 2-1, 2-2, 2-3). With mild disease, the dicrotic notch is blunted. As the disease progresses, the change in volume, and hence the amplitude of the tracing, is diminished. In very severe obstructive lesions, the wave is almost flat, indicating no significant change in limb volume during systole (21). Pulse volume recordings provide a qualitative assessment of flow-mediated changes and when combined with segmental blood pressures are a very useful tool to assess the lower extremity circulation (22,23).

Exercise Testing

Similar to cardiac stress testing, the purpose of exercise testing in the evaluation of PAD is to reproduce the physiologic conditions that result in intermittent claudication. The treadmill exercise protocol may be either constant-grade (i.e., speed of 2 miles per hour and 12% incline, for 5 minutes) or variable-grade (2 miles per hour and 0% incline increasing by 2% every 2 minutes). Performance parameters that are monitored include the following: (1) the development of symptoms, (2) the duration of exercise, and (3) the change in ankle systolic pressure with exercise.

A normal individual should be able to perform this level of exercise for the 5-minute duration without developing claudication and with no or little drop in the ankle pressure (24). A small drop in pressure (less than 20 mmHg) may be noted, but is expected to return to pre-exercise levels within 2 to 3 minutes. A patient who stops exercise within the first minute due to leg symptoms usually has severe disease. If symptoms develop after 3 to 5 minutes, the disease is milder in severity and the patient's lifestyle should be factored in any decision regarding the need for revascularization. A drop in ankle pressure of more than 20 mmHg (or a significant reduction in pulse amplitude by PVR) at the end of the exercise is considered positive for obstructive disease (17,25). The time to recovery of systolic pressure at the ankle to pre-exercise levels is also proportional to the severity of obstruction (26). Development of leg pain without a drop in ankle pressure is almost always due to causes other than ischemia (27).

Exercise testing has several advantages; it establishes the diagnosis of PAD in patients with normal or mildly reduced resting ABI, but with significant symptoms. It is also a valuable objective measure of the functional impairment that the patient is experiencing. The comparison of the patient's performance before and after treatment (medical, endovascular or surgical) is a good measure of treatment success, and may be used as an objective assessment in follow-up.

Duplex Ultrasonography

As the name implies, Duplex imaging involves 2 modalities: brightness, or B-mode imaging, and

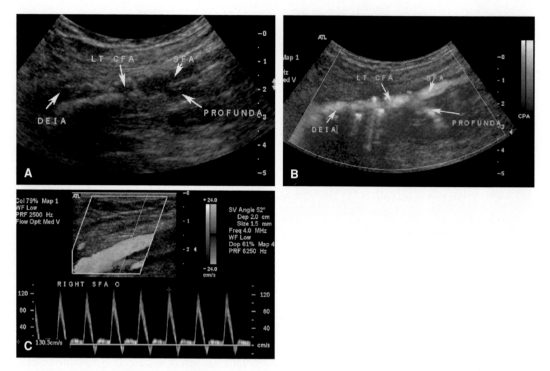

FIGURE 2-5 ● **Duplex ultrasonography of the common femoral artery (CFA) bifurcation. A:** B-mode ultrasound image showing limited detail of the arterial lumen and wall. **B:** Color power image from the same site clearly showing the lumen of the distal external iliac artery (DEIA), the CFA, and the proximal portions of the superficial femoral (SFA) and profunda arteries. **C:** Routine color Doppler of the CFA bifurcation facilitating sampling of Doppler waveform from the SFA.

pulsed-wave Doppler ultrasonography. B-mode or gray-scale imaging displays a 2-dimensional (2D) image of the arterial wall and lumen within the surrounding tissue, using transducers of variable frequencies (i.e., 2 MHz to 3 MHz, for iliac arteries; 5.0 MHz to 7.5 MHz for femoral and more distal arteries) (Figs. 2-5A and 2-5B).

Due to the difference in acoustic properties of the arterial wall layers and components of atherosclerotic plaques, the ultrasound reflections may be reconstructed into different shades of gray scale. The resolution of the gray-scale image permits a rough evaluation of the lesion and atheroma characteristics, but does not allow an accurate assessment of stenosis severity. Gray-scale imaging is also important in the identification and measurement of aortic and peripheral aneurysms, hematomas and false aneurysms.

The addition of pulsed-wave Doppler ultrasound resulted in a dramatic improvement of the sensitivity and specificity of the technique (28).

Pulsed-wave Doppler ultrasound complements the 2D imaging by providing a Doppler waveform of the flow within the lumen. The angle of insonation must be 60° or less. This allows analysis of direction, velocity and pattern of arterial flow. Color-coding the Doppler signal facilitates the examination of a specific arterial segment (Fig. 2-5C).

As color-coding allows interrogation of specific segments surveyed by B-mode imaging, waveforms of flow from the segment of interest are obtained and compared to waveforms from adjacent segments. At a stenotic segment, flow velocity increases to a degree proportional to the severity of the stenosis. Thus, diagnostic criteria have been developed that allow an estimation of the stenosis severity based on the Doppler waveforms obtained at the segment of interest and comparing it with waveforms obtained in a more proximal apparently normal segment (29). More recently, a simpler but more reliable classification has been adopted by most clinicians, in which arteries are classified into patent with mild disease, patent with at least 50% or more stenosis, and occluded. The main criterion for diagnosis of a hemodynamically significant lesion (angiographic diameter stenosis of 50% or more) is doubling of the peak systolic velocity (PSV) at the lesion site, compared to the proximal segment and a PSV of more than 200 cm per second with turbulence demonstrated on color Doppler (30,31). With less significant stenoses, the increase in PSV is less pronounced, the reverse-flow component of the triphasic wave is preserved, and the spectral broadening is less apparent (29).

Compared to digital subtraction imaging, Duplex imaging is an accurate tool in the detection of significant stenoses (more than 50% diameter reduction) and totally occluded vessels. The sensitivity and specificity of Duplex imaging in the detection of significant lesions are 92% and 97%, respectively. For total occlusions, the sensitivity and specificity are 95% and 99%, respectively (30,32,33). In general, more than 95% of the lower extremity arterial segments may be adequately visualized, with the exception of the peroneal artery, which may be examined in about 82% of patients (30).

Duplex imaging is also valuable in identifying the exact site of obstruction in patients with multiple diseased segments. This is critical in planning potential interventional or surgical therapies. Moreover, it is useful in the follow-up monitoring of patients who have undergone endovascular or surgical revascularization. In those situations, the segments of interest are well defined and baseline studies performed before and after the procedure serve as a useful reference.

Magnetic Resonance Arteriography

Magnetic Resonance Arteriography (MRA) of the peripheral arteries was previously performed without the use of contrast, using what was known as the 2D time-of-flight (2D TOF) technique. This approach had several technical limitations; acquisition times were lengthy, motion artifacts resulted in image degradation, and image quality was adversely affected when severely stenosed lesions resulted in diminished velocity of arterial flow and retrograde filling of occluded vessels occurred via collateral flow.

Contrast-enhanced (CE) three-dimensional (3D) peripheral MRA has supplanted this technique and overcome many of its technical limitations. Acquisition times are fast; with high-performance systems it may be as short as a breath hold. For a complete peripheral MRA study, imaging is sequentially performed on 3 overlapping fields: the aortoiliac region, the femoral-popliteal region and below-knee run-off vessels. Paramagnetic contrast agents are necessary for this fast, gradient-echo sequence acquisition. Gadolinium, the most commonly used contrast agent for this purpose, has no nephrotoxicity as compared to the iodinated contrast agents used with CT scanning or digital subtraction angiography (DSA). It is given as a peripheral intravenous bolus or as a slow infusion. The purpose of administering the agent is to shorten the T-1 relaxation time of blood, thus accentuating the signal-to-noise ratio within the lumen and eliminating the flow-related artifacts that plagued 2D-TOF imaging. The contrast agent is "chased" down the arterial tree by synchronizing table translation and image acquisition with arterial transit time. By acquiring volumetric 3D-data sets, it is possible to process the images on independent workstations, postprocedurally (34–36).

Using current technology, CE 3D MRA has a sensitivity of approximately 90% and specificity of about 97% in detection of hemodynamically significant stenoses in any of the lower extremity arteries, as compared to DSA (37–40). In patients presenting for surgical revascularization, MRA may identify small runoff vessels that were not visualized using mid-stream aortic DSA. This most typically occurs in patients with severe stenoses on multiple levels, which hinders adequate opacification of runoff vessels on DSA. Adequate visualization of run-off vessels may be extremely beneficial in planning limb salvage surgery (41,42).

Computerized Tomographic Angiography

Building on the advances provided by helical CT technology, the availability of multidetector-row CT (MDCT) has dramatically improved the ability of CT angiography to image the arteries of the lower extremities. Current MDCT scanners have 16 rows of detectors, and newer 64-row scanners have been developed. Using the 16-row MDCT, and customized protocols for the injection of contrast and acquisition of axial images, the abdominal aorta and vasculature of the entire lower extremity may be imaged in approximately 45 seconds. Contrast is injected at approximately 1.5 mL per second to 3 mL per second, for a total of 100 mL to 150 mL through a superficial vein in the upper extremity, using a power injector. Sophisticated postprocessing methods have been developed that provide a more meaningful 3D representation of the axial images acquired. These include: maximum intensity projection (MIP), which produces images similar to digital subtraction angiography, and volume rendering (VR), which is the most computer intensive method that maintains the highest fidelity to the original data set acquired (43,44).

Compared with DSA, computerized tomographic angiography (CTA) has less spatial resolution and has limited accuracy in vessels with heavy calcification, especially in below knee arteries. However, CTA is superior to DSA in other respects: it is non-invasive, less expensive, requires less radiation exposure and has better contrast resolution (45). Compared to MRA, CTA has the disadvantages of radiation exposure and the need for nephrotoxic contrast agents. However, diagnostic accuracy and reproducibility are similar, with better patient satisfaction with CTA. In addition, the accuracy of CTA is not affected by metallic stents or surgical clips and the technique may be safely offered to claustrophobic patients or those with electronic pacemakers (44,46).

Sensitivity for the detection of >50% stenoses in peripheral limb vessels by CTA exceeds 90% (47). In other series, there was a 100% concordance between CTA and DSA in the assessment of lesion severity, with CTA identifying a significant number of additional segments that could not be visualized by DSA due to inadequate opacification caused by inflow vessel disease.

UPPER EXTREMITY ISCHEMIA

General principles governing the evaluation of ischemia in the lower limbs may be applied

to the upper limbs. However, important differences need to be recognized. As a general rule, atherosclerosis does not occur distal to the subclavian artery. Exceptions to this rule occur in patients with diabetes and end-stage renal disease. Distally, small- and medium-sized arteries are more prone to a variety of vasculitides associated with the following conditions: thromboangiitis obliterans, scleroderma, CREST syndrome, and mixed connective tissue disease.

Subclavian artery disease is easily detected and evaluated by conventional testing and duplex scanning. Measuring the blood pressures in both arms is a useful screen, and measuring segmental pressures along the length of the arm will help localize the diseased segment to the subclavian artery (and innominate artery on the right side). While the origin of the left subclavian artery below the clavicle is not accessible for Doppler duplex imaging, all of the right subclavian artery and the remaining sections of the left are typically amenable. Duplex imaging of the subclavian artery provides the same information as that described with lower limb arterial imaging. The Doppler waveforms obtained from a normal subclavian artery are identical to that described earlier for lower limb arteries (i.e., triphasic). Guidelines for estimating the severity of subclavian obstructive lesions based on peak systolic velocities are similar to those used for the lower limbs. Similarly, qualitative changes in the waveform (e.g., loss of reversal of flow, monophasic morphology) infer similar conclusions regarding the hemodynamic significance of obstructive disease. MRA and CTA are very useful adjunctive imaging modalities for the diagnosis of aortic arch and subclavian artery disease, yielding very high sensitivity and specificity for the detection of significant lesions in the arch and its branches (48,49). Distal to the subclavian artery, segmental pressure measurements may be applied, as well as duplex imaging. It is important to note that the reversal-flow phase of the Doppler signal obtained from brachial, ulnar or radial arteries is absent in up to 50% of healthy individuals. Palmar arch flow and digital arterial flow are best evaluated using Doppler. The contribution of the ulnar and radial arteries to palmar arch flow may be assessed using the Doppler device with sequential occlusion of the arteries.

CEREBROVASCULAR DISEASE

Most patients with cerebrovascular disease are asymptomatic. In addition, physical examination is not sensitive enough to reliably detect cases with occult carotid disease (50). Several imaging modalities have therefore been developed to enable the accurate diagnosis of cerebrovascular disease, with carotid duplex scanning being the most commonly employed modality. Other modalities available for extracranial and intracranial arterial imaging include MRA and CT angiography.

Duplex Ultrasonography

This technique has several advantages in the evaluation of the cerebrovascular disease: it is noninvasive, widely available, without known risk, involves minimal inconvenience, and above all, is accurate and reproducible when performed by an experienced sonographer.

The Examination

The patient is placed in the supine position, turning the neck away from the side of the examination. Transducers with frequencies of 5 MHz to 7.5 MHz are most commonly used. Initially, the common carotid artery (CCA) is identified at the base of the neck and then traced cephalad to identify the bifurcation and both internal and external carotid arteries (ICA and ECA). After the initial scan for orientation, the CCA, carotid bulb and ICA are then examined more closely, using B-mode or gray-scale imaging (in both the longitudinal and transverse planes) for identification of normal segments, ulcers, plaques and plaque characteristics. Doppler waveforms are obtained from all the arterial segments; the peak systolic velocity (PSV) and end diastolic velocity (EDV) at each site are recorded. Doppler color-coding may identify segments with flow turbulence, which facilitates the identification of segments with the highest velocities (51). It is important to sweep the Doppler through the entire vessel so as not to miss a high velocity jet.

Normal Doppler Velocity Patterns

It is imperative to distinguish between the ICA and ECA early on in the examination process. The ICA is usually larger in size, has no branches in the neck, and courses posteriorly towards the mastoid process. However, most importantly, the ICA has a low resistance Doppler signature since it feeds a low resistance vascular bed in the brain. The characteristic flow pattern shows high forward flow velocity during systole with continuing forward flow during diastole (albeit at a lower velocity) (Fig. 2-6A). The diastolic flow is

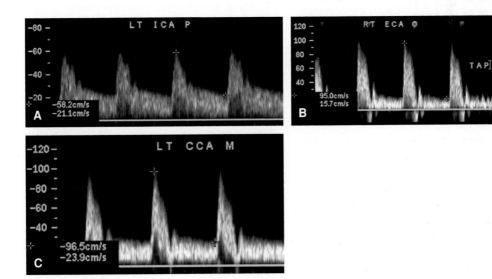

FIGURE 2-6 ● **Normal Doppler waveforms from carotid artery. A:** Internal carotid artery (ICA). **B:** External carotid artery (ECA). Note the typical effect of tapping on the superficial temporal artery on the Doppler waveform. **C:** Common carotid artery (CCA).

therefore above the baseline and no flow reversal is seen.

The ECA, on the other hand, supplies a high-resistance peripheral vascular bed in the neck and face. Its typical waveform has a high-velocity forward flow, followed by a prominent dicrotic notch with possible flow reversal, and minimal diastolic flow (Fig. 2-6B). However the most accurate way to discriminate the external carotid artery is to perform a temporal tap. Tapping one's finger over the superficial temporal artery (just anterior to the external auditory meatus) produces a characteristic appearance indicating that the Doppler is in the ECA (Fig. 2-6B). As the temporal artery is a branch of the ECA, velocity deflections caused by the tapping should be seen on the ECA waveform (17,51). Physiologically, approximately 80% of CCA flow is directed to the brain, therefore the normal Doppler CCA has characteristics of both the ICA and ECA (Fig. 2-6C). A CCA that has the appearance of an ECA usually indicates the presence of an ipsilateral ICA occlusion.

Gray-Scale Imaging

The initial part of the Duplex examination of the carotid arteries is usually spent surveying the arterial segments by B-mode imaging. In clinical settings, the extent and severity of plaque is presented in descriptive or semiquantitative terms. For example, plaques maybe described as extending from the CCA to the proximal third of the ICA and may be further labeled as mild, moderate, or severe. Furthermore, atherosclerosis may be circumferential or localized. As will be discussed later, it is generally possible to use the gray-scale image of the arterial wall and plaque in conjunction with color-coded flow in the lumen to have a rough estimate of the degree of diameter reduction (e.g., more or less than 50%, near total or total occlusion) (52) (Fig. 2-7).

Echogenicity of the plaque has been proposed as an indicator of plaque composition. Low echogenicity suggests a high-lipid content. Some lipid-laden plaques may be of such low echogenicity that they may not be visualized on gray-scale imaging. They are identified as a flow void, on color imaging. Marked echogenicity with shadowing suggests calcification. The shadowing may be sufficiently extensive to

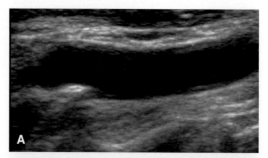
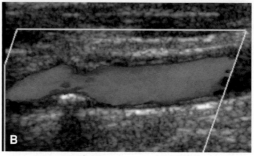

FIGURE 2-7 ● B-mode image and color Doppler of the common carotid artery showing localized echogenic plaque producing mild degree of stenosis.

preclude Doppler interrogation of the arterial segment, under the area of calcification. Plaques predominantly composed of fibrous tissue will have an intermediate echogenicity comparable to surrounding muscular tissue, but less echogenic than the arterial adventitia (52,53).

When the echogenicity of the plaque is variable, it is described as heterogenous. This is possibly caused by intra-plaque hemorrhage and/or necrosis (54). Some studies have suggested that heterogenous plaques and intraplaque hemorrhage identified by gray-scale imaging are more frequently encountered in patients with clinical evidence of cerebral ischemia (55). Although surface ulceration of the plaque as detected by 2D ultrasound has been suggested as a risk factor for cerebral ischemic events (56), the data are inconsistent, and the reproducibility of this ultrasonographic finding is moderate (54,57).

Difficulties in Defining Carotid Stenosis Severity

Prior to discussing the different Doppler criteria used to define carotid stenosis severity, it is important to understand the methodology of

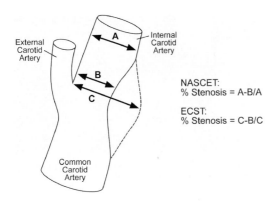

NASCET:
% Stenosis = A-B/A

ECST:
% Stenosis = C-B/C

FIGURE 2-8 ● Illustration of methodology used to define the severity of internal carotid-artery stenosis in the NASCET and ECST trials.

the angiographic 'gold-standard' assessment of lesion severity. As will be discussed in Chapter 6, the indications for carotid endarterectomy were defined by large clinical trials: NASCET and ECST for symptomatic patients, and ACAS for the asymptomatic individuals (58–60). The angiographic methods for measuring the degree of stenosis in these studies were different (Fig. 2-8).

In NASCET, the minimal lumen diameter at the point of maximal stenosis was compared to the diameter of the distal internal carotid artery, where the walls become parallel (i.e., stenosis at the bifurcation was referenced to a normal-looking segment in the ICA). In the ECST trial, the stenosis at the bifurcation was calculated as the diameter of the contrast-filled lumen divided by an extrapolated diameter representing the original size of the bulb, and without consideration of the size of the ICA. The NASCET method appeared more objective and reproducible, although it is somewhat illogical when there is moderate disease at the bifurcation (e.g., a 50% stenosis using the carotid bulb as a reference point would be a 0% stenosis using the NASCET method).

This variability in angiographic methods created confusion because the validity of the Duplex criteria published prior to NASCET and ACAS came into question, and the Duplex equivalent of the stenosis cutoffs, as defined by these trials, became unclear. Thus, the original standards developed in the 1980s had to be revised; new criteria were developed to correspond to the 50%

and 60% stenosis cutoff points, defined angiographically in NASCET and ACAS, as being the cutoff values that defined a benefit for surgical therapy.

In addition to the discrepancies in the methods of stenosis measurement among trials, there is inherent variability in angiographic measurement as well (61). Although reproducibility in large trials is usually high, the rigor of the methods and the use of core laboratories may not be extrapolated to everyday clinical practice.

Duplex evaluation carries its own set of variabilities. Technical variability exists among different laboratories and even among sonographers in the same laboratory. This may be related to a number of technical issues that are beyond the scope of this chapter. However, the importance of a correct Doppler angle, and the location of the cursor, in relation to the point of maximum velocity, may not be overemphasized.

Doppler Criteria for Stenosis Severity

Several Doppler measurements may aid in defining the severity of stenosis. The main variables are: the ICA peak systolic velocity (PSV), ICA end diastolic velocity (EDV), and the ratio of PSV of the ICA to that of the CCA (ICA/CCA PSV).

The rationale for using these measurements is dependent on two pathophysiologic facts. First, the velocity of flow increases within a stenotic arterial segment, compared to the velocity of flow in a more proximal and relatively disease-free lumen. Although not linear, this relationship is proportional, such that certain ranges of flow velocities may be used to estimate the degree of diameter reduction. This applies to both the PSV and the EDV. Second, the atherosclerosis of the carotid arteries predominantly affects the carotid bifurcation, at the junction of the CCA and the ICA, and the proximal portion of the ICA. Normally, with laminar flow, there is no difference between CCA- and ICA-flow velocity. As the stenosis at the bifurcation becomes more severe, the velocity of the ICA at the stenosis but not that of the CCA velocity increases, which in turn, leads to a higher ICA/CCA PSV ratio (Fig. 2-9).

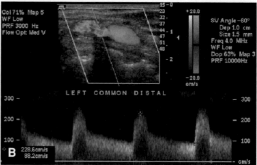

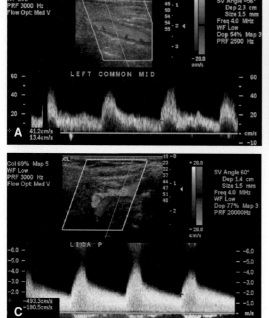

FIGURE 2-9 ● Duplex examination in a patient with a severe internal carotid-artery (ICA) stenosis. Doppler waveforms from **(A)** mid- common carotid artery (CCA), **(B)** distal CCA, and **(C)** ICA. Note the increase in peak systolic flow from the normal level in the mid- CCA to the ICA, caused by the stenosis. The resultant ratios of these velocities is thus 12. The ICA end-diastolic velocity is also significantly increased. Note the appearance of the ICA Doppler waveform as being completely filled, indicating the severe turbulence of flow in the ICA.

Others have also examined the ICA/CCA EDV ratio, as well as the severity of spectral broadening in the ICA Doppler signal, which indicates more turbulent flow and hence, is considered a sign of more severe stenosis.

Several sets of criteria have been proposed by leading vascular laboratories. The criteria most commonly followed are those proposed by Strandness and Zwiebel (62,63). The Cleveland Clinic and Mount Sinai vascular medicine laboratories follow a slightly different set of criteria. Recently, the Society of Radiologists in Ultrasound proposed a consensus set of criteria, based on the large body of evidence accumulated over the last 2 decades (64) (Table 2-1).

Despite the publication of these criteria for defining lesion severity, it is critical for each laboratory to establish and validate its own criteria. The aforementioned sources of variability, both in the angiogram and in the duplex assessment, may not be overemphasized. The published cri-

teria may be a starting point that is fine tuned after internal quality control and correlation with CTA, MRA, angiography, and surgical specimens. Therefore, physicians caring for patients with carotid disease should be familiar with the laboratory standards and criteria used to make the diagnosis. It is also imperative that angiographers and surgeons provide feedback to the vascular laboratory, in a continuous effort to improve the accuracy of reporting.

Caveats and Special Situations

A commonly encountered limitation of the standard sets of Doppler criteria is the existence of a contralateral ICA occlusion (Fig. 2-10).

In these cases, there is increased flow in the patent ICA and the vertebral arteries, to maintain adequate cerebral arterial blood supply. With the increased flow, the Doppler velocities in the patent ICA are elevated, giving the false

TABLE 2-1

Ultrasound Criteria For Diagnosis of Internal Carotid Artery Stenosis Severity

Cleveland Clinic	Strandness	Zwiebel	Consensus Panel
Normal —PSV <105 —No SB —No or minimal plaque	**Normal** —PSV <125 —No SB —Flow reversal in bulb	**Normal** —PSV <110 —EDV <40 —PSV ICA/CCA <1.8 —EDV ICA/CCA <2.4 —SB <30	**Normal** —PSV <125 —No plaque —PSV ICA/CCA <2.0 —EDV <40
1% to 15% —PSV <105 —SB —Visible plaque	**1% to 39%** —PSV <125 —No or minimal SB —No flow reversal	**<50%** —PSV <110 —EDV <40 —PSV ICA/CCA <1.8 —EDV ICA/CCA <2.4 —SB <40	**<50%** —PSV <125 —Plaque <50% DS —PSV ICA/CCA <2.0 —EDV <40
16% to 49% —PSV 105–159 —SB —Visible plaque	**40% to 59%** —PSV ≤125 —Marked SB	**50% to 69%** —PSV <130 —EDV <40 —PSV ICA/CCA <1.8 —EDV ICA/CCA <2.4 —SB <40	**50% to 69%** —PSV 125–230 —Plaque ≥50% DS —PSV ICA/CCA 2.0–4.0 —EDV 40–100
50% to 79% —PSV >160 —EDV <135 —SB —Visible plaque ***>70%** —if PSV ICA/CCA >4.0	**60% to 79%** —PSV >125 —EDV <140	**≥ 70% (but not near occlusion)** —PSV >130 —EDV >40 —PSV ICA/CCA >1.8 —EDV ICA/CCA >2.4 —SB >40	**≥ 70% (but not near occlusion)** —PSV >230 —Plaque ≥50% DS —PSV ICA/CCA >4.0 —EDV >100
80% to 99% —PSV >240 —EDV ≥135	**80% to 99%** —PSV >125 —EDV >140	**Near occlusion** —PSV >250 —EDV >100 —PSV ICA/CCA >3.7 —EDV ICA/CCA >5.5 —SB >80	**Near occlusion** —PSV variable —Plaque: visible, subtotal —PSV ICA/CCA: variable —EDV: variable
Total Occlusion No flow signal	**Total Occlusion** No flow signal	**Total Occlusion** No flow signal	**Total Occlusion** —No flow signal —No visible lumen

PSV, Peak systolic velocity and EDV, end-diastolic velocity are measured in cm/sec.
Spectral broadening (SB) is assessed qualitatively or quantitatively (cm/sec).
ICA, internal carotid artery; CCA, common carotid artery.

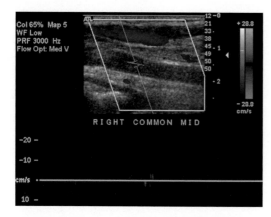

FIGURE 2-10 ● **Duplex ultrasound from a patient with occlusion of the common carotid artery (CCA).** There is no color or Doppler from the CCA. Note the presence of color signal from the adjacent internal jugular vein.

impression of obstructive disease. The exact degree to which the ICA flow velocity increases in this setting is difficult to ascertain, but may be dependent on the adequacy of the Circle of Willis, the contribution of vertebral flow, and the presence or absence of scar tissue in the distribution of the occluded ICA. Several investigators have modified existing Doppler cut-off values to define lesion severity of a patent ICA, in the presence of a contralateral occlusion. For lesions 50% to 79%, a PSV of at least 140 cm per second and EDV of less than 140 cm per second were suggested, whereas 80% to 99% lesions were present if the PSV was greater than 140 cm per second and EDV was more than 140 cm per second (70). Other proposed criteria in this setting use the same PSV cut-off value of more than 140 cm per second, but add an EDV of less than 155 cm per second, for 50% to 79% lesions, and of more than 155cm per second for 80% to 99% lesions (71). Both of these adjusted Doppler criteria sets had approximately 97% accuracy.

In order to determine how much of the increase in PSV is due to stenosis of the ICA and how much is due to compensatory flow, it may be useful to compare the velocities in the CCA. If there is a significant increase in the CCA velocities, contralateral to an occluded ICA, then compensatory flow is contributing to the high velocity in the contralateral ICA. In patients with bilateral 80% to 99% stenosis who are undergoing carotid

endarterectomy or stenting on one side, it is important to recheck the duplex ultrasound on the contralateral side soon after the operation, to be certain that the stenosis is real and not due to compensatory flow (72).

The usual Doppler criteria may also create a false impression of obstructive disease following carotid stenting. In this situation, the ICA compliance is significantly reduced by the stent and thus the flow velocity increases to a range that may be interpreted as a significant stenosis. Duplex examination of patients with carotid stents within days of a successful procedure (i.e., when the residual stenosis is minimal) identifies a significant proportion of patients in whom the PSV is more than 125 cm per second (31%) or the ICA/CCA is more than 2.0 (11%), suggesting a moderate stenosis. Recently, Lal et al proposed new criteria to define a stenosis of at least 20%, after carotid stenting: PSV of at least 150 cm per second and ICA/CCA PSV ratio of at least 2.16 (73). Although these preliminary data require further validation in larger data sets, it is clear that caution is warranted when interpreting Doppler velocities following carotid stenting.

CCA STENOSIS

Atherosclerotic obstructive disease may affect the CCA, more often at its origin. In these cases and in the case of brachiocephalic stenosis, the CCA waveform may be dampened or its amplitude diminished (74). This is important because there is no direct, gray-scale visualization of the origin of the CCA, and the changes in the waveform may represent the only clue to the diagnosis as determined by Duplex imaging. Another clue to the diagnosis is the difference between the velocity and waveform patterns of the two common carotid arteries. Although there may be some minor differences in the normal individual, significant differences should alert the examiner to the possibility of CCA disease. Ultrasonography should include Doppler waveforms taken as proximally as possible, using the linear transducer. If there is the suggestion that a stenosis may be present, a low-frequency transducer should be used to sample the origin of the innominate and left common carotid arteries, directly.

There are no well defined criteria for the assessment of common carotid artery stenosis. In cases of total ICA occlusion, when there is reduced ipsilateral flow, the CCA signal amplitude may be diminished as well. If the changes are seen bilaterally, that points to a systemic phenomenon (e.g., low cardiac output or severe aortic stenosis) (75).

VERTEBRAL ARTERIAL DISEASE

Examination of the vertebral arteries usually accompanies Duplex evaluation of the carotid arteries. The vertebral arteries are located posteriorly to the CCA, and slightly medially. They may be visualized on gray-scale imaging from the origin to the point of entry into the skull, although the origin is technically challenging to examine. It is usually easy to obtain a Doppler signal from the vertebral artery and the velocity ranges between 20 cm per second and 40 cm per second (Fig. 2-11A).

In presence of significant disease, the signal is damped distally to the obstruction, and the velocity is less than 20 cm per second. Although the criteria for diagnosis of vertebral lesions are not as robust as those published for carotid

lesions, the accuracy of Duplex in identifying severe lesions and total occlusions is quite high, approximately 95%. Duplex imaging, however, is not so accurate with lesions at the origin of the vertebral artery.

When the signal of vertebral flow is unusually strong and the velocity is more than 40 cm per second, this raises the suspicion that there is increased ipsilateral flow. This may be the result of contralateral vertebral occlusion, contralateral subclavian steal, or severe carotid disease, with the ipsilateral vertebral artery contributing significantly to the collateral flow (Fig. 2-11B). In cases of subclavian steal, the direction of flow signal in the vertebral artery is reversed and indicates a severe stenosis in the innominate or subclavian artery (76,77).

TRANSCRANIAL DOPPLER EXAMINATION

Transcranial Doppler (TCD) is a technique to examine the intracranial arteries using ultrasonography. It may be performed using blind Doppler probes to detect velocity signals but currently, it is possible to obtain the standard, spectral-Doppler signals, gray-scale images, and color-coded Doppler images, as well. Direct visualization using Duplex scanners is important, as it reduces the possibility of error in identifying specific vessels. The examination requires an acoustic window through which it is possible to isolate the intracranial vessels. The middle (MCA), anterior (ACA), and posterior cerebral arteries (PCA) are usually identified through a transtemporal window (above the zygomatic arch). The ophthalmic artery and the ICA siphon are approached via a transorbital window. The vertebral and basilar arteries are reached via a suboccipital window.

Identification of the different arteries is based on prior knowledge of their expected depth and direction of flow. For example, the normal MCA is located at a depth of 40 mm to 50 mm, its normal flow is towards the transducer, and its mean velocity is 30 cm per second to 80 cm per second. The ACA is slightly deeper, and flow is directed away from the transducer in the transtemporal window. Both vertebral and basilar arterial flow is away from the transducer, with velocities

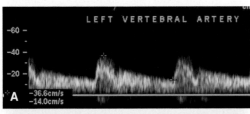

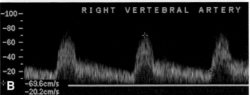

FIGURE 2-11 ● **Doppler waveforms from left (A) and right (B) vertebral arteries of the patient shown in Figure 2-10.** The flow velocities in the left vertebral artery are normal. The flow velocities in the right vertebral artery are increased compared to the left because the right common carotid artery occlusion has resulted in collateral flow from the vertebral artery to the ipsilateral carotid system.

ranging between 30 cm per second and 40 cm per second. Obstructive lesions are diagnosed when there is focal turbulence and velocity increase in a specific segment of an artery, together with a drop in distal velocity. Reversal of expected direction of flow and evidence of collateral circulation development are other clues to obstructive disease.

CEREBROVASCULAR MAGNETIC RESONANCE ANGIOGRAPHY

Magnetic resonance angiography (MRA) has been used for the evaluation of extracranial and intracranial arterial disease for about a decade. It provides highly accurate images of the whole cerebral circulation, without the use of ionizing radiation or nephrotoxic contrast agents. As discussed previously, there are several MRA techniques, each with its advantages and limitations. TOF-MRA imaging modalities have a tendency to overestimate the severity of carotid stenosis, owing to turbulent flow and signal dropout. The 3D-TOF method is more accurate in defining lumen and plaque morphology, and is less susceptible to turbulence artifacts (78). A meta-analysis of a large number of MRA studies demonstrated the accuracy of MRA in determining carotid-lesion severity. For total occlusions, sensitivity and specificity was 0.84 and 0.98 respectively, compared to angiography. For the 70% diameter stenosis cutoff, sensitivity and specificity of MRA were greater than 0.9 and 0.89, respectively (79). In addition to the usual limitations against using MR imaging (e.g., patients with pacemakers, metallic clips, claustrophobia), TOF techniques have the additional limitations of relatively long acquisition times and the potential for motion artifacts. Contrast-enhanced (usually with gadolinium) 3D MRA provides high-quality images while avoiding most of the limitations of TOF techniques. The acquisition times are much shorter, therefore limiting motion artifacts. With 3D MRA, there are fewer dephasing effects (and thus less signal dropout), which is the primary difficulty in distinguishing between stenosis and occlusion using TOF imaging. Using maximum intensity projection (MIP) algorithms, 3D MRA is more accurate in defining stenosis severity and identification of plaque morphology (80). The technique has been compared to conventional subtraction angiography, with very good agreement: the category of lesion severity was identical in 89% of all lesions, and 93% in the category of 70% to 99%. All total occlusions and near-occlusions were correctly identified by CE 3D MRA in this study (81). A more recent systematic review of MRA and Duplex studies, for evaluation of carotid-arterial disease, confirmed the very high sensitivity and specificity of MRA for diagnosis of lesions with at least 70% stenosis (95% and 90%, respectively) (82). In the same review, the authors calculated the sensitivity and specificity of Duplex imaging to be 86% and 87%, respectively. Both imaging modalities were slightly more accurate and equivalent in identification of total occlusions, with a specificity of 100% for both (82). CE MRA also has the advantage of accurate depiction of the intracranial circulation and brain imaging, all in the same session.

CEREBROVASCULAR COMPUTERIZED TOMOGRAPHIC ANGIOGRAPHY

In computerized tomographic angiography (CTA) evaluation of cerebrovascular disease, images are acquired in a continuous fashion using 1.25-mm to 2-mm section images. Volumetric data are obtained before and after injection of a contrast bolus, timed to achieve maximum arterial opacification. Images are examined in the axial plane and 3D reconstructions (i.e., maximum intensity projection [MIP] and volume rendering [VR]). Suboptimal images and inaccurate interpretation may result from the administration of inadequate volume or inaccurate timing of the contrast bolus, the presence of calcifications (seen especially with MIP reconstruction), and the numerous vascular structures in the neck, which are opacified simultaneously.

Compared to DSA of the carotid arteries, CTA is highly sensitive and specific in defining carotid stenosis (83,84). However, the accuracy varies according the severity of stenosis and the location of the lesion (84–88). However, the sensitivity of the technique in defining lesion severity may be less impressive when lesions are in the range of 50% to 69% or 70% to 99% (87). In other series, CTA was 100% sensitive in detection of total occlusions and near occlusions (89). It is particularly useful in identifying stenoses at the origin of the vertebral artery (90) and in thoracic CCA lesions that may not be visualized on Duplex imaging.

RENAL ARTERIAL DISEASE

Renal artery stenosis (RAS) is difficult to diagnose on clinical grounds alone. Duplex ultrasonography, MRA and CTA, and captopril nuclear scans are the most commonly utilized testing modalities.

Duplex Ultrasonography

This technique has several advantages in the evaluation of RAS. In addition to providing a 2D image of the renal arteries from the aorta to the hilum, duplex imaging also provides information on the flow velocity patterns in the different segments of the artery, as well as in the parenchyma of the kidney poles. Adjunctive information that helps in making the diagnosis includes the measurement of kidney size. Other abnormalities or pathology in the abdominal aorta or the kidney may also be identified.

Renal artery duplex scanning is the most technically demanding of all vascular beds. The arteries arise from the aorta posteriorly. Thus, the renal arteries are separated from the ultrasound transducer by the anterior abdominal wall, its muscles, visceral fat and the peritoneal cavity with its contents, most importantly the gas-filled bowel loops. In experienced hands, the incidence of technically suboptimal examinations is 5% to 12% (76). The examination is ideally performed as early in the day as possible, following 12 hours of fasting to minimize the amount of bowel gas. Owing to the depth at which the renal arteries lie from the surface, the optimal transducer frequency is low (2.25 MHz to 3.0 MHz). The examination begins with the patient in the supine position by obtaining a Doppler waveform from the abdominal aorta at the level of the renal artery (Fig. 2-12A).

Using B-mode imaging, the main renal artery and accessory renal artery, if present, should be identified (Fig. 2-12B). Identified arteries are examined from the aortic origin to the hilum of the kidney (Fig. 2-12C). Pulsed-wave Doppler and color-coding are utilized to obtain Doppler signals from all segments of the artery (Fig. 2-12D). If there is bowel gas interference, the patient is turned to a lateral position. Alternatively, the renal arteries may be identified at the hilum of the kidney, and traced back to the aortic origin, to obtain the same information. In addition, kidney size is measured from pole-to-pole (Fig. 2-12E) and Doppler signals are obtained from the interlobar branches to calculate indirect measurements of renal arterial flow (Fig. 2-12F) (17,76).

The PSV in the abdominal aorta at the level of the renal arteries is normally 100 ± 20 cm per second (Fig. 2-12A). The normal renal artery has a low resistance Doppler wave (i.e., flow continues throughout diastole and there is no reversal-flow phase) (Fig. 2-12D). Under normal conditions, the PSV in the renal artery is between 80 cm per second and 120 cm per second, the EDV/PSV ratio is approximately 0.33, and the ratio of the PSV in the renal artery to that in the aorta at the renal level is between 1.1 ± 0.3.

Several Doppler criteria have been proposed to diagnose the presence of RAS (Table 2-2). To avoid errors caused by the large variability in normal renal artery PSV, a ratio between the PSV in the renal artery and the aorta was devised (i.e., Renal Aortic Ratio [RAR]) (Fig. 2-4) (91). A RAR of at least 3.5 correlates with a significant stenosis (at least 60% diameter reduction). This cut-off value has a sensitivity of 84% and a specificity of 97% (92). A cut-off PSV value of more than 180 cm per second has been proposed to define renal artery stenosis, with an accuracy exceeding 90% (93). Sensitivity and specificity are improved if there is a significant reduction in the distal velocity, in addition to the proximal PSV of more than 180 cm per second (94).

A more commonly accepted velocity cut-off is a PSV of at least 200 cm per second, in the presence of turbulent flow by color Doppler, which corresponds to a 60% diameter reduction with very high sensitivity and specificity (Fig. 2-13) (95).

In a large prospective study to compare duplex imaging to renal DSA, the diagnosis of significant RAS (i.e., corresponding to more than

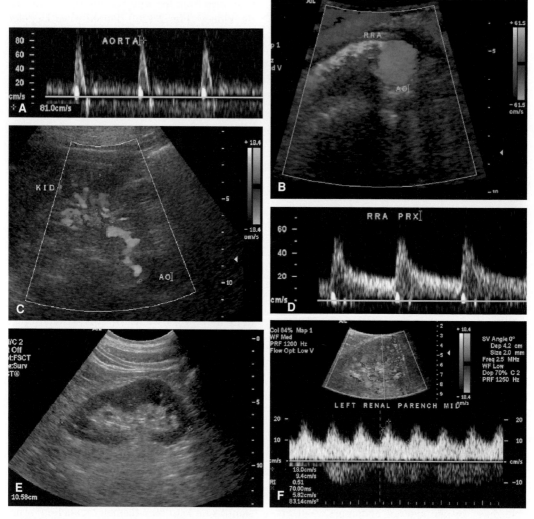

FIGURE 2-12 ● **Components of the duplex ultrasound examination of the renal arteries. A:** Doppler waveform obtained from aorta, at the level of the renal arteries. **B:** B-mode and color Doppler allow identification of origin of the right renal artery. **C:** Path of right renal artery is shown from the origin to hilum of kidney. **D:** Doppler waveform obtained from origin, proximal, mid-, and distal sections of the artery. **E:** Right kidney size measured, using B-mode image. **F:** Doppler signals obtained from segmental arteries in the upper, mid-, and lower poles of the kidney.

60% diameter stenosis, by DSA) was achieved by demonstrating one or both of the following Doppler findings: a RAR of at least 3.5 and/or a PSV of at least 200 cm per second (Fig. 2-13). Both sensitivity and specificity of the duplex criteria in this study were 98% (96). Other findings that are helpful in making the diagnosis include an end-diastolic velocity (EDV) equal to or greater than 150 cm per second, which corresponded to an RAS of at least 80% (96). A simple measurement of the kidney length demonstrating diminished size (i.e., less than 10 cm, or significantly smaller than the contralateral kid-

ney) is also another clue to RAS of more than 60% or total occlusion, since such a degree of reduced arterial flow is often accompanied by loss of renal mass (97).

The most commonly used indirect measure of RAS is the renal resistive index (RI). After a Doppler signal is obtained from the interlobar arteries in the renal parenchyma, the RI is calculated as the average of $\left(1 - \frac{EDV}{PSV}\right)$(98) (Figure 2-12F). RI is reduced in patients with RAS, but generally is not useful in distinguishing mild from severe stenosis (98). It does, however, have significant prognostic implications; the

TABLE 2-2

Duplex Criteria for Diagnosis of Renal Artery Stenosis*

Reference	Criteria	Sensitivity[†]	Specificity[†]	Comments
Taylor et al[110]	RAR >3.5	84	97	
Hoffman et al[111]	PSV >180 cm/sec	95	90	
Hansen et al[113]	PSV ≥200 cm/sec	93	98	Excluding kidneys with multiple vessels
	PSV ≥200 cm/sec	67	100	Including kidneys with multiple vessels
Olin et al[114]	PSV ≥200 cm/sec and/or RAR ≥3.5	98	98	
	EDV ≥150 cm/sec			RAS ≥80% by DSA
Radermacher et al[112]	PSV >180 cm/sec & distal velocity <25% of PSV	97	98	RAS ≥50% by DSA
Schwerk et al[115]	Delta RI >5%	100	94	Underestimates severity if bilateral RAS, RI better used for prognostication

* Renal artery stenosis (RAS) refers to diameter reduction of ≥60% by angiography, unless otherwise specified.
† Using angiography as the gold standard.
RAR, renal aortic ratio; EDV, end-diastolic velocity; PSV, peak systolic velocity; DSA, digital subtraction angiography; RI, renal resistive index; RAS, renal artery stenosis.

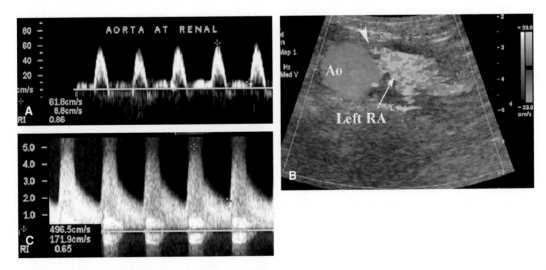

FIGURE 2-13 ● **Doppler examination from patient with severe left renal artery stenosis. A:** Doppler waveform obtained from abdominal aorta at the level of the aorta. **B:** Color Doppler image showing marked turbulent flow, at the origin of the left renal artery indicative of a severe stenosis. **C:** Doppler waveform from the proximal left renal artery. This waveform meets all the criteria for the diagnosis of severe renal artery stenosis, specifically: PSV >200 cm/sec (496 cm/sec), EDV >150 cm/sec (171 cm/sec), and RAR >3.5 (8.1).

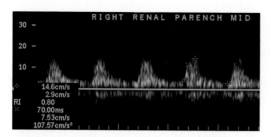

FIGURE 2-14 ● **Doppler waveform from segmental artery in mid-pole of right kidney.** Compare this waveform with that in Figure 2-12F. Note that the ratio of the EDV to the PSV is much lower in this waveform, with a resistive index of 0.8, suggesting the presence of small-vessel disease in the kidney.

likelihood of improvement in blood pressure or renal function after renal artery revascularization is very small if the preprocedural RI was more than 0.8 (94). The very high RI is considered a marker of structural small-vessel changes that are unlikely to be reversed by large vessel intervention (Fig. 2-14).

In another study assessing the prognostic value of Doppler findings, patients who were likely to exhibit blood pressure or renal function improvement after revascularization were identified by a preprocedural EDV of more than 90 cm per second and an RI of less than 0.75 (99).

There are few limitations to Duplex imaging of renal arteries. In addition to the technical difficulties posed by bowel gas and obesity, most studies have shown a limited sensitivity in detection of accessory renal arteries (i.e., approximately 60%). The presence of RAS in an accessory artery is the most common explanation, in cases in which duplex imaging is falsely negative (95). Renal artery duplex imaging is very useful in follow-up monitoring after revascularization procedures (100). With the increasing use of metallic stents in renal artery revascularization procedures, MR and CT angiography often provide inadequate image quality, resulting from artifacts caused by the metal.

Magnetic Resonance Arteriography

MRA is an excellent imaging modality for evaluation of the visceral arteries, in general. The accuracy of CE 3D MRA in identification of significant RAS is excellent, with a sensitivity of 100%

and specificity of more than 92%, compared to DSA. In a recent meta-analysis, CE 3D MRA and CTA were identified as the most accurate tests for evaluation of renovascular hypertension (101). Acquisition time is less than a minute and there is no concern about nephrotoxicity with the use of gadolinium, the most commonly employed paramagnetic contrast agent. Supplementing the CE 3D MRA images with phase contrast (PC) MRA may display segments of turbulent flow, thus confirming the findings of contrast MRA. In general, MRA is less sensitive in identifying fibromuscular dysplasia than it is for atherosclerosis (36). In addition, MRA may not be feasible in patients with prosthetic implants such as mechanical valves and pacemaker/defibrillator devices.

CT Angiography

Multidetector-row CT angiography (CTA) has an excellent spatial resolution and is very useful in delineating visceral arteries. Renal arteries are small in diameter, so axial tomographic slices must be 1 mm to 2 mm in thickness. Postprocessing is performed to display 3D reconstructed and axial or coronal images (e.g., perpendicular to the long axis of the renal artery). It is, in fact, preferable to review the study on workstations that allow scrolling through the images, since using hard copy cut films requires sampling of the data set, which in turn may lead to less accurate interpretations (102).

Sensitivity and specificity of CTA for detection of RAS producing more than 50% diameter stenosis is approximately 95%. The very thin, 1-mm to 2-mm slices that are obtained by multidetector CT, the use of 3D reconstruction, and reviewing the whole data set on computer workstations also allows very accurate identification of accessory renal arteries (i.e., greater than 95% correlation between findings by CTA and operative findings) (103). This is a significant advantage of CTA over duplex scanning, in which a very common cause of false negative studies is missed disease in accessory arteries. A major limitation to CTA in the evaluation of RAS is the need for iodinated contrast agents, which makes MRA a more suitable modality in patients with renal insufficiency.

It is important to recognize that MRA and CTA provide an anatomic assessment of the renal artery, as opposed to Doppler ultrasonography and captopril scintigraphy, which assess the hemodynamic significance of the stenosis. Since the gold standard (i.e., DSA) also assesses the anatomic severity of disease, this may represent a bias favoring MRA and CTA.

Captopril Nuclear Scanning

The test is based on the asymmetric effects of angiotensin-converting enzyme inhibitors (ACE-I), such as captopril, on kidneys with normal and abnormal renal flow. In the normal kidney, captopril induces an increase in glomerular flow rate (GFR) and urine output, despite a decrease in systemic blood pressure. In cases with significant RAS, the affected kidney secretes more renin, resulting in higher levels of angiotensin II. This, in turn, causes efferent-arteriolar vasoconstriction, which maintains the GFR despite the lower afferent arteriolar flow caused by RAS. Captopril interferes with efferent arteriolar vasoconstriction, and GFR in the affected kidney drops by up to 30% (104).

Captopril renal scans consist of a standard, nuclear-renographic scan performed using a GFR tracer (e.g., ^{99m}Tc-DTPA) given at baseline, and again 60 minutes after oral administration of 25 mg to 50 mg of captopril. Scintigraphic images and time activity curves are generated. Diagnosis of RAS depends on demonstrating an asymmetric effect on GFR between the affected and the normal kidney. The diagnostic criteria include (a) delayed time to peak activity (i.e., longer than 10 minutes), (b) significantly lower peak activity in the affected kidney, (c) marked retention of activity after captopril, and (d) greater than 40% reduction in GFR in the affected kidney, after captopril (97). Although the test has very high sensitivity and specificity in research settings, its performance in the clinical setting has proved disappointing. The rate of false negatives and false positives is unacceptably high, at least in comparison to other testing modalities. In addition, the test is not suitable for patients with bilateral RAS, since it is based on demonstrating a disparity in function between both kidneys. It is also not feasible in those with azotemia, since their GFRs are already below the normal range (100).

MESENTERIC ISCHEMIA

The gut is supplied by three main arteries that arise directly from the abdominal aorta: the celiac trunk, the superior mesenteric artery (SMA), and the inferior mesenteric artery (IMA). All of these aortic branches are susceptible to atherosclerotic disease, particularly at their origins. Acute mesenteric ischemia usually results from thrombosis or embolism to one of those arteries, which leads to a life-threatening situation in which there is rarely any time for noninvasive testing. In cases of chronic, progressive atherosclerosis, intestinal ischemia generally does not develop unless both the celiac and superior mesenteric arteries (and possibly the inferior mesenteric artery as well) are significantly obstructed. This is attributed to the very rich network of collaterals that prevents the development of clinically significant ischemia, if the obstructive disease is only limited to one arterial bed. Similar to the renal arteries, several noninvasive modalities (e.g., duplex imaging, MRA and CTA) are available to image the mesenteric arteries in patients with suspected symptoms of gut ischemia.

Duplex Ultrasonography

Patients are required to fast for at least 6 hours prior to mesenteric artery imaging. In addition to eliminating bowel gases, this practice is critically important in the case of SMA imaging, since the Doppler velocity pattern is entirely different in the fasting and postprandial states. Technically, patients are imaged in the supine position, using a 2.0-MHz to 3.0-MHz transducer placed in the epigastrium. B-mode and color imaging allow identification of the arteries as they arise from the abdominal aorta (Fig. 2-15), and the Doppler waveforms are obtained after ensuring the angle of insonation is no more than 60° (Fig. 2-16) (76).

In the fasting state, SMA flow is typical of a high-resistance arterial bed (Fig. 2-16A). Within 1 minute of eating, and for about 6 hours afterwards, the SMA arterial bed dilates significantly and turns into a low-resistance system with a

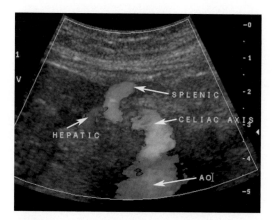

FIGURE 2-15 ● Axial view of the celiac trunk with color Doppler imaging clearly showing the origin of celiac trunk and its main branches. This image allows appropriate sampling of Doppler waveforms from the vessel of interest.

low-resistance waveform (i.e., no reversal in direction of flow following systole, continuous diastolic flow, and a relatively high end-diastolic velocity). Since the majority of celiac-trunk flow supplies two low-resistance beds (i.e., liver and spleen), the normal velocity pattern in that artery is that of a low-resistance circulation (Fig. 2-16B) (17,76,105). The Doppler velocity pattern of the IMA is normally triphasic, typical of high-resistance vascular beds (Fig. 2-16C). It is not usual for IMA flow to change to a low-resistance pattern in the postprandial setting, since the resistance in the capillary bed

of the colon is not as variable, as is the case with the small bowel and SMA flow (17).

Several cut-off PSV and EDV values have been suggested to define hemodynamically significant celiac and SMA stenosis. For the celiac trunk, an EDV of at least 55 cm per second, or the absence of flow signal, had 95% accuracy in identifying stenoses causing at least a 50% angiographic diameter reduction. A PSV cut-off value 200 cm per second, or no flow signal, had 93% accuracy (Fig. 2-17). In addition, retrograde flow in the hepatic artery was 100% predictive of severe celiac stenosis or occlusion (106).

For SMA stenoses of at least 50%, an EDV equal to or greater than 45 cm per second had the best sensitivity (90%) and specificity (91%). A PSV cut-off value of at least 300 cm per second was highly specific (100%), but less sensitive (60%), with an overall accuracy of 89% (106) (Fig. 2-18).

Other laboratories use a cut-off PSV of at least 275 cm per second, or the absence of flow, to diagnose SMA stenosis in the 70% to 100% range. These criteria have a sensitivity and specificity of 89% and 92%, respectively (107). A comparison of fasting and postprandial PSV in the SMA may provide some further insight into the significance of obstructive disease. Patients with a severe (i.e., 70% to 99%) SMA stenosis have a blunted postprandial rise in PSV, as compared to those with no disease or mild-to-moderate disease. However, the response to ingestion is quite

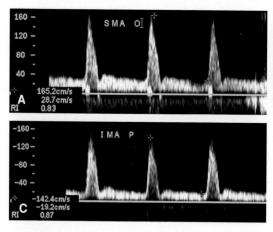

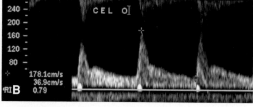

FIGURE 2-16 ● **Normal Doppler waveforms from mesenteric vessels. A:** Superior mesenteric artery in the fasting state, with high resistance pattern. **B:** Celiac artery in the fasting state, low-resistance pattern with continued diastolic flow. **C:** Inferior mesenteric artery with high-resistance pattern.

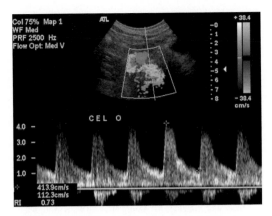

FIGURE 2-17 ● **Doppler waveform from celiac artery.** The PSV is >200 cm/sec and the EDV is >55 cm/sec indicating the presence of severe stenosis. Note the marked turbulence of flow demonstrated in the color Doppler picture above consistent with the presence of stenosis.

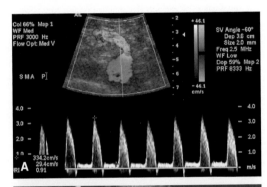

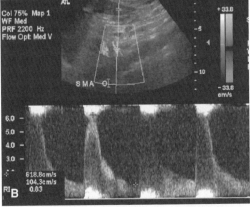

FIGURE 2-18 ● **Two examples of Doppler waveforms from patients with superior mesenteric artery stenosis. A:** The PSV is >275 cm/sec and there is turbulence of flow in the color Doppler image. **B:** The PSV is >300 cm/sec, the EDV is >45 cm/sec, and there is turbulence of flow in the color Doppler image.

variable, and it only marginally improves the accuracy of duplex imaging in identifying significant lesions (108).

In addition to the usual technical difficulties, there are two main limitations to duplex imaging of mesenteric arteries. The IMA is not easy to image, owing to its relatively small size and course, although efforts are improved with modern scanners. The IMA contributes to the arterial supply of the gut, and to the rich collateral network of the other mesenteric vessels, which makes its examination an important part of the overall evaluation of the patient with suspected mesenteric ischemia. Finally, identification of anatomic variations of arterial supply may be extremely important. This is not uncommon; up to 20% of patients may have one or more anomalies in the origins of arteries that may influence interpretation of duplex data. For example, the hepatic artery may arise from the SMA, leading to a biphasic pattern in the fasting state, even in absence of stenosis (106).

Magnetic Resonance Angiography

Most recent techniques of MRA result in excellent resolution and diagnostic accuracy in identifying significant mesenteric lesions. The principles of imaging are very similar to those described for renal MRA. CE 3D MRA images may be acquired very rapidly while avoiding motion artifacts related to peristalsis, and images are usually evaluated in a sagittal slab, unlike the renal arteries, which are routinely examined in axial or coronal slabs. The CE images may be supplemented by PC MRA, which allows evaluation of flow volume and velocity. MRA is excellent in identifying significant lesions, with reported 100% sensitivity and 95% specificity compared to DSA. Its accuracy is limited with IMA disease and in branch stenoses, as well as in the rare cases of nonatherosclerotic disease of the mesenteric arteries (109).

CT Angiography

As discussed with RAS, CTA is a very accurate tool to evaluate visceral arteries. The technical details are very similar in evaluation of renal and mesenteric arterial disease. However, the image orientation that best delineates mesenteric artery lesions is the sagittal plane, in addition to the 3D reconstructed images. As with any CTA, the relative timing of the contrast bolus and the image acquisition is critical in obtaining accurate information.

Coupled with visceral CT changes, CTA has been used to diagnose acute mesenteric occlusion with great accuracy. The very high spatial resolution, thin slices, and the feasibility of 3D reconstruction makes multidetector row CTA ideal for diagnosis of chronic mesenteric ischemia as well. These features also allow the identification of more distal lesions in the SMA or celiac trunk branches. The IMA is easier to identify with CTA. Congenital anomalies in the origins of different mesenteric branches have been identified with CTA as well.

REFERENCES

1. McDermott MM, Greenland P, Liu K, et al. Leg symptoms in peripheral arterial disease: associated clinical characteristics and functional impairment. *JAMA*. 2001;286:1599–1606.
2. McDermott MM, Greenland P, Liu K, et al. The ankle brachial index is associated with leg function and physical activity: the Walking and Leg Circulation Study. *Ann Intern Med*. 2002;136:873–883.
3. Carter SA. Clinical measurement of systolic pressures in limbs with arterial occlusive disease. *JAMA*. 1969;207:1869–1874.
4. Yao JST. Hemodynamic studies in peripheral arterial disease. *Br J Surg*. 1970;57:761.
5. Taylor MG. Wave travel in arteries and design of the cardiovascular system. In: E.O. A, ed. *Pulsatile Blood Flow*. New York: McGraw-Hill Book Co.; 1964.
6. Hobbs JT, Yao ST, Lewis JD, et al. A limitation of the Doppler ultrasound method of measuring ankle systolic pressure. *VASA*. 1974;3:160–162.
7. Raines JK, Darling RC, Buth J, et al. Austen WG. Vascular laboratory criteria for the management of peripheral vascular disease of the lower extremities. *Surgery*. 1976;79:21–29.
8. Carter SA. Indirect systolic pressures and pulse waves in arterial occlusive diseases of the lower extremities. *Circulation*. 1968;37:624–637.
9. Jaff MR. Lower extremity arterial disease. Diagnostic aspects. *Cardiol Clin*. 2002;20:491–500, v.
10. Hirsch AT, Criqui MH, Treat-Jacobson D, et al. Peripheral arterial disease detection, awareness, and treatment in primary care. *JAMA*. 2001;286:1317–1324.
11. Diehm C, Schuster A, Allenberg JR, et al. High prevalence of peripheral arterial disease and co-morbidity in 6880 primary care patients: cross-sectional study. *Atherosclerosis*. 2004;172:95–105.
12. Criqui MH, Langer RD, Fronek A, et al. Mortality over a period of 10 years in patients with peripheral arterial disease. *N Engl J Med*. 1992;326:381–386.
13. Kornitzer M, Dramaix M, Sobolski J, et al. Ankle/arm pressure index in asymptomatic middle-aged males: an independent predictor of ten-year coronary heart disease mortality. *Angiology*. 1995;46:211–219.
14. Newman AB, Sutton-Tyrrell K, Vogt MT, et al. Morbidity and mortality in hypertensive adults with a low ankle/arm blood pressure index. *JAMA*. 1993;270:487–489.
15. Newman AB, Siscovick DS, Manolio TA, et al. Ankle-arm index as a marker of atherosclerosis in the Cardiovascular Health Study. Cardiovascular Heart Study (CHS) Collaborative Research Group. *Circulation*. 1993;88:837–845.
16. Chiu JH, Topol EJ, Whitlow PL, et al. Peripheral vascular disease and one-year mortality following percutaneous coronary revascularization. *Am J Cardiol*. 2003;92:582–583.
17. Strandness DEJ. Noninvasive vascular laboratory and vascular imaging. In: Young JR, O, JW, Bartholomew JR, eds. *Peripheral Vascular Diseases*. St. Louis: Mosby; 1996:33–64.
18. Holstein P, Lassen NA. Healing of ulcers on the feet correlated with distal blood pressure measurements in occlusive arterial disease. *Acta Orthop Scand*. 1980;51:995–1006.
19. Cutajar CL, Marston A, Newcombe JF. Value of cuff occlusion pressures in assessment of peripheral vascular disease. *Br Med J*. 1973;2:392–395.
20. Strandness DE Jr, Schultz RD, Sumner DS, et al. Ultrasonic flow detection. A useful technic in the evaluation of peripheral vascular disease. *Am J Surg*. 1967;113:311–320.
21. Darling RC, Raines JK, Brener BJ, et al. Quantitative segmental pulse volume recorder: a clinical tool. *Surgery*. 1972;72:873–877.
22. MacDonald NR. Pulse volume plethysmography. *J Vasc Tech*. 1994;18:241–248.
23. Raines JK. Use of pulse volume recorder in peripheral arterial disease. In: Bernstein EF, ed. *Noninvasive Diagnostic Techniques in Vascular Disease*. 3rd ed. St Louis: Mosby; 1985.
24. King LT, Strandness DE Jr, Bell JW. The hemodynamic response of the lower extremities to exercise. *J Surg Res*. 1965;148:167–171.
25. Wolf EA Jr, Sumner DS, Strandness DE Jr. Correlation between nutritive blood flow and pressure in limbs of patients with intermittent claudication. *Surg Forum*. 1972;23:238–239.
26. Sumner DS, Strandness DE Jr. The relationship between calf blood flow and ankle blood pressure in patients with intermittent claudication. *Surgery*. 1969;65:763–771.
27. Strandness DE Jr, Zierler RE. Exercise ankle pressure measurements in arterial disease. In: Bernstein EF, ed. *Noninvasive Diagnostic Techniques in Vascular Disease*. 3rd ed. St Louis: Mosby; 1985.
28. Hatsukami TS, Primozich JF, Zierler RE, Harley JD, Strandness DE Jr. Color Doppler imaging of infrainguinal arterial occlusive disease. *J Vasc Surg*. 1992;16:527–531; discussion 531–533.
29. Jager KA, Ricketts HJ, Strandness DE Jr. Duplex scanning for the evaluation of lower limb arterial disease. In: Bernstein EF, ed. *Noninvasive Diagnostic Techniques in Vascular Disease*. 3rd ed. St. Louis: Mosby; 1985.
30. Moneta GL, Yeager RA, Antonovic R, et al. Accuracy of lower extremity arterial duplex mapping. *J Vasc Surg*. 1992;15:275–283; discussion 283–284.
31. Ligush J Jr, Reavis SW, Preisser JS, et al. Duplex ultrasound scanning defines operative strategies for

patients with limb-threatening ischemia. *J Vasc Surg.* 1998;28:482–490; discussion 490–491.

32. Kohler TR, Nance DR, Cramer MM, et al. Duplex scanning for diagnosis of aortoiliac and femoropopliteal disease: a prospective study. *Circulation.* 1987;76:1074–1080.

33. Whelan JF, Barry MH, Moir JD. Color flow Doppler ultrasonography: comparison with peripheral arteriography for the investigation of peripheral vascular disease. *J Clin Ultrasound.* 1992;20:369–374.

34. Goyen M, Ruehm SG, Debatin JF. MR angiography for assessment of peripheral vascular disease. *Radiol Clin North Am.* 2002;40:835–846.

35. Rofsky NM, Adelman MA. MR angiography in the evaluation of atherosclerotic peripheral vascular disease. *Radiology.* 2000;214:325–338.

36. Ho VB, Corse WR. MR angiography of the abdominal aorta and peripheral vessels. *Radiol Clin North Am.* 2003;41:115–144.

37. Carpenter JP, Owen RS, Holland GA, et al. Magnetic resonance angiography of the aorta, iliac, and femoral arteries. *Surgery.* 1994;116:17–23.

38. Quinn SF, Sheley RC, Szumowski J, et al. Evaluation of the iliac arteries: comparison of two-dimensional time of flight magnetic resonance angiography with cardiac compensated fast gradient recalled echo and contrast-enhanced three-dimensional time of flight magnetic resonance angiography. *J Magn Reson Imaging.* 1997;7:197–203.

39. Ruehm SG, Hany TF, Pfammatter T, et al. Pelvic and lower extremity arterial imaging: diagnostic performance of three-dimensional contrast-enhanced MR angiography. *AJR Am J Roentgenol.* 2000;174:1127–1135.

40. Meaney JF, Ridgway JP, Chakraverty S, et al. Stepping-table gadolinium-enhanced digital subtraction MR angiography of the aorta and lower extremity arteries: preliminary experience. *Radiology.* 1999;211:59–67.

41. Owen RS, Carpenter JP, Baum RA, et al. Magnetic resonance imaging of angiographically occult runoff vessels in peripheral arterial occlusive disease. *N Engl J Med.* 1992;326:1577–1581.

42. Rofsky NM, Johnson G, Adelman MA, et al. Peripheral vascular disease evaluated with reduced-dose gadolinium-enhanced MR angiography. *Radiology.* 1997;205:163–169.

43. Rubin GD, Shiau MC, Leung AN, et al. Aorta and iliac arteries: single versus multiple detector-row helical CT angiography. *Radiology.* 2000;215:670–676.

44. Lawler LP, Fishman EK. Multidetector row computed tomography of the aorta and peripheral arteries. *Cardiol Clin.* 2003;21:607–629.

45. Bluemke DA, Chambers TP. Spiral CT angiography: an alternative to conventional angiography. *Radiology.* 1995;195:317–319.

46. Rubin GD, Schmidt AJ, Logan LJ, et al. Multidetector row CT angiography of lower extremity arterial inflow and runoff: initial experience. *Radiology.* 2001;221:146–158.

47. Ofer A, Nitecki SS, Linn S, et al. Multidetector CT angiography of peripheral vascular disease: a prospective comparison with intraarterial digital subtraction angiography. *AJR Am J Roentgenol.* 2003;180:719–724.

48. Carpenter JP, Holland GA, Golden MA, et al. Magnetic resonance angiography of the aortic arch. *J Vasc Surg.* 1997;25:145–151.

49. Matsumura JS, Rilling WS, Pearce WH, et al. Helical computed tomography of the normal thoracic outlet. *J Vasc Surg.* 1997;26:776–783.

50. Olin JW. Evaluation of peripheral circulation. In: Izzo JL, Black HR, eds. *Hypertension Primer.* 3rd ed. Dallas, TX: American Heart Association; 2003:361–365.

51. Zwiebel WJ. Normal carotid arteries and carotid examination technique. In: Zwiebel WJ, ed. *Introduction to Vascular Ultrasonography.* 4th ed. Philadelphia: WB Saunders; 2000:113–124.

52. Zwiebel WJ. Ultrasound assessment of carotid plaque. In: Zwiebel WJ, ed. *Introduction to Vascular Ultrasonography.* 4th ed. Philadelphia: WB Saunders; 2000:125–135.

53. Widder B, Paulat K, Hackspacher J, et al. Morphological characterization of carotid artery stenoses by ultrasound duplex scanning. *Ultrasound Med Biol.* 1990;16:349–354.

54. Bluth EI, Kay D, Merritt CR, et al. Sonographic characterization of carotid plaque: detection of hemorrhage. *AJR Am J Roentgenol.* 1986;146:1061–1065.

55. Imparato AM, Riles TS, Mintzer R, et al. The importance of hemorrhage in the relationship between gross morphologic characteristics and cerebral symptoms in 376 carotid artery plaques. *Ann Surg.* 1983;197:195–203.

56. O'Donnell TF Jr, Erdoes L, Mackey WC, et al. Correlation of B-mode ultrasound imaging and arteriography with pathologic findings at carotid endarterectomy. *Arch Surg.* 1985;120:443–449.

57. Ratliff DA, Gallagher PJ, Hames TK, et al. Characterization of carotid artery disease: comparison of duplex scanning with histology. *Ultrasound Med Biol.* 1985;11:835–840.

58. Beneficial effect of carotid endarterectomy in symptomatic patients with high-grade carotid stenosis. North American Symptomatic Carotid Endarterectomy Trial Collaborators. *N Engl J Med.* 1991;325:445–453.

59. MRC European Carotid Surgery Trial: interim results for symptomatic patients with severe (70%–99%) or with mild (0%–29%) carotid stenosis. European Carotid Surgery Trialists' Collaborative Group. *Lancet.* 1991;337:1235–1243.

60. Endarterectomy for asymptomatic carotid artery stenosis. Executive Committee for the Asymptomatic Carotid Atherosclerosis Study. *JAMA.* 1995;273:1421–1428.

61. Pan XM, Saloner D, Reilly LM, et al. Assessment of carotid artery stenosis by ultrasonography, conventional angiography, and magnetic resonance angiography: correlation with ex vivo measurement of plaque stenosis. *J Vasc Surg.* 1995;21:82–88; discussion 88–89.

62. Strandness DE Jr. Extracranial arterial disease. In: Strandness DE Jr, ed. *Duplex Scanning in Vascular Disorders.* 2nd ed. New York: Raven Press; 1993:113–158.

63. Zwiebel WJ. Doppler evaluation of carotid stenosis. In: Zwiebel WJ, ed. *Introduction to Vascular Ultrasonography.* 3rd ed. Philadelphia: WB Saunders; 1992:123–132.

64. Grant EG, Benson CB, Moneta GL, et al. Carotid artery stenosis: gray-scale and Doppler US diagnosis–Society of Radiologists in Ultrasound Consensus Conference. *Radiology.* 2003;229:340–346.

65. Moneta GL, Edwards JM, Chitwood RW, et al. Correlation of North American Symptomatic Carotid Endarterectomy Trial (NASCET) angiographic definition

of 70% to 99% internal carotid artery stenosis with duplex scanning. *J Vasc Surg.* 1993;17:152–157; discussion 157–159.

66. Faught WE, Mattos MA, van Bemmelen PS, et al.
Color-flow duplex scanning of carotid arteries: new velocity criteria based on receiver operator characteristic analysis for threshold stenoses used in the symptomatic and asymptomatic carotid trials. *J Vasc Surg.*
1994;19:818–827; discussion 827–828.

67. Neale ML, Chambers JL, Kelly AT, et al. Reappraisal
of duplex criteria to assess significant carotid stenosis with special reference to reports from the North
American Symptomatic Carotid Endarterectomy Trial
and the European Carotid Surgery Trial. *J Vasc Surg.*
1994;20:642–649.

68. Moneta GL, Edwards JM, Papanicolaou G, et al.
Screening for asymptomatic internal carotid artery
stenosis: duplex criteria for discriminating 60% to 99%
stenosis. *J Vasc Surg.* 1995;21:989–994.

69. AbuRahma AF, Robinson PA, Strickler DL, et al. Proposed new duplex classification for threshold stenoses
used in various symptomatic and asymptomatic carotid
endarterectomy trials. *Ann Vasc Surg.* 1998;12:349–
358.

70. AbuRahma AF, Richmond BK, Robinson PA, et al. Effect of contralateral severe stenosis or carotid occlusion on duplex criteria of ipsilateral stenoses: comparative study of various duplex parameters. *J Vasc Surg.*
1995;22:751–761; discussion 761–762.

71. Fujitani RM, Mills JL, Wang LM, et al. The effect of unilateral internal carotid arterial occlusion upon contralateral duplex study: criteria for accurate interpretation.
J Vasc Surg. 1992;16:459–467; discussion 467–468.

72. Sachar R, Yadav JS, Roffi M, et al. Severe bilateral
carotid stenosis: the impact of ipsilateral stenting on
Doppler-defined contralateral stenosis. *J Am Coll Cardiol.* 2004;43:1358–1362.

73. Lal BK, Hobson RW II, Goldstein J, et al. Carotid artery
stenting: is there a need to revise ultrasound velocity
criteria? *J Vasc Surg.* 2004;39:58–66.

74. Hriljac I, Gustavson S, Olin JW. Images in vascular
ultrasound. Stenosis of the innominate or left common
carotid artery origin diagnosed on carotid ultrasound
examination. *Vasc Med.* 2003;8:287–288.

75. Zwiebel WJ. Doppler evaluation of carotid stenosis. In:
Zwiebel WJ, ed. *Introduction to Vascular Ultrasonography.* 4th ed. Philadelphia: WB Saunders; 2000:137–
154.

76. Zwolak RM. Arterial duplex imaging. In: Rutherford
RB, ed. *Vascular Surgery.* 5th ed. Philadelphia: WB
Saunders; 2000:192–214.

77. Ricci MA, Knight SJ. The role of noninvasive studies in the diagnosis and management of cerebrovascular disease. In: Rutherford RB, ed. *Vascular Surgery.*
5th ed. Philadelphia: WB Saunders; 2000:1775–1789.

78. Anderson CM, Haacke EM. Approaches to diagnostic
magnetic resonance carotid angiography. *Semin Ultrasound CT MR.* 1992;13:246–255.

79. Blakeley DD, Oddone EZ, Hasselblad V, et al. Noninvasive carotid artery testing. A meta-analytic review.
Ann Intern Med. 1995;122:360–367.

80. Willig DS, Turski PA, Frayne R, et al. Contrast-
enhanced 3D MR DSA of the carotid artery bifurcation: preliminary study of comparison with unenhanced
2D and 3D time-of-flight MR angiography. *Radiology.*
1998;208:447–451.

81. Remonda L, Senn P, Barth A, et al. Contrast-enhanced

3D MR angiography of the carotid artery: comparison with conventional digital subtraction angiography.
AJNR Am J Neuroradiol. 2002;23:213–219.

82. Nederkoorn PJ, van der Graaf Y, Hunink MG. Duplex ultrasound and magnetic resonance angiography compared with digital subtraction angiography in
carotid artery stenosis: a systematic review. *Stroke.*
2003;34:1324–1332.

83. Simeone A, Carriero A, Armillotta M, et al. Spiral CT
angiography in the study of the carotid stenoses. *J Neuroradiol.* 1997;24:18–22.

84. Randoux B, Marro B, Koskas F, et al. Carotid
artery stenosis: prospective comparison of CT, three-
dimensional gadolinium-enhanced MR, and conventional angiography. *Radiology.* 2001;220:179–185.

85. Sameshima T, Futami S, Morita Y, et al. Clinical usefulness of and problems with three-dimensional CT angiography for the evaluation of arteriosclerotic stenosis of the carotid artery: comparison with conventional
angiography, MRA, and ultrasound sonography. *Surg
Neurol.* 1999;51:301–308; discussion 308–309.

86. Marcus CD, Ladam-Marcus VJ, Bigot JL, et al.
Carotid arterial stenosis: evaluation at CT angiography with the volume-rendering technique. *Radiology.*
1999;211:775–780.

87. Anderson GB, Ashforth R, Steinke DE, et al. CT angiography for the detection and characterization of
carotid artery bifurcation disease. *Stroke.* 2000;31:
2168–2174.

88. Patel SG, Collie DA, Wardlaw JM, et al. Outcome, ob-
server reliability, and patient preferences if CTA, MRA,
or Doppler ultrasound were used, individually or together, instead of digital subtraction angiography before
carotid endarterectomy. *J Neurol Neurosurg Psychiatry.*
2002;73:21–28.

89. Chen CJ, Lee TH, Hsu HL, et al. Multi-Slice CT angiography in diagnosing total versus near occlusions
of the internal carotid artery: comparison with catheter
angiography. *Stroke.* 2004;35:83–85.

90. Farres MT, Grabenwoger F, Magometschnig H, et al.
Spiral CT angiography: study of stenoses and calcification at the origin of the vertebral artery. *Neuroradiology.*
1996;38:738–743.

91. Kohler TR, Zierler RE, Martin RL, et al. Noninvasive
diagnosis of renal artery stenosis by ultrasonic duplex
scanning. *J Vasc Surg.* 1986;4:450–456.

92. Taylor DC, Kettler MD, Moneta GL, et al. Duplex ultrasound scanning in the diagnosis of renal artery stenosis: a prospective evaluation. *J Vasc Surg.* 1988;7:363–
369.

93. Hoffmann U, Edwards JM, Carter S, et al. Role of duplex scanning for the detection of atherosclerotic renal
artery disease. *Kidney Int.* 1991;39:1232–1239.

94. Radermacher J, Chavan A, Bleck J, et al. Use of Doppler
ultrasonography to predict the outcome of therapy for
renal-artery stenosis. *N Engl J Med.* 2001;344:410–417.

95. Hansen KJ, Tribble RW, Reavis SW, et al. Renal duplex
sonography: evaluation of clinical utility. *J Vasc Surg.*
1990;12:227–236.

96. Olin JW, Piedmonte MR, Young JR, et al. The utility
of duplex ultrasound scanning of the renal arteries for
diagnosing significant renal artery stenosis. *Ann Intern
Med.* 1995;122:833–838.

97. Olin JW, Begelman SM. Renal artery disease. In: Topol
EJ, ed. *Textbook of Cardiovascular Medicine.* 2nd ed.
Philadelphia: Lippincott Raven; 2002:2139–2159.

98. Schwerk WB, Restrepo IK, Stellwaag M, et al. Renal

artery stenosis: grading with image-directed Doppler US evaluation of renal resistive index. *Radiology.* 1994;190:785–790.

99. Mukherjee D, Bhatt DL, Robbins M, et al. Renal artery end-diastolic velocity and renal artery resistance index as predictors of outcome after renal stenting. *Am J Cardiol.* 2001;88:1064–1066.

100. Olin JW. Atherosclerotic renal artery disease. *Cardiol Clin.* 2002;20:547–562, vi.

101. Vasbinder GB, Nelemans PJ, Kessels AG, et al. Diagnostic tests for renal artery stenosis in patients suspected of having renovascular hypertension: a meta-analysis. *Ann Intern Med.* 2001;135:401–411.

102. Fillinger MF. Computed tomography and three dimensional reconstruction in evaluation of vascular disease. In: Rutherford RB, ed. *Vascular Surgery.* 5th ed. Philadelphia: WB Saunders; 2000:230–269.

103. Beregi JP, Elkohen M, Deklunder G, et al. Helical CT angiography compared with arteriography in the detection of renal artery stenosis. *AJR Am J Roentgenol.* 1996;167:495–501.

104. Nally JV Jr, Clarke HS Jr, Grecos GP, et al. Effect of captopril on 99mTc-diethylenetriaminepentaacetic acid renograms in two-kidney, one clip hypertension. *Hypertension.* 1986;8:685–693.

105. Jager KA, Fortner GS, Thiele BL, Strandness DE Jr. Noninvasive diagnosis of intestinal angina. *J Clin Ultrasound.* 1984;12:588–591.

106. Zwolak RM, Fillinger MF, Walsh DB, et al. Mesenteric and celiac duplex scanning: a validation study. *J Vasc Surg.* 1998;27:1078–1087; discussion 1088.

107. Moneta GL, Yeager RA, Dalman R, et al. Duplex ultrasound criteria for diagnosis of splanchnic artery stenosis or occlusion. *J Vasc Surg.* 1991;14:511–518; discussion 518–520.

108. Gentile AT, Moneta GL, Lee RW, et al. Usefulness of fasting and postprandial duplex ultrasound examinations for predicting high-grade superior mesenteric artery stenosis. *Am J Surg.* 1995;169:476–479.

109. Meaney JF, Prince MR, Nostrant TT, et al. Gadolinium-enhanced MR angiography of visceral arteries in patients with suspected chronic mesenteric ischemia. *J Magn Reson Imaging.* 1997;7:171–176.

110. Fleischmann D. Multiple detector-row CT angiography of the renal and mesenteric vessels. *Eur J Radiol.* 2003;45(suppl 1):S79–S87.

CHAPTER 3

General Angiographic and Interventional Principles

Kent W. Dauterman, Ivan P. Casserly, and Christopher J. Bajzer

Peripheral angiography specialty suites have evolved over the last decade to contain a number of features that are important in performing high-quality peripheral vascular angiography and intervention. The purpose of this chapter is to provide a description and discussion of these unique features, since most operators are familiar with the basic workings of radiographic imaging systems. In addition, an overview of the equipment most commonly used during peripheral diagnostic and interventional studies, and a description of some of the fundamental principles involved in these procedures, are provided.

RADIOGRAPHIC IMAGING

The interactive components of a radiographic imaging system are shown in Figure 3-1.

Image Intensifier

In the peripheral intervention laboratory, the diameter of the image intensifier is 15″, or occasionally 12″, providing a large field of view. This is particularly important when imaging the aorta or lower extremities. The smaller image intensifier in most cardiac catheterization laboratories (i.e., 9″) is adequate for diagnostic angiography and intervention of the carotid, vertebral, subclavian, renal, and iliac arteries.

Examination Console

During peripheral angiography, a variety of settings (i.e., kVp, mA, frames per second) will vary automatically, depending on the vascular territory of interest. These territories are usually divided as follows: cerebral, thorax, abdomen, upper extremity, and lower extremity. The tube kilovoltage will be set highest for cerebral and abdominal angiography, and lowest for angiography of the extremities, with the thorax having an intermediate setting. Frame rates for peripheral angiography are generally 2 to 3 per second, but this may be adjusted for specific circumstances (e.g., increased for angiography with gadolinium contrast, or decreased for venous studies in which the cineangiographic runs are long). These vascular package options may be found in the room examination console controls that programs the x-ray generator.

Digital Subtraction Angiography vs. Cineangiography

Cineangiography simply takes multiple x-ray pictures of the contrast-filled vessel as well as the surrounding tissue (Fig. 3-2A). For rapidly moving structures with a radiolucent background, such as the coronary arteries moving with the beating heart, this 15 to 30 frames per second imaging modality is ideal (1).

For static vascular structures that are surrounded by radiodense structures (e.g., bone), digital subtraction angiography (DSA) is the ideal imaging modality (2). With this technique, the initial images obtained when stepping on the x-ray pedal are used to generate the baseline image from which all radio-opaque structures are subtracted. Subsequent images obtained

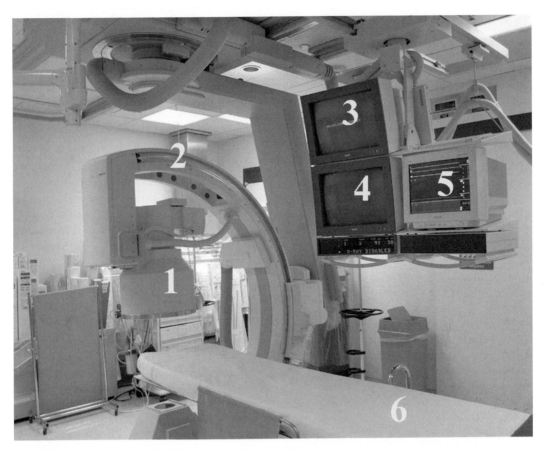

FIGURE 3-1 ● **Peripheral angiographic suite. 1:** 15″ Image intensifier; **2:** Multiplane C-arm, mounted on overhead track; **3:** Saved-image monitor; **4:** Image monitor; **5:** Hemodynamic monitor; and **6:** Long patient bed.

following contrast injection will be the subtracted images and will, therefore, demonstrate only the contrast-filled vascular structures (Fig. 3-2B).

The DSA imaging modality requires that the patient not move during image acquisition. In vascular territories where the vessels may move during respiration or swallowing (e.g., carotid, vertebral), the patients must also suspend these activities during image acquisition.

Trace Subtract Fluoroscopy or Road Mapping

Trace-subtract fluoroscopy is the fluoroscopic equivalent of DSA. Like DSA, the initial few seconds of this mode are used to obtain a fluoroscopic image that is then subtracted (2). Once the subtracted image is seen on the screen, contrast agent is injected to completely fill the vessel. The pedal is then released and the subtracted im-

age with the contrast-filled vessel remains on the screen (Figure 3-3A).

In contrast to DSA, the contrast-filled vessel will appear white, as opposed to black. Subsequent activation of the fluoroscopy pedal allows visualization of catheters, wires, and interventional equipment superimposed on the saved image of the contrast-filled vessel (Figure 3-3B).

When used correctly, this technique may improve the safety of various maneuvers (e.g., advancement of wires and catheters) and help to minimize contrast use. For optimal results, the patient must remain perfectly still between the time of contrast agent injection and the completion of any intended maneuver.

Leg Imaging Capability

The ability to perform lower extremity angiography requires that the image intensifier should be able to travel on an overhead track, to the patient's

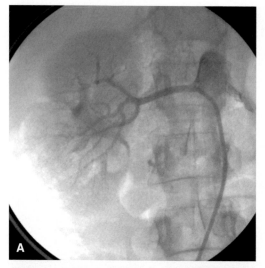

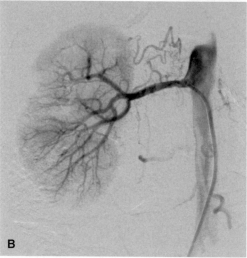

FIGURE 3-2 ● **A:** Cineangiogram of right renal artery showing vascular and surrounding structures. **B:** Digital subtraction angiogram of right renal artery showing vascular structures with background subtracted.

feet. In addition, the table should be sufficiently long to provide working space caudal to the feet since the image intensifier is placed over the legs, thereby eliminating the usual workspace. Long wires (260 cm to 300 cm) are frequently used, so it is important to have plenty of workspace.

Interactive Mode vs. Stepped Mode with Multiple Injections

When performing a run-off of the arterial system in the legs, traditional practice has been to obtain sequential, stepped, static angiographic im-

ages (i.e., external iliac, SFA, popliteal, anterior tibial/posterior tibial/peroneal, and foot) using bolus contrast injections. This may be time consuming and requires selective cannulation of the respective common and external iliac arteries.

The interactive mode permits complete imaging of one or both lower extremities, with a single bolus given in the external iliac artery or distal abdominal aorta respectively. The first step is to engage the interactive mode in the control room and establish the beginning and end positions of the table. The bolus is then given, cineangiography commences simultaneously, and the bolus is chased by moving the table proximally, relative to the image intensifier. The table is then brought back to the starting position automatically, and a dry cineangiographic run is performed at the same table movement rate. The latter images are used to subtract from the initial contrast agent containing images. Multiple digital subtraction images are then obtained from the interactive run, and stored. Currently, it is not possible to obtain new DSA images from the interactive run, once the case has been transferred from local storage.

Problems arise if a patient has trouble holding still for the 1 to 2 minutes that it takes to complete an interactive run. Additionally, severe stenosis or occlusion in one extremity often results in unequal rates of contrast run-off in both extremities requiring that the operator prioritize imaging from the leg of interest, and compromise on the image quality from the contralateral leg.

Minimizing Radiation Exposure

Peripheral vascular interventions may take a long time and involve significant radiation exposure for the operator, laboratory staff, and patient. For the operator, maintaining distance from the x-ray source is the best advice. When performing power injections, step away from the table and stand in the control room or behind a lead screen. Stand back one step during cine runs. Wear an appropriate lead apron that is checked annually for its integrity, maximize your shielding (e.g., screens, acrylic leaded shields, thyroid collars, lead glasses), collimate when possible, and use low-dose pulse fluoroscopy. Wear your monitoring badge. If the readings are high,

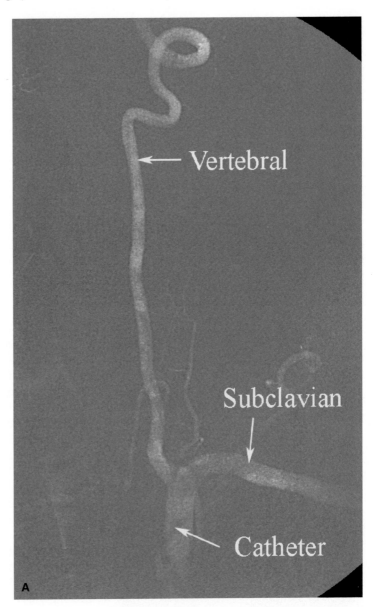

FIGURE 3-3 ● **Trace subtract fluoroscopic image of left vertebral artery. A:** Note that vascular structures appear white with this fluoroscopic technique. (*continued*)

you may often take steps to decrease your exposure.

ACCESS

One of the first steps of any endovascular procedure is determining the most appropriate site for arterial access. The following sites are considered.

Common Femoral Artery

This is the most common access site used for peripheral diagnostic angiography and interven-

tion. The CFA artery is centrally located and all vascular arterial systems may be reached barring occlusive and tortuous peripheral vascular disease. The advantage of this access site is the size of the CFA, which may accommodate sheath sizes of 12 Fr to 14 Fr with minimal risk for ischemia. Most equipment has been developed for the femoral approach and the femoral artery approach also provides greater distance from the x-ray source and a more spacious workplace compared to the arm. On the other hand, CFA access is associated with an increased bleeding risk and delayed ambulation (3,4).

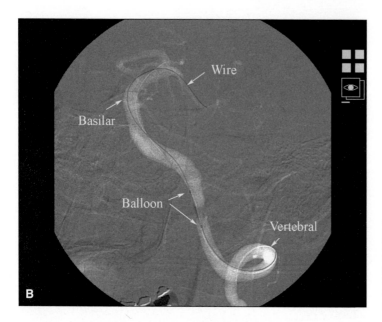

FIGURE 3-3 ● (Continued)
B: Trace subtract fluoroscopic image of intracerebral portion of the left vertebral and basilar arteries demonstrating the usefulness of this technique for wiring vessels and positioning equipment.

In peripheral angiography, the CFA may be accessed in an antegrade (toward the foot) or retrograde (toward the iliac artery) fashion, which impacts the access technique. In the retrograde approach, puncture of the CFA should be performed proximal to its bifurcation with an 18-gauge or 19-gauge access needle, using the front-wall technique (Fig. 3-4).

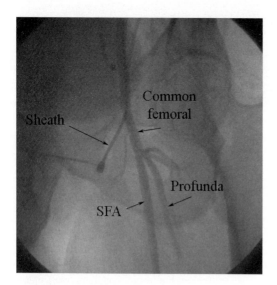

FIGURE 3-4 ● Common femoral artery (CFA) angiogram demonstrating correct position of CFA sheath proximal to the CFA bifurcation at the level of the middle of the femoral head.

The bifurcation usually occurs proximal to the level of the mid-femoral head. We would advocate always using fluoroscopic guidance to help ensure the appropriate location of the puncture. Having obtained pulsatile backflow with the needle, our practice is to use a 0.035″ soft-tipped wire to wire the iliac vessels and aorta and exchange the needle for the femoral sheath. We would specifically warn against using J-tipped or straight wires for this purpose, since there is a high incidence of previously unrecognized iliac artery disease in patients undergoing peripheral vascular procedures and dissections may easily be created by the unsuspecting operator.

The antegrade approach requires careful attention, particularly in obese patients, where the bleeding risk is significantly increased. For right-handed individuals, the operator generally stands on the right-hand side of the table. In order to puncture the CFA above the bifurcation, the skin-puncture site of the needle is often much higher than would be anticipated by the inexperienced operator. There is a compromise between entering the CFA at the typical 45° and puncturing the skin below the inguinal ligament. This usually results in a needle angle of at least 60°, which often makes introduction of the sheath more difficult. Our practice is to use a micropuncture access set (i.e., with a long 21-guage needle) and to perform the puncture under direct fluoroscopic guidance. One must ensure that the 0.018″ wire is

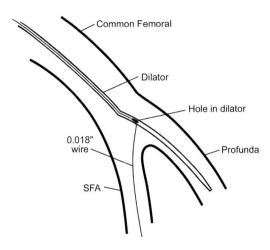

FIGURE 3-5 ● Use of Cope–Saddekni superficial femoral artery access dilator to wire the SFA during an antegrade access of the common femoral artery.

in the SFA before advancing the sheath. If there is prominent calcification in the SFA, this may be straight forward. Otherwise, a useful rule-of-thumb is to visualize the wire crossing the border of the femur in the typical location of Hunter's canal. Introducing the sheath over the 0.018″ wire may be challenging because of the angulation issue described above. When the wire persistently goes into the profunda branch, the use of an angulated dilator with an opening approximately 4 cm proximal to the tip, may be helpful in directing the wire into the SFA (Fig. 3-5).

Using stiffer sheaths with a longer taper on the introducer and a smooth introducer-sheath transition will help. Once a small sheath or dilator has been advanced over the 0.018″ wire, exchanging for a stiff wire and sequentially increasing the sheath size will usually allow the operator to deliver the desired sheath size.

Upper Extremity Access: Brachial and Radial

Access from the upper extremity arteries offers the advantage of early ambulation and a reduced risk of bleeding complications. The downside of these access sites is the limited sheath sizes that may be used (5 Fr to 6 Fr at radial, 6 Fr to 7 Fr at brachial), particularly in smaller patients, and the increased risk of ischemic complications (5). Even more serious is the risk of embolization to the cerebral circulation that may occur from instrumentation of the aortic arch, or passage of equipment across the origin of the vertebral or right common carotid arteries.

Brachial artery puncture is performed with the arm and forearm extended and slightly abducted. The site of puncture should be in the area of maximal arterial pulsation but care should be taken not to stick the brachial artery significantly above the antecubital crease, as it increases the risk of bleeding (Fig. 3-6).

Radial artery puncture is performed with the wrist extended and the forearm and hand supinated. The site of puncture is generally approximately 1 cm to 2 cm proximal to the wrist crease. We would recommend the use of a micropuncture access set (i.e., 21-guage needle, 0.018″ guide wire) for all radial and brachial artery punctures. Both vessels are prone to significant spasm and thrombosis in response to instrumentation. Aggressive administration of vasodilators (e.g., nitroglycerin, verapamil) and

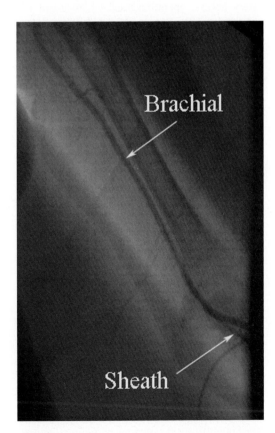

FIGURE 3-6 ● Angiogram of left brachial artery demonstrating typical location of the brachial artery sheath during brachial artery access.

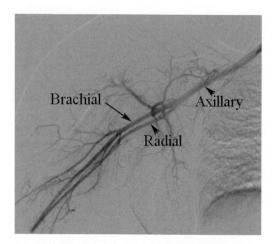

FIGURE 3-7 ● Right axillary artery angiogram demonstrating anomalous origin of the radial artery from the axillary artery.

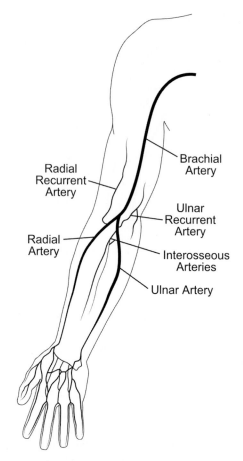

FIGURE 3-8 ● **Schematic of right upper extremity arterial supply.** Note the recurrent radial branch which can be entered by wires and catheters during use of the radial artery access site and may be subject to trauma.

heparin (at least 3,000 units) directly into the sheath is recommended, following sheath insertion, to minimize these risks. During brachial artery access, operators must be aware of the potential for anomalous origin of the radial or ulnar arteries from the axillary or high brachial artery (Fig. 3-7).

In addition, the potential for wires and catheters to track along the course of the recurrent radial branch when using radial artery access should be appreciated, as this may result in trauma to this branch and hematoma formation (Fig. 3-8).

Popliteal Artery

In a small number of specific situations during lower extremity interventions, the popliteal artery may be accessed. The patient is placed in the prone position on the table. The puncture may be performed using fluoroscopic guidance alone or alternatively, access may be guided by injection of contrast from another arterial site, using the road mapping function to help guide the puncture (Fig. 3-9). A micropuncture access set is recommended and using sheath sizes greater than 6 Fr in this location should be avoided.

Decision-Making Considerations for Access

The choice of access site for a particular diagnostic study or interventional procedure will be outlined in the various chapters to follow. However,

a number of principles are worth highlighting at this point, as follows.

Vascular Anatomy

One must always be aware of the vascular anatomy of the patient. This may be gleaned from previous angiographic studies, as well as from noninvasive studies (e.g., ultrasound, CT angiography, MR). Important things to look for include: known occlusions; significant stenoses; or tortuosity proximal to a potential access site (e.g., subclavian artery, iliac arteries). The angulation of the aortic bifurcation (i.e., acute angulation) increases the difficulty in performing cross-over techniques, and the presence of known aortic arch or great vessel disease increases the risk of cerebral embolization during upper extremity

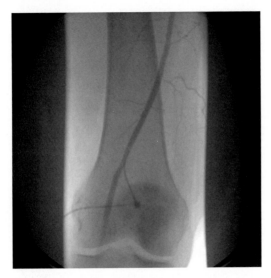

FIGURE 3-9 ● Popliteal artery angiogram demonstrating typical location of popliteal artery sheath.

arterial access (Figs. 3-10A and 3-10B). In addition, it is imperative to document carefully the palpable pulses present both at the various potential access sites and distal to these sites, prior to the procedure.

Previous Revascularization

The timing and nature of previous surgical revascularization procedures need to be defined clearly. For example, knowing that a patient had a femoral-femoral bypass is insufficient. Knowing the direction of flow in the graft is important, since a left common femoral artery (CFA) to right CFA bypass will necessitate access on the left side (usually above the graft). The timing of any previous surgery is important, as percutaneous puncture of grafts is generally avoided in the first 6 to 12 months.

Clinical History

One must be aware of the patient's clinical history and noninvasive evaluation. For example, in lower extremity diagnostic studies, one generally obtains access from the CFA contralateral to the extremity with the most symptoms, since this still allows for a subsequent cross-over technique to be employed if an intervention is indicated.

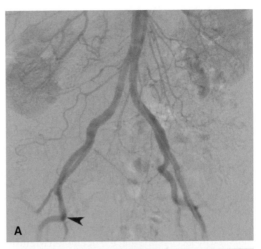

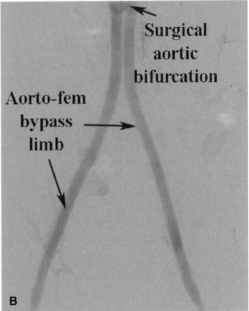

FIGURE 3-10 ● **A: Pelvic angiogram from patient with right superficial femoral artery occlusion.** The aortic bifurcation demonstrates an acute angle between the two common iliac arteries. The additional presence of tortuosity in the right external iliac artery (arrowhead) resulted in an antegrade common femoral artery (CFA) approach as opposed to a contralateral CFA approach. **B: An extreme example of an acute angle at the aortic bifurcation created by a surgical aorto-bifemoral bypass procedure.** This anatomy makes a contralateral common femoral artery approach for lower extremity intervention extremely difficult and argues in favor of a brachial artery approach or an antegrade CFA approach.

Access Appropriate to Site of Intervention

One should be aware that owing to the limitations of the length of interventional equipment, below-knee interventions are generally not possible from the brachial access. However, the left brachial access will allow about 10 cm greater reach for lower extremity intervention, compared to right brachial access.

Anatomy of the Occlusion

The anatomy of an occlusion is often critical in determining the access approach. The points to consider are: (1) Is there enough running room between the access site and the occlusion to allow safe placement of the sheath and to provide sufficient support for wiring the lesion and delivering equipment (Fig. 3-11A).

(2) It is important to assess from which side the occlusion should be approached. Generally, the chances of success will be greatest where there is a tapered stump without collaterals (Fig. 3-11B).

Sheath Sizes and Arterial Access

When considering an intervention, one should always be aware of the sheath sizes required to deliver the equipment that will be required to complete an intervention. For example, if the equipment requires a sheath size of at least 8 Fr or larger, femoral access will generally be required.

CHOICE OF CONTRAST AGENT

Ionic contrast is no longer used for peripheral angiography owing to its high osmolality.

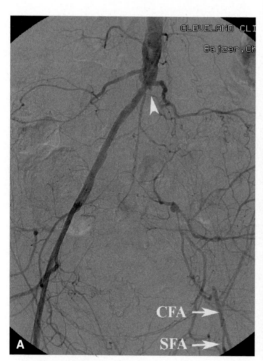
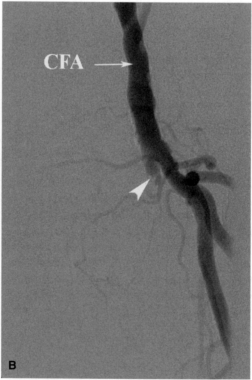

FIGURE 3-11 ● **A: Pelvic angiogram demonstrating a long occlusion extending from the origin of the left common iliac artery to the proximal left common femoral artery (CFA).** There is inadequate space to allow an access sheath to be safely placed in the left CFA. The ostial location of the occlusion in the left common iliac artery will likely result in very poor support if access is obtained from the contralateral CFA. The ideal initial access site for this case is the brachial artery. **B: Common femoral artery angiogram demonstrating an occlusion of the superficial femoral artery (SFA) (arrowhead).** This occlusion is favorable in that there is a clearly defined stump with no collaterals, similar to the occlusion in figure 3-11A. Note that angulated views may be required to fully define the anatomy of the stump.

During cerebral angiography, this type of contrast agent has been associated with transient blindness, and injection into the extremities is often excruciatingly painful. Its use is limited to inflation of angioplasty balloons and balloon-expandable stents, during interventions. Owing to the large size of peripheral balloons and balloon-expandable stents, a mixture of 70% saline and 30% contrast agent is used, in order to decrease the viscosity and facilitate balloon emptying following inflation.

The best tolerated and least nephrotoxic contrast agent for peripheral vascular interventions appears to be iodixanol, which is a nonionic, isosmolar contrast agent (1). Patients rarely have any discomfort when iodixanol is injected in the peripheral circulation. However, when a catheter is placed in the mid-to-distal arm and a manual injection is performed, a 50:50 mixture of saline and contrast agent is used to avoid discomfort for the patient.

For patients with chronic renal insufficiency, the optimal strategy for avoiding renal failure appears to be preprocedural hydration with normal saline, giving N-acetylcysteine 600 mg by mouth, twice daily, one day prior to the procedure, and minimizing the amount of contrast injected. Iodixanol should be used if possible. Gadolinium and carbon dioxide are both options for these patients but vascular imaging is often suboptimal. There is some evidence that doses greater than 60 mL of gadolinium may have the same nephrotoxicity as iodinated contrast agents.

MANIFOLD AND HEMODYNAMIC MONITORING

A pressure/saline/contrast manifold allows continuous pressure measurement during diagnostic and interventional procedures. Any dampened waveform suggests that the catheter end hole is against a vessel wall and an injection may cause vessel dissection. The system also minimizes the risk of air embolization. Continuous monitoring of the electrocardiogram (EKG), heart rate, blood pressure, and oxygen saturation often helps to detect any life-threatening issues, such as anaphylaxis, hemorrhage, pulmonary edema, oversedation, etc., that may arise during a procedure.

WIRE SELECTION (0.035″, 0.018″, 0.014″)

The three primary 0.035″ wires used in peripheral endovascular interventions at the Cleveland Clinic are the Wholey®, Magic Torque®, and Stiff-Angled Glide® wires (Table 3-1).

The Wholey® wire has good directional control and is quite safe, but sometimes does not track very well in tortuous vessels. During interventions, the white portion of the wire seems to swell making over-the-wire balloon exchanges somewhat difficult. The Magic Torque® wire provides good support and the over-the-wire balloon exchanges are easy. However, it sometimes requires a degree of magic to torque it. The Stiff-Angled Glide® wire is very controllable and trackable, and provides good support. Owing to its hydrophilic nature, great care and attention must be paid to its tip, since it may dissect or perforate more easily than the other two wires. Where directional control and tracking is required and support is not an issue, a floppy glide wire is safer than the stiff glide wire. Wires of 0.035″ diameter are typically used for subclavian, innominate, iliac, superficial femoral, and popliteal artery interventions.

Table 3-1 lists 0.014″ wires that are suitable for carotid, vertebral, renal, and below knee interventions. A long list of 0.014″ wires have been developed for percutaneous coronary intervention and may be applied safely in peripheral vascular intervention. It is wise to become familiar with a short list of wires that will be sufficient for the majority of procedures. This should include low-, moderate-, and high-support nonhydrophilic and hydrophilic wires (Table 3-1). For peripheral interventions, largely, moderate or high-support wires will be used. In addition, some niche wires, such as the Synchro® wire for intracerebral procedures, may be stocked. Less commonly, 0.018″ wires may be used for renal, subclavian, and popliteal interventions.

DIAGNOSTIC CATHETERS

Side-hole Diagnostic Catheters

These catheters permit large volumes of contrast agent to be infused safely in a large artery at a rapid rate via power injection (e.g., Pig,

TABLE 3-1

Wires

Wire Diameter	Directional Control	Tracking Capability	Support	Length (cm)	Company
WIRES 0.035"					
Stiff Angled Glidewire (3 cm or 5 cm flexible tip)	Excellent	Excellent	Good	260	Boston Scientific
Amplatz Extra Stiff w/ J-tip	Poor	Fair	Very Good	260	Boston Scientific
Amplatz Super Stiff (1 cm, 3.5 cm, 6 cm, and J-tip)	Poor	Poor	Excellent	260	Boston Scientific
Magic Torque	Fair	Good	Good	300	Boston Scientific
Wholey	Excellent	Good	Fair	260	Mallinckrodt
Lunderquist	Fair	Poor	Excellent	260	Cook
WIRES 0.018"					
Flex-T	Good	Good	Good	295	Mallinckrodt
Glidewire Gold (45 or 70 degree angle) with GT Leggiero Hydrophilic Microcatheter	Good	Excellent	Poor*	180	Boston Scientific
WIRES 0.014"					
Balance Trek	Good	Good	Fair	190, 300	Guidant
Balance Middle Weight	Good	Good	Moderate	190, 300	Guidant
Iron Man	Fair	Fair	Excellent	190, 300	Guidant
Platinum Plus	Poor	Poor	Excellent	300	Boston Scientific
Sparta Core	Fair	Fair	Good	130, 190, 300	Guidant
Whisper (hydrophilic)	Good	Excellent	Fair	190, 300	Guidant
Shinobi (hydrophilic)	Excellent	Good	Excellent	190, 300	Cordis
Synchro Wire (hydrophilic)	Excellent	Good	Fair	300	Boston Scientific

*advise exchange of Glidewire Gold for other supportive wire via microcatheter

Omniflush, Grollman, Universal Flush, Multi-purpose). The authors use the Pig catheter for ascending and arch aortography, abdominal aortography, and bilateral lower extremity run-offs (i.e., with catheter in distal abdominal aorta) (Fig. 3-12).

Flush catheters are often used for imaging the contralateral external iliac artery with runoff to the leg. For example, if the right leg arterial circulation needs to be studied and the left common femoral artery is accessed, then the flush catheter is advanced to the abdominal aorta. The flush catheter is then slowly pulled back to the aortic bifurcation where the wire and catheter hook the contralateral common iliac artery. The wire and flush catheter are then

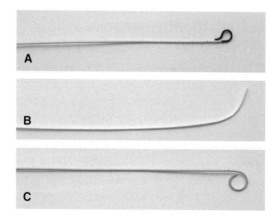

FIGURE 3-12 ● Sample of side-hole catheters. A: Omni Flush; B: Multipurpose; and C: Pigtail.

advanced to the contralateral external iliac artery, where power injection is performed.

End-hole Diagnostic Catheters

Selective diagnostic angiography is performed using manual injections of contrast agent through end-hole catheters. Good studies may be obtained with 5 Fr catheters when using digital subtraction angiography (Table 3-2).

The 5F JR4 catheter is our workhorse catheter for imaging the carotid, vertebral, subclavian, and renal arteries (Fig. 3-13).

Care must be taken with the use of Simmons, Amplatz Left, Newton, Vitek, and SOS catheters since they require forming the catheter in the aorta, proximal to the artery of interest. These catheters are then pulled distally, with care, (to-

ward the sheath and operator) with the intention of hooking the catheter tip into the artery of interest. Embolization and dissection are real concerns and heparin should be considered when these catheters are used.

GUIDING CATHETER VS. SHEATH (FIG. 3-14 AND 3-15)

Peripheral interventions may be performed using either a sheath or guide-based system. Straight or shaped sheaths (Table 3-3) are most commonly used.

One of the major advantages of sheaths over guides is that a smaller sheath (e.g., 6 Fr) has the same internal diameter as a guiding catheter two French sizes larger (i.e., 8 Fr). However, generally, it is not possible to maneuver

TABLE 3-2

Diagnostic Catheters

End-Hole Catheters

Vascular Bed	Name	Size (Fr)	Length (cm)	Comments
Cerebral, Carotid, Vertebral, Subclavian, and Innominate	Angled Glide	5	100, 120	Great tracking ability in tortuous vessels. Soft atraumatic catheter tip
	Berenstein	5	90	Not as versatile as the JR4
	JR4	5	100, 125	Primary catheter
	Newton (HN2, HN4, HN5)	5	100	Similar to Vitek
	Simmons 1, Simmons 1.5, Simmons 2, Simmons 3	5	100	Requires care with catheter manipulation
	Vitek	5	125	Softer than the Simmons. First choice if JR4 is unsuccessful. Excellent for Type 3 and bovine arches
Upper Extremity	Angled Glide	4, 5	100, 120	
Renal	JR4	5	100, 125	
	SOS Omni	5	80	Requires care with catheter manipulation
Mesenteric	Cobra (C1, C2, C3)	5	65	
	SOS Omni	5	80	
Leg	IM (approach from contralateral leg)	5	100	Use to cross from ipsilateral iliac to contralateral iliac artery
	Multipurpose	5	125	

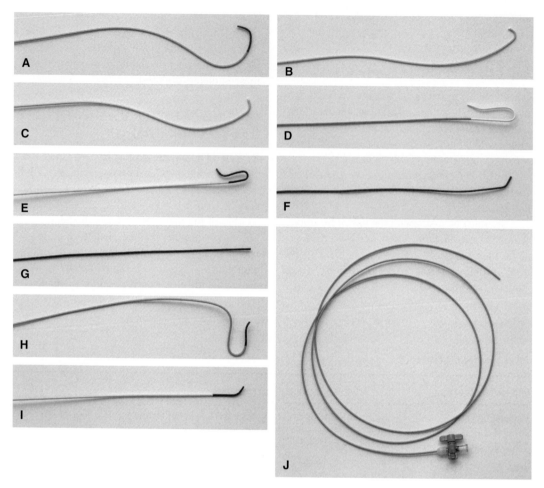

FIGURE 3-13 ● Sample of end-hole catheters. A: Cobra; B: IMA; C: Judkins Right; D: Simmons;
E: SoS; F: angled glide; G: straight glide; H: Vitek; I: Berenstein; and J: red rubber.

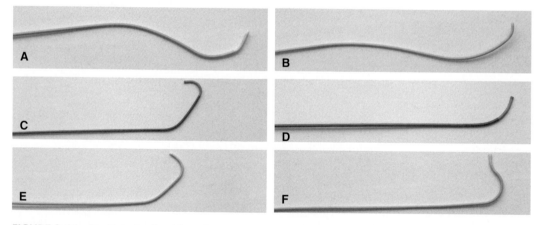

FIGURE 3-14 ● Sample of guide catheters. A: Headhunter (H-1); B: Judkins Right (JR4); C: Renal Standard
(RES); D: Renal Multipurpose; E: Renal Double Curve (RDC); and F: Amplatz Right (AR1).

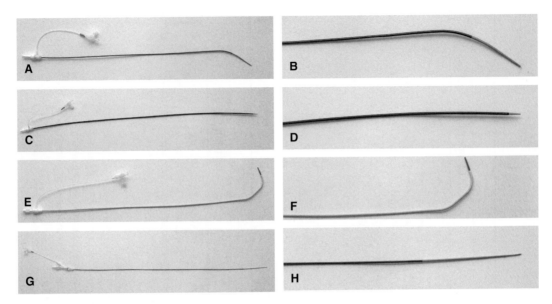

FIGURE 3-15 ● **Sample of sheaths. A:** and **B:** Low and high magnification view of Ansel sheath; **C:** and **D:** Low and high magnification view of Raabe sheath; **E:** and **F:** Low and high magnification view of Renal Double Curve guide sheath; and **G:** and **H:** Low and high magnification view of Shuttle sheath.

the direction of the sheath tip, which reduces some flexibility during interventional procedures. Additionally, sheaths do not offer the same degree of support as guide catheters.

Sheath: Diaphragm vs. Rotating Hemostatic Valve

Sheaths are designed with either a simple diaphragm or a hemostatic valve at their ends. These serve as the access points for delivery of equipment. A hemostatic valve allows blood to bleed back when the valve is open, thereby reducing the risk of air and atherosclerotic debris embolization. This device should be in place when working in the aortic arch vessels and the renal and mesenteric arteries. It is less critical during lower extremity intervention. Guiding catheters always require hemostatic valves be attached at their ends to allow delivery of equipment.

Telescoping Technique

Advancing large guiding catheters and sheaths into certain arteries may often be quite challenging and is often made simpler by telescoping the larger guide or sheath over a smaller diameter catheter (Fig. 3-16).

For example, placing an 8 Fr Headhunter-1 (8F H-1) guiding catheter into the distal right common carotid artery is made possible with the assistance of a stiff-angled glide wire and a long 5F JR4 diagnostic catheter. It is important to be aware that this technique requires the use of 125 cm length catheters, since most guides and sheaths are approximately 100 cm in length. Currently, only a small number of catheters are commercially available in this longer length.

The JR4 catheter is advanced through a hemostatic valve that is placed at the end of the 8F H-1 guiding catheter, such that its tip extends distal to the tip of the H-1 guide. The catheter-guide combination is then delivered to the aortic arch over a soft-tipped 0.035″ wire. The JR4 tip is engaged in the innominate artery and a stiff-angled glide wire is advanced to the distal right common carotid artery, over which the JR4 catheter is then advanced. Finally, the H-1 guide is advanced over the JR4 catheter-angled glide wire combination, which provides excellent support for the maneuver. The wire and JR4 guide catheter are removed and the H-1 guide catheter is left in place. This maneuver may also be used for straight sheaths when advancing them to the subclavian or carotid arteries, or when engaging renal sheaths in

TABLE 3-3

Guiding Catheters and Sheaths

A: Interventional Guiding Catheters

Vascular Bed	Name	Size (Fr)	Length (cm)	Comments
Carotid, Vertebral, Subclavian, Innominate	Headhunter (H1)	8, 9	90 cm	Primary guide
	Judkins Right (JR4)	8, 9	110 cm	Good for vertebral and subclavian arteries
	Amplatz Left (AL1)	8, 9	110 cm	Useful for performing carotid intervention when not possible to delivery sheath or guide to distal CCA (i.e. Type III arch and marked tortuosity of CCA). Procedure may be attempted with AL-1 guide at ostium of CCA.
Renal/Mesenteric	Renal Standard Curve	7, 8	55 cm	Short tipped RES guide may also be useful
	Renal Double Curve	7, 8	55 cm	Primary guide
	Renal Multipurpose	7, 8	55 cm	Excellent when used from the arm
	JR4	7, 8	110 cm	Good for small, heavily diseased aorta. Provides little back-up
	Hockey Stick	7, 8	55 cm	Infrequent use
Iliac	Multipurpose	7, 8	110 cm	When access is from the brachial artery
Femoral, Popliteal, Below Knee	Multipurpose	6, 7, 8	110 cm	Place inside Balkan sheath

B: Interventional Sheaths

Vascular Bed	Name	Size (Fr)	Length (cm)	Company	Comments
Carotid, Vertebral, Subclavian, Innominate	Ansel (AN1, AN2, AN3)	6, 7	45	Cook	For subclavian/innominate interventions from the brachial artery
	Raabe	6, 7, 8, 9	55, 70, 80, 90	Cook	Good sheath for subclavian/ vertebral intervention from the leg
	Shuttle Sheath	6, 7, 8, 9	80, 90	Cook	Excellent tracking sheath with smooth dilator-sheath transition. Carotid sheath of choice. Also can be used in innominate and subclavian arteries.
Renal	Renal Standard Curve	7, 8	55	Cordis	
	Renal Double Curve	7, 8	55	Cordis	
	Renal Multipurpose	7, 8	55	Cordis	Typically used from brachial artery access site
Iliac	Balkin	6, 7, 8	40	Cook	Primary sheath for contralateral iliac intervention
	Brite Tip	6, 7, 8	35, 55, 90	Cordis	Primary sheath for ipsilateral iliac intervention
Femoral, Popliteal, Below Knee	Balkin	6, 7, 8	40	Cook	Primary sheath for contralateral leg intervention. Wire initially advanced to contralateral iliac via diagnostic catheter. Heavy support wire may be required to advance sheath from ipsilateral to contralateral iliac.

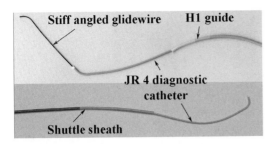

FIGURE 3-16 ● **Telescope technique.** A long diagnostic catheter is advanced through the interventional guide or sheath and is used to facilitate delivery of the guide or sheath to the desired location.

the renal arteries. It is quite important to have a smooth transition between the guide or sheath and the telescoping catheter when advancing these devices around corners, and in tortuous diseased vessels, in order to minimize vessel trauma and embolization (Fig. 3-2).

BALLOONS

Most peripheral balloons are compliant with rated-burst pressures somewhat lower than their coronary counterparts (Table 3-4). Thus, they are slower to inflate and deflate. To help these balloons fill and empty more effectively, a mixture of 70% saline and 30% contrast agent is used. All balloons should be adequately aspirated prior to use, especially during cerebrovascular procedures, where the consequence of air embolization may be catastrophic. Peripheral balloons come in varying lengths (up to 135 cm). The longer balloons are important when performing an SFA intervention from the brachial access site.

STENTS: BALLOON EXPANDABLE VS. SELF-EXPANDING, STENT GRAFTS

Balloon-expandable stents require positive pressure for expansion and are typically rigid with high radial strength (Table 3-5). These stents are ideal for immobile areas of the body, such as the subclavian, renal, mesenteric, and iliac arteries, and at ostial locations.

Other arteries such as the carotid, axillary, and superficial femoral flex and twist whenever the neck, shoulder, and leg move. Deploying rigid stents in these arteries would eventually lead to the stent being deformed and crushed. A flexi-

ble stent with "memory" is therefore required at these sites. The memory refers to the ability of these stents to regain their original shape after being deformed (e.g., when the artery flexes).

Nitinol is currently the metal that best provides this flexibility and memory. Nitinol stents do not require positive pressure balloon inflation for deployment. The stent is simply compressed over a stent-delivery catheter at the factory, and covered with a sheath. Stent deployment is achieved by pulling back the sheath to allow stent expansion (like a coiled spring). It is important that the stent diameter chosen is 1 mm to 2 mm larger than the actual diameter of the vessel, to ensure adequate stent apposition with the vessel wall.

Stent grafts (Table 3-5) are used to exclude aneurysms and to treat perforations when other more conservative options fail (e.g., prolonged balloon inflation). The JOMED GraftMaster® is a balloon expandable stent with diameters ranging from 3.0 mm to 5.0 mm that has recently become available premounted on a balloon delivery system. The self-deploying Wallgraft® and Viabahn® stents are the two options currently available for treatment of perforations or aneurysms in larger vessels. Both require larger sheaths for delivery, compared to balloon-expandable stents.

INTRAVASCULAR ULTRASOUND

Intravascular ultrasound (IVUS) is used infrequently during peripheral vascular procedures, except during percutaneous abdominal aortic-aneurysm repair. IVUS may be helpful for vessel sizing, ensuring good stent apposition, and to clarify anatomic issues when angiography is indeterminate (Table 3-6). Owing to the larger vessel sizes involved in peripheral vascular procedures, peripheral IVUS catheters use lower-frequency transducers (i.e., typically 15MHz or less) compared to coronary IVUS catheters (i.e., typically 30 MHz to 40MHz).

ADDITIONAL PEARLS

Surgical Back-up System

It is wise to establish a system for surgical back-up protection during peripheral vascular

TABLE 3-4

Balloons

Name	Wire Compatibility	Delivery	Shaft Length (cm)	Minimum Sheath Size (Fr)	Balloon Compliance	Balloon Diameter (mm)	Balloon Length (mm)	Company
Aviator	0.014″	RX	75, 135	4-6	Compliant	4-7	15, 20, 30, 40	Cordis
Viatrac	0.014″	RX	80, 135	4-5	Compliant	4.0-6.5	20, 30	Guidant
Agiltrac	0.018″	OTW	80, 135	5-7	Compliant	4-7	15, 20, 30, 40	Guidant
Gazelle	0.018″	RX	90, 135	4-5	Compliant	2-6	20	Boston Scientific
Slalom	0.018″	OTW	80, 120, 135	4-6	Compliant	3-8	20, 40	Cordis
Talon	0.018″	OTW	90, 135	5-6	Non-compliant	4-7	15, 20, 40	Boston Scientific
Ultra-Soft SV	0.018″	RX	90, 150	4-5	Compliant	4-7	15, 20	Boston Scientific
Agiltrac	0.035″	OTW	55, 80, 135	5-7	Compliant	4-14	20, 40, 60, 80, 100	Guidant
Opta PRO	0.035″	OTW	80, 110, 135	5-8	Compliant	3-10 and 12	10, 15, 20, 40, 60, 80, 100	Cordis
Optiplast	0.035″	OTW	75, 100, 120	5-8	Compliant	3-12	15-100	Bard
Powerflex P3	0.035″	OTW	40, 65, 80, 110, 135	5-8	Non-compliant	4-10 and 12	10, 15, 20, 40, 60, 80, 100	Cordis
Powerflex Extreme	0.035″	OTW	40, 80, 120	5-6	Non-compliant	4-10	20, 40, 60	Boston Scientific
Ultra-Thin SDS	0.035″	OTW	50, 75, 90, 135, 150	5-7	Non-compliant	4-10	15, 20, 30, 40, 60, 80	Boston Scientific
XXL	0.035″	OTW	120	7-8	Non-compliant	12, 14, 16, 18	20, 40	Boston Scientific

RX: Monorail delivery system, OTW: over-the-wire delivery system.

TABLE 3-5

Stents

A: Self-Expanding Stents

Name	Wire Compatibility	Delivery	Shaft Length (cm)	Diameter (mm)	Stent Length (mm)	Company
Dynalink	0.018″	OTW	80, 120	5–10	28, 38, 56, 80, 100	Guidant
Precise	0.018″	OTW	135	5–10	20, 30, 40	Cordis
Zilver	0.018″	OTW	125	5–9	20, 30, 40, 50, 60	Cook
Dynalink	0.035″	OTW	55, 80, 120	5–10, 12, 14	28, 38, 56, 80, 100 80, 120	Guidant
Smart	0.035″	OTW	80, 120	6–14	20, 40, 60, 80, 100, 120	Cordis
Luminex	0.035″	OTW	80, 135	4–14	20–120	Bard

B: Balloon Expandable Stents

Name	Wire Compatibility	Delivery	Shaft Length (cm)	Diameter (mm)	Stent Length (mm)	Company
Genesis	0.014″	RX	75, 135	5–9	12, 15, 18, 24	Cordis
Herculink	0.014″	RX	80, 135	4–7	12, 18	Guidant
Racer	0.014″/0.018″	OTW	130	4, 5, 6, 7	12, 18	Medtronic
Genesis	0.018″	RX	80, 135	3–8	12, 15, 18, 24, 29, 39	Cordis
Express Biliary LD	0.035″	OTW	75	5–9	17, 27, 37, 57	Boston Scientific
Genesis	0.035″	OTW	80, 135	4–10	12, 15, 18, 19, 24, 29, 39, 59, 79	Cordis
Omnilink	0.035″	OTW	80, 125	5-10	18, 28 38, 58	Guidant

C: Stent Grafts

Name	Wire Compatibility	Delivery	Shaft Length (cm)	Type	Diameter (mm)	Stent Length (mm)	Company
JOSTENT GraftMaster	0.014″	OTW	>100	Balloon Expansion	3.0, 3.5, 4.0, 4.5, 5.0	12, 16, 19, 26	Abbott Vascular
Viabahn	0.035″	OTW	110	Self-Expansion	5–13	25, 50	Gore
Wallgraft	0.035″	OTW	90	Self-Expansion	6–14	20, 30, 50, 70	Boston Scientific

RX: Monorail delivery system, OTW: over-the-wire delivery system

TABLE 3-6

Intravascular Ultrasound

Catheter	Console	Maximum Guide Wire (OD)	Minimum Sheath Size (Fr)	Image Depth (mm)	Transducer Frequency (MHz)	Company
Atlantis ®PV Peripheral Imaging Catheter	Galaxy™ Galaxy™²	0.035″	8	24	15	Boston Scientific
Visions™ PV 018 IVUS Imaging Catheter	In Vision	0.018″	4	24	15	Volcano Therapeutics
Visions™ PV 8.2F IVUS Imaging Catheter*	Gold™	0.038″	8	60	10	

* Designed specifically for assessment of abdominal aortic aneurysms
OD: Outer diameter, Fr: French

procedures, particularly with those procedures deemed high risk (e.g., common iliac artery or subclavian artery occlusions). Similarly, having neurovascular back-up protection with the capability of treating intracranial complications during extracranial cerebrovascular procedures is appropriate.

Vascular Anatomy

One should be thoroughly familiar with the vascular anatomy of the vessel(s) on which the diagnostic or interventional procedures are being performed. Know which problems will arise if the artery occludes or if distal embolization occurs. For example, left subclavian stenting, in a patient with a patent left internal mammary artery (LIMA) graft to the left anterior descending artery, could compromise the left vertebral artery, the LIMA graft, and arterial flow to the left hand.

Key Points

1. Raising the table to its maximum height and minimizing the distance between the image intensifier and the patient will maximize the field of view.
2. When performing a power injection, always use a side-hole catheter to minimize the risk of vessel perforation or dissection.
3. Do not inject through end-hole catheters if you have a dampened-pressure tracing.
4. For diagnostic angiography, obtain orthogonal views of suspected lesions, and identify the view that produces the least foreshortening of the lesion.
5. Always advance catheters and sheaths over a wire.
6. At the beginning of a peripheral intervention, be aware of the vessel diameter being treated and the balloon and/or stent planned for use. One should then be aware of the outer diameter of these balloons/stents, since this will determine the minimum size sheath or guide catheter that will be required to deliver this equipment. An assessment of the distance of the lesion from the access site will determine the appropriate length of equipment to choose. This forward planning will help ensure that an appropriate access site is used and that the right equipment to complete a successful procedure is ready.
7. When performing an intervention, try to have the guide catheter or sheath near the lesion (e.g. proximal SFA for mid-SFA lesion; distal common carotid for internal carotid lesion). This provides for better visualization and improved support.
8. When advancing guiding catheters and sheaths, try to have a tapered leading edge

in order to prevent vessel trauma (e.g., dissection, embolization). For sheaths, use the dilator. For guiding catheters, consider telescoping with a 5 Fr diagnostic catheter.

9. Avoid deploying stents in vessels that vascular surgeons use for anastomotic sites. These vessels include the common femoral artery and popliteal artery.

10. After crossing an occlusion in peripheral vessels, the presence of blood back flow from an over-the-wire balloon or catheter does not necessarily indicate an intraluminal position. The easy movement of the wire, distally, into branch vessels is a better indicator of intraluminal position. A gentle manual injection of a contrast agent: saline mixture (i.e., 50:50) is the gold standard to confirm intraluminal position.

REFERENCES

1. Baim DS. Proper use of cineangiographic equipment and contrast agents. In: Baim DS, Grossman W, eds. *Cardiac Catheterization, Angiography, and Intervention.* 6th ed. Philadelphia: Lippincott, Williams, and Wilkins; 2000: 15–34.
2. Wahl SI, Zinn KM. Filming and injection techniques. In: Bakal CW, Silberzweig JE, Cynamon J, Sprayregen S, eds. *Vascular and Interventional Radiology: Principles and Practice.* New York: Thieme Medical Publishers; 2002: 17–24.
3. Khoury M, Batra S, Berg R, et al. Influence of arterial access sites and interventional procedures on vascular complications after cardiac catheterizations. *Am J Surg* 1992;164(3):205–209.
4. Kiemeneij F, Laarman GJ, Odekerken D, et al. A randomized comparison of percutaneous transluminal coronary angioplasty by the radial, brachial and femoral approaches: the access study. *J Am Coll Cardiol* 1997;29(6):1269–1275.
5. Campeau L. Entry sites for coronary angiography and therapeutic interventions: from the proximal to the distal radial artery. *Can J Cardiol* 2001;17(3):319–325.

CHAPTER 4

Peripheral Arterial Thrombolysis

Kenneth Ouriel

Acute limb ischemia develops when a peripheral arterial occlusion occurs abruptly and in the absence of preexisting collateral channels. The underlying etiology is usually thrombosis of a native artery or bypass graft, but embolic events continue to account for 10 to 20% of cases (1). Irrespective of etiology, the acute occlusive event may be catastrophic for the patient; with great risk to the patient's limb and life. A now-classic study by Blaisdell, published over 20 years ago, documented amputation and mortality rates, in excess of 25% each, following open surgical repair for acute leg ischemia (2). Despite improvements in operative technique and postoperative patient care, more recent series continue to verify unacceptably high rates of morbidity. Jivegård and colleagues observed a 20% mortality rate in patients treated operatively. Even recent prospective studies of patients treated operatively documented rates of limb loss and death that exceeded desired targets (3).

There is some evidence to confirm the impression that a less invasive intervention is better tolerated in this very ill group of patients who develop acute limb ischemia (4). Poor technique, inadequate devices, and inferior agents colored the initial experiences with catheter-directed thrombolytic therapy. For instance, the now well accepted principle of ensuring infusion of the thrombolytic agent directly into the substance of the occluding thrombus was not always ardently followed. End-hole catheters were employed; it was not until the late 1980s

that multisided-hole catheters were available. Lastly, streptokinase was the most frequently used thrombolytic agent until the landmark article of McNamara, in 1985, documented improved results with locally administered high-dose urokinase (5).

CHOICE OF CANDIDATES FOR THROMBOLYTIC THERAPY

Decisions regarding the choice of optimal management for a patient are founded upon a fundamental knowledge base and the personal experiences that a clinician gains over the course of his or her clinical practice. There exist some data in the literature to suggest which patients do best with thrombolytic therapy, in comparison to other options (e.g., open surgical revascularization), but much of the decision-making process must be intuitive and based on something less than objective information.

Most importantly, thrombolytic therapy is contraindicated in patients with bleeding diatheses. Thus, patients with a history of gastrointestinal bleeding, recent major surgery, or stroke should normally not be considered for pharmacologic thrombolysis (Table 4-1).

As well, patients with contraindications to the angiographic procedures inherent in thrombolytic therapy may represent poor candidates for thrombolysis. Specifically, patients with impaired renal function should be treated with caution. Open surgery, mechanical thrombolysis, or if the ischemia is not severe, anticoagulation

TABLE 4-1

Contraindications for Pharmacologic Thrombolysis*

Absolute Contraindications

Cerebrovascular accident	Within 6 months
Intracranial surgery	Within 6 months
Gastrointestinal hemorrhage	Within 10 days
Major surgical procedure or trauma	Within 10 days
Uncontrolled hypertension	>180/110
Puncture of a non-compressible site	Within 48 hours
Intracranial neoplasm, aneurysm, AVM	

Relative Contraindications

Renal insufficiency (contrast load)	Creatinine >2.5**
Hepatic insufficiency	Enzymes >3 × normal
Transient ischemic attack	Within 3 months
Diabetic retinopathy	
Pregnancy	
Thrombocytopenia	>100,000/dl
Elevated prothrombin time	INR >1.5

*The table is not complete and many of the contraindications and timeframes are not based on objective clinical data; rather, each represents the standard of care.
**Unless patient is on dialysis
AVM, Arteriovenous malformation
INR, International normalized ratio

alone, may be more appropriate options in these cases.

Certain clinical variables have been identified as predictors of outcome with thrombolytic therapy. In a series of 80 patients undergoing arterial thrombolysis, success was defined by the complete (i.e., greater than 80% volume) dissolution of thrombus and the absence of the need for open surgical intervention (6). Success was more frequent in prosthetic graft (78%) and native arterial (72%) occlusions than in vein graft occlusions (53%, $P = 0.017$) and in nondiabetics than in diabetics (80% vs. 52%, $P = 0.031$). Lysis was dependent on placement of the catheter into the substance of the thrombus (85% vs. 0% success, $P = 0.004$) and passage of a guidewire through the occlusive process (92% vs. 10% success,

$P = 0.001$). The only parameter independently predictive of successful outcome, without the use of adjuvant procedures, was the location of the occlusion; additional procedures were necessary in 88% of aortoiliac and 82% of infrainguinal occlusions vs. only 17% of upper-extremity occlusions ($P = 0.005$).

The Surgery or Thrombolysis for the Ischemic Lower Extremity (STILE) trial randomized 393 patients with lower extremity ischemia to thrombolysis (i.e., urokinase or rt-PA, 1:2 ratio) or primary surgical intervention (7). Subsequent to the primary publication, two subgroup analyses were published. These studies confirmed the finding that patients with bypass graft occlusions had improved outcome with thrombolysis, compared with results of primary surgical intervention (8). The amputation rate at 1 year was significantly lower in patients treated with thrombolysis, compared with primary surgical revascularization ($P = 0.02$). By contrast, patients with native artery occlusions had better outcomes with surgical treatment, with a 1-year amputation rate of 0% versus 10% ($P = 0.002$) (9). While these data do not exclude the appropriate use of thrombolysis for native artery occlusions, the threshold for using a percutaneous means of restoring arterial perfusion in these cases should be higher than for bypass graft occlusions. Specifically, surgical management should be the primary consideration in patients with more chronic native artery occlusions (e.g., older than 14 days) and those with a reasonable, open surgical option (e.g., those patients with an adequate autogenous saphenous vein conduit).

In a multivariable analysis of the 544 patients randomized to thrombolytic therapy or open surgery in the Thrombolysis Or Peripheral Arterial Surgery (TOPAS) trial, 28 variables predictive of amputation-free survival were evaluated (10). Among these, eight main effects were predictive of amputation-free survival. These included two demographic factors: white race (risk ratio [RR] = 1.75; $P = 0.003$), and younger age (RR = 1.015; $P = 0.046$). Comorbidities comprised four of the eight main effects: history of central nervous system disease (RR = 1.726; p = 0.005), history of malignancy (RR = 1.615; $P = 0.024$); congestive heart failure (RR = 2.202; $P < 0.001$); or low body weight (RR = 1.007 per pound; $P = 0.006$). The severity of the process was also predictive, as gauged by the presence of skin color changes (RR = 1.585, P = 0.007) or pain at rest (RR = 0.503; P = 0.003). All eight effects were similar in the two treatment groups; none of these variables predicted improved outcome with one form of initial therapy over the other (i.e., there was no therapy-by-variable interaction). The length of occlusion, however, predicted whether a patient would fare better with thrombolysis or operation. With a threshold occlusion length of 30 cm, the RR for longer occlusions to shorter occlusions was 43% better in patients who received thrombolysis, whereas the situation was reversed for those who were randomized to surgery.

CHOICE OF THE THROMBOLYTIC AGENT

There exist four clinically available thrombolytic agents: streptokinase (SK), urokinase (UK), alteplase (rt-PA) and reteplase (r-PA). Of interest, streptokinase is the only agent to have been approved for peripheral vascular indications by the U.S. Food and Drug Administration (FDA), although streptokinase is rarely used, clinically, today. Urokinase holds FDA indications for pulmonary embolism, rt-PA for coronary occlusion and pulmonary embolism, and r-PA for coronary occlusion, alone. Nevertheless, each agent has been used with success for peripheral artery occlusions; albeit being offlabel use for urokinase, rt-PA, and r-PA (11).

The history of the development of pharmacologic thrombolysis began over 70 years ago. In 1933, Tillett and Garner at the Johns Hopkins Medical School discovered that filtrates of broth cultures of certain strains of hemolytic streptococcus bacteria had fibrinolytic properties (12). This streptococcal byproduct was originally termed *streptococcal fibrinolysin*. The purity of this agent was poor, however. Clinical use, of necessity, awaited adequate purification. Tillett and Sherry administered streptokinase intrapleurally, to dissolve loculated hemothoraces, in the late 1940s, (13) but intravascular administration was not attempted until the following decade. Tillett first reported intravascular administration of a thrombolytic agent in an article published in 1955 (14). A concentrated and partially purified SK was injected into 11 patients. This investiga-

tion was performed with the intent to gain data on the safety of the agent in volunteers; in no case was the SK administered to dissolve pathologic thrombi. Fever and hypotension developed as the amount of SK approached therapeutic levels. Whereas fever was generally mild and controllable with antipyretics, hypotension was sometimes prominent. The mean fall in systolic pressure was 31 mmHg and three of the patients manifested systolic pressures below 80 mmHg. These untoward reactions were more likely a result of contaminants in the preparation, rather than in the SK itself. Despite these reactions, systemic proteolysis was observed, with a decrease in fibrinogen and plasminogen, concurrent with a mild increase in the prothrombin time.

These early studies were followed by reports on the use of SK in patients with occluding vascular thrombi. In 1956, E. E. Cliffton, at the Cornell University Medical College in New York, was responsible for the first brief description of the clinical effectiveness of intravascular thrombolytic administration (15). The following year, Cliffton published his results in 40 patients with occlusive thrombi treated with a SK-plasminogen in combination (16). The locations of the thrombi were diverse, and included peripheral arterial thrombi, venous thrombi, pulmonary emboli, retinal occlusions, and in two patients, occlusive carotid thrombi. The Cliffton clinical results were far from exemplary; recanalization was not uniform and bleeding complications were frequent. Nevertheless, he must be credited with the first use of thrombolytic agents for the treatment of pathologic thrombi, as well as with the first use of catheter-directed administration of a thrombolytic agent.

Several schemes may be used to classify thrombolytic agents. The agents may be grouped by their mechanisms of action (i.e., those that directly convert plasminogen to plasmin versus those that are inactive zymogens and require transformation to an active form before they may cleave plasminogen). Thrombolytic agents may be grouped by their mode of production (i.e., those manufactured via recombinant techniques and those of bacterial origin). Of interest, recombinant agents harvested from a bacterial-expression system, such as *Escherichia coli*, do not contain carbohydrates, while products of mammalian hybridoma (e.g., recombinant prourokinase from mouse hybridoma SP2/0 cells) are fully glycosylated. Thrombolytic agents may be classified by their pharmacologic actions (i.e., those that are fibrin specific, binding to fibrin but not fibrinogen, versus nonspecific, as well as those that have a great degree of fibrin affinity, binding avidly to fibrin, versus those that do not. The authors and their colleagues have found it most useful to classify thrombolytic agents into groups based on the origin of the parent compound. It is most efficient to divide the agents into four groups: the streptokinase compounds, the urokinase compounds, the tissue-plasminogen activators, and then an additional, miscellaneous group, consisting of novel agents distinct from agents in the three other groups.

Streptokinase Compounds

Streptokinase (SK), originating from the streptococcus bacteria, was the first thrombolytic agent to be described. SK is a 50 kDa molecule with a biphasic half-life comprising a rapid $t1/2$ of 16 minutes, and a second, slower $t1/2$ of 90 minutes (17). Whereas the initial half-life is accounted for by the complex of the molecule with SK antibodies, the second half-life represents the actual biologic elimination of the protein. SK differs from other thrombolytic agents with respect to the stoichiometry of plasminogen binding. Whereas other agents directly convert plasminogen to plasmin, SK must form an equimolar stoichiometric complex with a plasmin or plasminogen molecule, to gain activity. Only then may this SK-plasmin(ogen) complex activate a second plasminogen molecule to form active plasmin; thus, two plasminogen molecules are used in SK-mediated plasmin generation. Unfortunately, SK suffers from the limitation of antigenic potential. Preformed antibodies exist, to a certain extent, in all patients who have been infected with the streptococcus bacterium. Similarly, patients with exposure to streptokinase may have high antibody titers on repeat exposure. These neutralizing antibodies inactivate exogenously administered streptokinase. SK antibodies may be overwhelmed through the use of a large, initial bolus of drug, and a large, initial SK loading dose may be employed in this regard. Some investigators have recommended measurement of antibody titers prior to beginning SK

therapy, gauging the loading dose on the basis of this titer (18).

SK administration is complicated by allergic reactions in approximately 2% of patients treated, with the development of urticaria, periorbital edema and bronchospasm. Pyrexia may also occur, but is usually adequately treated with acetaminophen. The major untoward effect associated with SK is hemorrhage. SK-associated hemorrhage may be no different than bleeding associated with any thrombolytic agent. The primary cause is likely the actions of the systemic agent on the thrombi, sealing the sites of vascular disintegrity. The generation of free plasmin, however, may contribute to the problem, with degradation of fibrinogen and other serum clotting proteins, as well as the release of fibrin(ogen)-degradation products that are potent anticoagulants and exacerbate the coagulopathy.

Recognizing potential limitations with SK, anisoylated plasminogen-streptokinase activator complex (APSAC) was developed by pharmacologists at Beecham Laboratories (19). APSAC has a longer half-life than SK, since acylation rendered the complex less susceptible to degradation. Owing to this property, it was anticipated that APSAC would be associated with a reduced risk of rethrombosis. Contrary to expectations, APSAC offered little clinical benefit over other agents, and at present, is not used to treat thrombi in the peripheral vasculature.

Urokinase Compounds

MacFarlane first described the fibrinolytic potential of human urine in 1947 (20). The active molecule was extracted, isolated, and named urokinase (UK) in 1952 (21). This urokinase-type plasminogen activator is a serine protease composed of two polypeptide chains, occurring in a low-molecular weight (32 kDa) and high-molecular weight (54 kDa) form. The high-molecular weight form predominates in UK isolated from urine, while the low-molecular weight form is found in UK obtained from tissue cultures of kidney cells. Unlike SK, UK directly activates plasminogen to form plasmin; prior binding to plasminogen or plasmin is not necessary for activity. Also in contrast to SK, preformed antibodies to UK are not observed. The agent is nonantigenic and untoward reactions of fever or hypotension are rare. Presently, the most commonly employed UK in the United States is of tissue-culture origin, manufactured from human neonatal kidney cells. UK has been fully sequenced, and a recombinant form of UK (r-UK) was tested in two multicenter trials of patients with peripheral arterial occlusion (4,22). r-UK is fully glycosylated, since it is derived from a murine hybridoma cell line. r-UK differs from UK in several respects. First, r-UK has a higher molecular weight than UK. Second, r-UK has a shorter half-life than its low-molecular weight counterpart. Despite these differences, however, the clinical effects of the two agents have been quite similar.

A precursor of UK was discovered in urine in 1979 (23). Prourokinase was characterized and subsequently manufactured by recombinant technology, using *Escherichia coli* (nonglycosylated) or mammalian cells (fully glycosylated) (24). This single-chain form is an inactive zymogen, inert in plasma, but may be activated by kallikrein or plasmin, to form active two-chain UK. This property accounts for amplification of the fibrinolytic process; as plasmin is generated, more prourokinase is converted to active urokinase, and the process is repeated. Prourokinase is relatively fibrin specific; that is, its fibrin degrading (*fibrinolytic*) activity greatly outweighs its fibrinogen degrading (*fibrinogenolytic*) activity. This feature is explained by the preferential activation of fibrin-bound plasminogen found in a thrombus over free plasminogen found in flowing blood. Nonselective activators, such as SK and UK, activate free and bound plasminogen equally, and induce systemic plasminemia with resultant fibrinogenolysis and degradation of factors V and VII. Given the potential advantages of prourokinase over urokinase, Abbott Laboratories produced a recombinant form of prourokinase (r-ProUK) from a murine hybridoma cell line. This recombinant agent is converted to active two-chain urokinase by plasmin and kallikrein. r-ProUK has been studied in the settings of myocardial infarction, stroke and peripheral arterial occlusion. To date, it appears that r-ProUK offers the advantages associated with an agent that does not originate from a human cell source. Fibrin specificity, however, may be lost at the higher dose levels necessary to effect more rapid thrombolysis than UK.

Tissue-Plasminogen Activators

Tissue-plasminogen activator (t-PA) is a naturally occurring fibrinolytic agent produced by endothelial cells and intimately involved in the balance between intravascular thrombogenesis and thrombolysis. Wild-type t-PA is a single-chain (527 amino acid) serine protease with a molecular weight of approximately 65 kDa. Plasmin hydrolyses the Arg275-Ile276 peptide bond, converting the single-chain molecule into a two-chain moiety. In contrast to most serine proteases (e.g., urokinase), the single-chain form of t-PA has significant activity. t-PA has potential benefits over other thrombolytic agents. The agent exhibits significant fibrin specificity (25). In plasma, the agent is associated with little plasminogen activation. At the site of the thrombus, however, the binding of t-PA and plasminogen, to the fibrin surface, induces a conformational change in both molecules, greatly facilitating the conversion of plasminogen to plasmin and resulting in dissolution of the clot. t-PA also manifests the property of fibrin affinity; it binds strongly to fibrin. Other fibrinolytic agents, such as prourokinase, do not share this property of fibrin affinity. Recombinant t-PA (rt-PA, alteplase) was produced in the 1980s after molecular cloning techniques were used to express human t-PA DNA (26). A predominantly single-chain form of rt-PA was eventually approved in the United States for the indications of acute myocardial infarction and massive pulmonary embolism. rt-PA has been studied extensively in the setting of coronary occlusion. In the GUSTO-I study of approximately 41,000 patients with acute myocardial infarction, rt-PA was more effective than SK in achieving vascular patency (27). Despite a slightly greater risk of intracranial hemorrhage with rt-PA, overall mortality was significantly reduced.

In an effort to lengthen the duration of bioavailability of t-PA, the molecule was systematically bioengineered. Initial investigations identified regions in kringle 1 and the protease portion of t-PA that mediated hepatic clearance, fibrin specificity, and resistance to plasminogen-activator inhibitor. Three sites were modified to create TNK-tPA, a novel molecule with a greater half-life and fibrin specificity (28). The longer half-life of TNK-t-PA allowed successful administration as a single bolus, in contrast to the requirement for an infusion with rt-PA. In addition, TNK-tPA manifests greater fibrin specificity than rt-PA, resulting in less fibrinogen depletion. In studies of acute coronary occlusion, TNK-tPA performed at least as well as rt-PA, concurrent with greater ease of administration (29).

Reteplase

Similar to TNK-tPA, the novel recombinant plasminogen activator, reteplase, comprises the kringle 2 and protease domains of t-PA. Reteplase was developed with the goal of avoiding the necessity of a continuous intravenous infusion, thereby simplifying ease of administration (30). Reteplase, produced in *Escherichia coli* cells, is nonglycosylated, demonstrating a lower fibrin-binding activity and a diminished affinity to hepatocytes (31). This latter property accounts for a longer half-life than rt-PA, potentially enabling bolus injection versus prolonged infusion. The fibrin affinity of reteplase was only 30% of that exhibited with t-PA, similar to UK. The decrease in fibrin affinity was hypothesized to reduce the incidence of distant bleeding complications, in a manner similar to that of SK over rt-PA, in the GUSTO trial. In fact, several properties of reteplase may account for a decreased risk of hemorrhage, including poor lysis of platelet-rich, older clots. Reteplase has demonstrated some benefit over rt-PA in the RAPID 1 and RAPID 2 studies, as well as in GUSTO III (32). To date, a handful of peripheral arterial and venous studies have been published (33–36).

Miscellaneous Agents

There exist a wide variety of novel thrombolytic agents, all of which have undergone extensive preclinical study but few of which have been adequately evaluated in patients. Vampire-bat plasminogen activator (*bat PA*) was cloned and expressed from the saliva of the vampire bat Desmodus rotundus (37). This agent manifests extraordinary fibrin specificity; the plasminogenolytic activity is over 100,000 times greater in the presence of fibrin. The half-life of bat PA is five to nine times slower than that of rt-PA, offering some potential advantages with

respect to ease of administration. Clinical trials were originally organized as a Phase I study with healthy volunteers (38).

Fibrolase is a metalloproteinase originating from venom of the southern copperhead snake (39). Fibrolase is a unique, fibrinolytic agent that does not require plasminogen for its activity (40). Rather, the agent directly degrades fibrin without the requirement of any other blood components. As well, the agent is rapidly inactivated through binding to the circulating protein alpha-2 macroglobulin. So long as the dose of the agent is kept below the threshold of available binding for alpha-2 macroglobulin, systemic activity should be nil, potentially decreasing the rate of distant hemorrhagic complications to near zero (41). Recently, a recombinant form of fibrolase, *alfimeprase,* has undergone a Phase I evaluation in patients with subacute and chronic peripheral arterial occlusive disease. The results are not yet available, but preliminary findings suggest that the agent is safe. A Phase II, international evaluation of alfimeprase for peripheral arterial occlusion is slated to begin.

Staphylokinase is a byproduct of *Staphylococcus aureus* bacterium, was originally mentioned in the classic streptococcal fibrinolysin paper of Tillett and Garner in 1933 (12). Staphylokinase has been produced by recombinant techniques and has been studied in the settings of myocardial infarction, peripheral arterial occlusion and deep venous thrombosis (42). Like SK, staphylokinase is inactive, and must bind to plasminogen to activate other plasminogen molecules. Unlike SK, staphylokinase is relatively fibrin specific and spares circulating plasminogen and fibrinogen. While staphylokinase is antigenic, antigenicity has been reduced with newer, recombinant mutants, and the initial clinical results have been quite acceptable in arterial and venous thrombotic occlusions (43,44).

Comparison of the Agents in Studies of Peripheral Vascular Disease

To date, there have been few well designed clinical comparisons of various thrombolytic agents in the peripheral vasculature. There exist a variety of in vitro studies and retrospective clinical trials, most pointing to improved efficacy and safety of UK and rt-PA over SK (45–47). In an analysis of data collected in a prospective, single institution registry at the Cleveland Clinic Foundation, UK demonstrated a diminished rate of bleeding complications when compared with rt-PA (48). Efficacy was not evaluated in this trial.

There have been two prospective, randomized comparisons of UK and rt-PA. Neither was blinded. Meyerovitz and associates from the Brigham and Women's Hospital (Massachusetts) randomized 32 patients with peripheral artery or bypass-graft occlusions, of less than 90 days duration, to rt-PA (10 mg bolus, 5 mg per hour to a maximum of 24 hours) or UK (60,000 IU bolus, 4,000 IU per minute for 2 hours, 2000 IU per minute for 2 hours, then 1000 IU per minute to a maximum of 24 hours, total administration) (49). There was significantly greater systemic-fibrinogen degradation in the rt-PA group ($P = 0.01$), indicating that the fibrin specificity of rt-PA was lost at this dosing regimen. rt-PA patients achieved more rapid initial thrombolysis, but efficacy was identical in the two groups, by 24 hours. The trade off to more rapid thrombolysis was a trend toward a higher rate of bleeding complications in the rt-PA treated patients ($P = 0.39$) The second, randomized comparison of UK and rt-PA was the STILE trial, a three-armed, multicenter comparison of UK (250,000 IU bolus, 4000 IU per minute for 4 hours, then 2000 IU per minute for up to 36 hours), rt-PA (0.05 to 0.1 mg/kg per hour, for up to 12 hours) and primary operation (7). There was one intracranial hemorrhage in the UK group (0.9%) and there were two in the rt-PA group (1.5%, no significant difference). Although actual rates of overall bleeding complications and efficacy were not reported for the two thrombolytic groups, the authors remarked that there were no significant differences detected in any of the outcome variables. In a subsequent reanalysis of the data, reported in 1999, the frequency of complete clot lysis was similar with urokinase and rt-PA, at the time of the early arteriographic study (50). These recent data suggest that the rate of thrombolysis may be quite similar, in direct contradiction to the popularly held view that rt-PA is a much more rapidly acting agent.

A multicenter, blinded trial compared the results of thrombolysis with UK vs r-UK in 300 patients with peripheral arterial occlusion (51). Despite a shorter half-life for r-UK, there were no significant clinical differences noted between the two agents. A North American multicenter trial compared three different doses of r-ProUK to UK in 241 patients with lower extremity arterial occlusions of less than 14 days duration (3). While the higher r-ProUK dose was associated with a slightly greater percentage of patients with complete (>95%) clot lysis at 8 hours, there was a mild increase in the rate of bleeding complications in this group, compared with either the UK or the lower-dose r-ProUK groups. The fibrinogen levels fell in the higher r-ProUK group, suggesting that fibrin specificity is lost at the higher-dose regimens for this compound.

TECHNIQUE FOR THROMBOLYSIS OF PERIPHERAL ARTERIAL OCCLUSIONS

Once the determination to implement thrombolytic therapy has been made, and the particular agent has been selected, several procedural issues must be resolved. Each of these issues plays an important role in achieving a therapeutic success. Precise attention to every clinical detail is imperative to accomplish reasonably rapid dissolution of the thrombus and normalization of arterial blood flow, without complications that may result in the loss of limb or life.

Management of the Anticoagulated Patient

At the outset, one must be cognizant of coagulation abnormalities that are frequent in patients with acute arterial occlusions. Many patients are on aspirin or clopidogrel, potentially increasing the risk of puncture site bleeding complications. A significant proportion of patients will be fully anticoagulated with warfarin at the time of presentation, prescribed and administered as a result of cardiac arrhythmia or a previous occlusive event. As well, patients with a distal bypass conduit, such as a prosthetic femoral-tibial graft, may be on long-term anticoagulation. There are two choices in such patients; either correct the international normalized ratio (INR) to acceptable levels (e.g., 1.5 or below) or proceed, using a micropuncture technique. In cases of severe ischemia, a micropuncture technique is elected, using a 4-Fr system and if necessary, ultrasound guidance, to ensure a single-wall puncture. In cases where an additional period of several hours between presentation and treatment may be tolerated, fresh frozen plasma is given to restore a normal INR. In general, refrain from the use of vitamin K to reverse anticoagulation, since the administration of more than trivial amounts of vitamin K makes subsequent reanticoagulation extremely difficult.

Choice for Arterial Access

The choice for the arterial access site is of great importance and is one of the primary determinants of complications associated with thrombolytic therapy. The peripheral pulse examination guides this decision. Access should be initially attempted through the contralateral (uninvolved) common femoral artery in patients with bilaterally palpable femoral pulses. If the contralateral femoral pulse is weak or absent, or in patients with an aortofemoral-bypass graft, a left brachial approach may be more appropriate. For femoral access, a single-wall puncture technique is important, with the placement of a short 5 Fr sheath into the iliac system, and a 5 Fr diagnostic catheter (pigtail or other variety) advanced into the abdominal aorta. For brachial access, one should maintain a low threshold for an open exposure of the artery. Direct cannulation of the brachial artery, just above the antecubital crease, may prevent complications such as brachial sheath hematoma and peripheral nerve palsies or brachial artery thrombosis.

Irrespective of the site of access, a complete diagnostic arteriogram is necessary in all patients with adequate renal function, obtaining full views of the run off paths in both legs. A complete interrogation of the lower extremity vessels will allow one to make an accurate assessment of whether or not the event is secondary to thrombosis or embolization, and to provide some indication of the chronicity of the problem. Lastly, it is important to image the ipsilateral outflow vessels adequately to provide baseline distal views, should subsequent distal embolization occur during thrombolysis.

Placement of the Infusion System

Just as gaining uncomplicated arterial access is the most important determinant of local bleeding complications (safety), accurate placement of the infusion system into the occluding thrombus is the primary determinant of successful and efficacious clot dissolution (Fig. 4-1).

In the case of occlusion of the superficial femoral artery or a bypass graft that originates from proximal femoral inflow, the contralateral femoral approach is best. The 5 Fr short sheath is exchanged for a 5.5 Fr or 6 Fr up-and-over sheath. When possible, it is best to place the distal tip of the sheath within the external iliac artery, to minimize contrast agent loss into the hypogastric (i.e., internal iliac) system.

Next, attempts are made to cannulate the occluded artery or bypass graft. Oblique views are helpful to find the orifice. One useful method is to use a 5 Fr, angled, hydrophobic catheter and an angled 0.035″ hydrophobic wire, placing the catheter just proximal to the expected occluded ostium with careful manipulation of the wire to gain access to the occlusion. Once access has been achieved, the wire is advanced well into the occlusion, so that the catheter may be advanced into the occluded artery or bypass graft. A small amount of contrast agent is injected through the catheter to confirm entry into the occlusion.

At this point, the hydrophobic guidewire may be exchanged for a stiffer wire (e.g., a 0.035″ Rosen). A sturdy wire is necessary to advance the thrombolytic infusion catheter into the occlusion, since the infusion catheters do not track as well as other, more flexible catheters. After estimating the length of the occlusion, an infusion catheter (usually 5 Fr but occasionally 4 Fr) with an appropriate length of side-holes is chosen and advanced into position.

An infusion wire will be necessary in cases when the thrombus is discontinuous (e.g., an occluded femoral-popliteal bypass graft, with an open popliteal artery but with thrombotic occlusion of the tibioperoneal trunk) or when the occlusion length is longer than the longest length of side-holes (i.e., usually 50 cm). The infusion wire may come with the particular thrombolytic infusion catheter, or if not, a Touhey-Borst connector may be necessary.

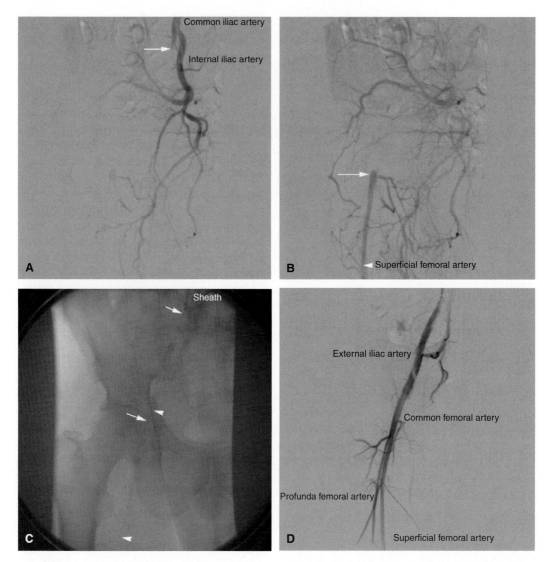

FIGURE 4-1 ● **Subacute thrombotic occlusion of the proximal right external iliac artery (*arrow*). A:** The origin of the external iliac vessel is best visualized in the right anterior oblique (RAO) view. **Proximal extent of thrombotic occlusion is demonstrated (*arrow*). B:** The distal common femoral artery (*arrow*) and superficial femoral artery fill by collaterals from the internal iliac vessel. **A 7 Fr cross-over sheath was positioned in the proximal right external iliac artery. C:** The position of the infusion catheter (*arrows*) and infusion wire (*arrowheads*) for administration of thrombolytic agent is demonstrated. t-PA was administered at a dose of 0.5 mg/hr through both the infusion catheter and wire, in addition to heparin at 500 units/hr via the side port of the femoral sheath. **D:** Final result following thrombolysis demonstrating near complete resolution of thrombus.

Some clinicians prefer to lace the thrombus with thrombolytic agent prior to instituting a slow infusion. There are several methods to accomplish this. The most common merely involves the use of the multiside-hole infusion catheter, manually injecting a dose of agent in a rapid, pulsed fashion into the thrombus. If the length of the thrombotic occlusion exceeds the length of the side-hole region of the catheter, the catheter may be repositioned one or more times to achieve an adequate distribution of thrombolytic agent throughout the thrombus. Other clinicians use a pulse-spray infusion, where a machine is used to provide rapid pulses of agent in attempts to provide better distribution into the thrombus, as well as some element of mechanical disruption

(52,53). The authors and others have not found the pulse-spray technique to offer significant advantages over a slow-drip method of administration (54). The infusion is begun once the catheter is in position. If an infusion wire is used, the dose of thrombolytic agent may be split between the catheter and the wire, in a ratio that is appropriate for the volume of thrombus addressed by the two systems. Concomitant heparin therapy, once a mainstay of thrombolysis, is now administered at a low dose—usually just a few hundred units per hour—through the sheath (35). Importantly, the heparin may never be mixed with the thrombolytic agent, as the low pH of the heparin solution may cause precipitation of the agent.

Once the infusion has begun, the patient is sent to an intensive care unit (ICU) or step-down unit for monitoring. The determination of when the patient is returned for a lytic check-up test is based on the severity of ischemia and the practicalities of the clinical schedule. In cases of severe ischemia, it is important to obtain an early angiogram, usually within 4 to 8 hours, with repositioning of the catheter if necessary. In less severely ischemic cases, the patient may be returned for a check at 12 hours, or even the next morning.

When distal embolization is heralded by the sudden development of worsening distal ischemia, continued upstream infusion usually suffices and the ischemia improves over an hour or two (Figure 4-2).

This represents the single example of when regional thrombolysis may be effective in dissolving a peripheral arterial thrombus, presumably because the embolized clot contains thrombolytic agent with active, ongoing thrombolysis. If improvement does not occur within a

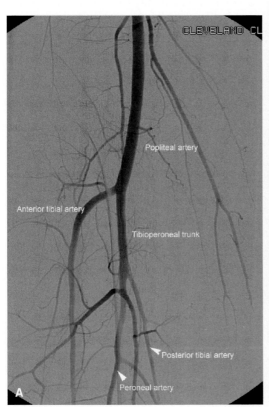
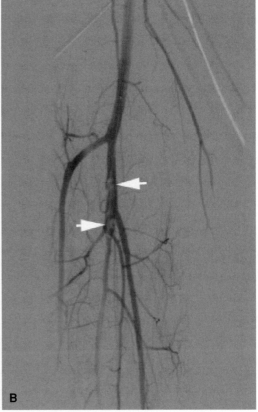

FIGURE 4-2 ● **A:** Baseline angiogram of the right popliteal artery and its branches prior to administration of thrombolysis for treatment of a proximal thrombotic occlusion **B:** Angiogram performed 12 hours post thrombolysis, demonstrating distal embolization to tibioperoneal trunk.

few hours, the patient should be returned to the angiography suite for repositioning of catheters and wires, in attempts to address the embolized fragments directly. Mechanical thrombectomy should also be considered when distal embolization is not resolved.

The decision to terminate thrombolytic therapy is not as simple as it may seem. One must often strike a risk:benefit balance between complete clot lysis and the risk of hemorrhagic complications. Although a longer infusion duration produces a more pristine angiographic appearance, the risk of hemorrhage rises over time. Traditionally, the cut-off time for discontinuation of thrombolytic administration has been 48 hours (55,56). The risk of hemorrhagic complications is said to increase dramatically beyond this time point, but there exist no objective data on which to base this contention. Some clinicians measure fibrinogen levels and terminate thrombolysis when the levels decline below 100 mg/dL (57). Fibrinogen, however, has been disappointing as a predictor of bleeding (4,58).

In practice, thrombolytic therapy should be terminated when there is antegrade flow through the target artery or bypass graft, when the amount of residual mural thrombus does not appear to be flow limiting, and when there is no significant thrombus in the out-flow bed. Thrombolytic administration should be terminated earlier if hemorrhagic complications arise. Consideration should be made to lower the infusion rate or to discontinue thrombolytic administration transiently, when precipitous fibrinogen decrements are noted, but this remains controversial. In most cases, thrombolysis should be terminated after no more than 48 hours of infusion, irrespective of the clinical course. Careful attention to these details will diminish the frequency of hemorrhagic complications.

Treatment After Thrombolysis

The objective of thrombolytic therapy is to dissolve the majority of intravascular thrombus and unmask any underlying arterial lesions that were responsible for the occlusive event. Thrombolysis, in and of itself, should never be considered sole therapy. Studies where thrombolysis was not routinely followed by correction of the underlying lesion, expectedly, found the therapy

to be of little use (59). In fact, despite complete thrombolytic dissolution of clot, the failure to find and correct an underlying culprit lesion is tantamount to failure. In a study of thrombolysed infrainguinal grafts, when a flow-limiting lesion was identified and corrected by angioplasty or surgery, the patency rate was significantly improved over those grafts without such lesions (79.0% versus 9.8% at 2 years, $P = 0.01$) (60).

Fortunately, most lesions may be addressed with contemporary percutaneous techniques. In the TOPAS trial, 46% of subjects treated with thrombolytic therapy left the hospital with nothing more than a percutaneous procedure (4). In the more recent study of recombinant prourokinase or acute limb ischemia, this ratio had increased to approximately 2/3 (3). The use of newer stents, and other percutaneous techniques with improved effectiveness for infrainguinal disease, will only increase the number of patients that may be treated with a fully percutaneous strategy. In this manner, it is hoped that the excessive morbidity and mortality associated with acute peripheral arterial occlusion may be lowered, dramatically.

REFERENCES

1. Dormandy J, Heeck L, Vig S. Acute limb ischemia. *Semin Vasc Surg*. 1999;12(2):148–153.
2. Blaisdell FW, Steele M, Allen RE. Management of acute lower extremity arterial ischemia due to embolism and thrombosis. *Surgery*. 1978;84:822–834.
3. Ouriel K, Kandarpa K, Schuerr DM, et al. Prourokinase vs. urokinase for recanalization of peripheral occlusions, safety and efficacy: the PURPOSE Trial. *J Vasc Intervent Radiol*. 1999;10:1083–1091.
4. Ouriel K, Veith FJ, Sasahara AA. A comparison of recombinant urokinase with vascular surgery as initial treatment for acute arterial occlusion of the legs. *N Engl J Med*. 1998;338:1105–1111.
5. McNamara TO, Fischer JR. Thrombolysis of peripheral arterial and graft occlusions: improved results using high-dose urokinase. *AJR Amer J Roentgenol*. 1985;144:769–775.
6. Shortell CK, Ouriel K. Thrombolysis in acute peripheral arterial occlusion: predictors of immediate success. *Ann Vasc Surg*. 1994;8(1):59–65.
7. The STILE Investigators. Results of a prospective randomized trial evaluating surgery versus thrombolysis for ischemia of the lower extremity. The STILE trial. *Ann Surg*. 1994;220(3):251–266.
8. Comerota AJ, Weaver FA, Hosking JD, et al. Results of a prospective, randomized trial of surgery versus thrombolysis for occluded lower extremity bypass grafts. *Amer J Surg*. 1996;172(2):105–112.
9. Weaver FA, Comerota AJ, Youngblood M, et al. Surgical revascularization versus thrombolysis for

nonembolic lower extremity native artery occlusions: results of a prospective randomized trial. The STILE Investigators. Surgery versus Thrombolysis for Ischemia of the Lower Extremity. *J Vasc Surg.* 1996;24(4):513–521.

10. Ouriel K, Veith FJ. Acute lower limb ischemia: determinants of outcome. *Surgery.* 1998;124(2):336–341.

11. Ouriel K. Urokinase and the US Food and Drug Administration. *J Vasc Surg.* 1999;30(5):957–958.

12. Tillett WS, Garner RL. The fibrinolytic activity of hemolytic streptococci. *J Exper Med.* 1933;58:485.

13. Tillett WS, Sherry S. The effect in patients of streptococcal fibrinolysin (streptokinase) and streptococcal desoxyribonuclease on fibrinous, purulent, and sanguinous pleural exudations. *J Clin Invest.* 1949;28:173.

14. Tillett WS, Johnson AJ, McCarty WR. The intravenous infusion of the streptococcal fibrinolytic principle (streptokinase) into patients. *J Clin Invest.* 1955;34:169–185.

15. Cliffton EE, Grunnet M. Investigations of intravenous plasmin (fibrinolysin) in humans. *Circulation.* 1956;14:919.

16. Cliffton EE. The use of plasmin in humans. *Ann NY Acad Sci.* 1957;68:209–229.

17. Reddy DS. Newer thrombolytic drugs for acute myocardial infarction. *Indian J Exper Biol.* 1998;36(1):1–15.

18. Jostring H, Barth U, Naidu R. Changes of antistreptokinase titer following long-term streptokinase therapy. In: Martin M, Schoop W, Hirsh J, eds. *New Concepts of Streptokinase Dosimetry.* Vienna: Hans Huber:1978: 110.

19. Smith RAG, Dupe RJ, English PD, et al. Fibrinolysis with acyl-enzymes: a new approach to thrombolytic therapy. *Nature.* 1981;290:505.

20. Macfarlane RG, Pinot JJ. Fibrinolytic activity of normal urine. *Nature.* 1947;159:779.

21. Sobel GW, Mohler SR, Jones NW, et al. Urokinase: an activator of plasma fibrinolysin extracted from urine. *Am J Physiol.* 1952;171:768–769.

22. Ouriel K, Veith FJ, Sasahara AA. Thrombolysis or peripheral arterial surgery: phase I results. TOPAS Investigators. *J Vasc Surg.* 1996;23(1):64–73; discussion 74–75.

23. Husain SS, Lipinski B, Gurewich V. Isolation of plasminogen activators useful as therapeutic and diagnostic agents (single-chair, high-fibrin affinity urokinase). Patent No. 4,381,346. 1979.

24. Gurewich V. Pro-urokinase: history, mechanisms of action, and clinical development. In: Loscalzo J, Sasahara AA, eds. *New Therapeutic Agents in Thrombosis and Thrombolysis.* New York: Marcel Dekker; 1997:539–559.

25. Tanswell P, Tebbe U, Neuhaus KL, et al. Pharmacokinetics and fibrin specificity of alteplase during accelerated infusions in acute myocardial infarction. *J Am Coll Cardiol.* 1992;19:1071–1075.

26. Hoylaerts M, Rijken DC, Lijnen HR, et al. Kinetics of the activation of plasminogen by human tissue plasminogen activator: role of fibrin. *J Biol Chem.* 1982;257: 2912.

27. The GUSTO Investigators. An angiographic study within the global randomized trial of aggressive versus standard thrombolytic strategies in patients with acute myocardial infarction. *N Engl J Med.* 1993;329:1615.

28. Cannon CP, McCabe CH, Gibson CM, et al. TNK-tissue plasminogen activator in acute myocardial infarction. Results of the Thrombolysis in Myocardial Infarction (TIMI) 10A dose-ranging trial. *Circulation.* 1997;95(2):351–356.

29. Cannon CP, Gibson CM, McCabe CH, et al. TNK-tissue plasminogen activator compared with front-loaded alteplase in acute myocardial infarction: results of the TIMI 10B trial. Thrombolysis in Myocardial Infarction (TIMI) 10B Investigators. *Circulation.* 1998;98(25):2805–2814.

30. Martin U. Clinical and preclinical profile of the novel recombinant plasminogen activator reteplase. In: Sasahara AA, Loscalzo J, eds. *New Therapeutic Agents in Thrombosis and Thrombolysis.* New York: Marcel Dekker; 1997:495–511.

31. Meierhenrich R, Carlsson J, Seifried E, et al. Effect of reteplase on hemostasis variables: analysis of fibrin specificity, relation to bleeding complications and coronary patency. *Internat J Cardiol.* 1998;65(1):57–63.

32. Anonymous. A comparison of reteplase with alteplase for acute myocardial infarction. The Global Use of Strategies to Open Occluded Coronary Arteries (GUSTO III) Investigators [see comments]. *N Engl J Med.* 1997;337(16):1118–1123.

33. Castaneda F, Li R, Young K, et al. Catheter-directed thrombolysis in deep venous thrombosis with use of reteplase: immediate results and complications from a pilot study. *J Vasc Interv Radiol.* 2002;13(6):577–580.

34. Drescher P, Crain MR, Rilling WS. Initial experience with the combination of reteplase and abciximab for thrombolytic therapy in peripheral arterial occlusive disease: a pilot study. *J Vasc Interv Radiol.* 2002;13(1): 37–43.

35. McNamara TO, Dong P, Chen J, et al. Bleeding complications associated with the use of rt-PA versus r-PA for peripheral arterial and venous thromboembolic occlusions. *Tech Vasc Interv Radiol.* 2001;4(2): 92–98.

36. Ouriel K, Katzen B, Mewissen MW, et al. Initial experience with reteplase in the treatment of peripheral arterial and venous occlusion. *J Vasc Interv Radiol.* 2000;11:849–854.

37. Hawkey C. Plasminogen activator in the saliva of the vampire bat *Desmodus rotundus. Nature.* 1966;211:434–435.

38. Verstraete M, Lijnen HR, Collen D. Thrombolytic agents in development. *Drugs.* 1995;50(1):29–42.

39. Randolph A, Chamberlain SH, Chu HL, et al. Amino acid sequence of fibrolase, a direct-acting fibrinolytic enzyme from Agkistrodon contortix venom. *Protein Science.* 1992;1(5):590–600.

40. Markland FS, Friedrichs GS, Pewitt SR, et al. Thrombolytic effects of recombinant fibrolase or APSAC in a canine model of carotid artery thrombosis. *Circulation.* 1994;90(5):2448–2456.

41. Ahmed NK, Tennant KD, Markland FS, et al. Biochemical characteristics of fibrolase, a fibrinolytic protease from snake venom. *Haemostasis.* 1990;20(3):147–154.

42. Collen D. Staphylokinase: a potent, uniquely fibrin-selective thrombolytic agent. *Nature Medicine.* 1998; 4(3):279–284.

43. Heymans S, Verhaeghe R, Stockx L, et al. Feasibility study of catheter-directed thrombolysis with recombinant staphylokinase in deep venous thrombosis. *Thromb Haemostasis.* 1998;79(3):517–519.

44. Heymans S, Vanderschueren S, Verhaeghe R, et al. Outcome and one year follow-up of intra-arterial staphylokinase in 191 patients with peripheral arterial occlusion. *Thromb Haemost.* 2000;83(5):666–671.

45. Ouriel K, Welch EL, Shortell CK, et al. Comparison of streptokinase, urokinase, and recombinant tissue plasminogen activator in an in vitro model of venous thrombolysis. *J Vasc Surg.* 1995;22(5):593–597.

46. Graor RA, Risius B, Denny KM, et al. Local thrombolysis in the treatment of thrombosed arteries, bypass grafts, and arteriovenous fistulas. *J Vasc Surg.* 1985;2(3):406–414.

47. Gardiner GA Jr, Koltun W, Kandarpa K, et al. Thrombolysis of occluded femoropopliteal grafts. *AJR Am J Roentgenol.* 1986;147(3):621–626.

48. Ouriel K, Gray B, Clair DG, et al. Complications associated with the use of urokinase and recombinant tissue plasminogen activator for catheter-directed peripheral arterial and venous thrombolysis. *J Vasc Interv Radiol.* 2000;11(3):295–298.

49. Meyerovitz M, Goldhaber SZ, Reagan K, et al. Recombinant tissue-type plasminogen activator versus urokinase in peripheral arterial and graft occlusions: a randomized trial. *Radiology.* 1990;175:75–78.

50. Comerota AJ. A re-analysis of the STILE data. Presented at the Annual VEITH symposium, 11-17-1999, New York, New York.

51. Credo RB, Burke SE, Barker WM, et al. Recombinant urokinase (r-UK): Biochemistry, pharmacology, and clinical experience. In: Sasahara AA, Loscalzo J, eds. *New Therapeutic Agents in Thrombosis and Thrombolysis.* New York: Marcel Dekker, Inc.; 1997:513–537.

52. Hye RJ, Turner C, Valji K, et al. Is thrombolysis of occluded popliteal and tibial bypass grafts worthwhile? *J Vasc Surg.* 1994;20(4):588–596.

53. Armon MP, Yusuf SW, Whitaker SC, et al. Results of 100 cases of pulse-spray thrombolysis for acute and subacute leg ischaemia. *Br J Surg.* 1997;84(1):47–50.

54. Kandarpa K, Chopra PS, Aruny JE, et al. Intraarterial thrombolysis of lower extremity occlusions: prospective, randomized comparison of forced periodic infusion and conventional slow continuous infusion. *Radiology.* 1993;188(3):861–867.

55. Thomas SM, Gaines P. Avoiding the complications of thrombolysis. *J Vasc Intervent Radiol.* 1999; 10(suppl):246.

56. Riggs P, Ouriel K. Thrombolysis in the treatment of lower extremity occlusive disease. *Surg Clin Nor Amer.* 1995;75(4):633–645.

57. Berni GA, Bandyk DF, Zierler RE, et al. Strandness DE, Jr. Streptokinase treatment of acute arterial occlusion. *Ann Surg.* 1983;198(2):185–191.

58. Sicard GA, Schier JJ, Totty WG, et al. Thrombolytic therapy for acute arterial occlusion. *J Vasc Surg.* 1985;2(1):65–78.

59. Faggioli GL, Peer RM, Pedrini L, et al. Failure of thrombolytic therapy to improve long-term vascular patency. *J Vasc Surg.* 1994;19(2):289–296.

60. Sullivan KL, Gardiner GAJ, Kandarpa K, et al. Efficacy of thrombolysis in infrainguinal bypass grafts. *Circulation.* 1991;83(2)(suppl):99–105.

CHAPTER 5

Percutaneous Mechanical Thrombectomy for Arterial Thrombus

Samir R. Kapadia and Stephen Ramee

HISTORICAL PERSPECTIVE

Since the introduction of the Fogarty catheter in early 1960s, extraction of thrombus from the artery has been performed in millions of patients worldwide (1). Although vascular access for these catheters was obtained surgically, balloon embolectomy catheters marked the beginning of minimally invasive, mechanical approaches to remove thrombi from the vasculature. Totally percutaneous thrombectomy was first implemented about 15 years ago, in the form of aspiration thrombectomy (2,3). Since then, many devices have been designed to remove thrombi from the arterial or venous circulation. The main aim of such device development has been to obviate the need for pharmacologic thrombolysis. However, over time, it has become apparent that mechanical and pharmacologic approaches to the treatment of thrombi are complimentary rather than competitive techniques. In this chapter, the indications for mechanical thrombectomy are discussed and details on various devices available for this purpose are provided.

INDICATIONS

The indications for thrombectomy in peripheral artery disease may be classified according to the circulation of interest (Table 5-1).

The major use of these devices has been in management of thrombosed dialysis fistulae (4). Most of the devices are actually approved for use for this indication. The second most common use of this procedure is in the management of acute limb ischemia.

Unlike the coronary circulation, where acute coronary syndromes are caused by formation of thrombus in situ, acute limb ischemia is most commonly caused by embolism from the heart or aorta. Acute thrombotic occlusion of grafts in patients with prior bypass surgery is also a common cause of acute limb ischemia. In all these instances, mechanical thrombectomy may be considered as a treatment option, either as an adjunct to fibrinolytic therapy or in some instances as stand-alone therapy with antithrombin or antiplatelet agents. The third common indication for mechanical thrombectomy is the management of embolization during endovascular procedures. Although pharmacologic therapy is most commonly used for this problem, mechanical removal of large emboli may help in some cases. The management of cerebrovascular thrombosis presents a unique challenge. Potential therapies include the use of small wires to physically move the thrombus toward distal smaller vessels, microsnares to mechanically remove the thrombus, and balloon dilation to displace the thrombus and restore blood flow that facilitates endogenous fibrinolysis. Adjunctive pharmacotherapy is essential, as in all other instances, for safe and sustained removal of thrombus (See Chapter 9A for additional details on the endovascular treatment of acute stroke).

DEVICES

The following paragraphs provide the functioning and technical specifications of the array of devices currently available, or under investigation,

TABLE 5-1

Indications for Mechanical Thrombectomy

Indication

Arterial Circulation
- Treatment of de novo emboli (usually cardiac)
- Management of acute vascular graft occlusion
- Management of acute native vessel occlusion (usually traumatic or iatrogenic)
- Cerebrovascular circulation (embolic or thrombotic occlusion)
- Management of distal embolization during endovascular intervention

Venous Circulation
- Acute ileocaval thrombosis
- Acute ileofemoral thrombosis
- Acute superior vena cava syndrome
- Management of massive pulmonary embolism
- Budd-Chiari syndrome

Arteriovenous Dialysis Fistulae
- Management of Thrombotic occlusion

TABLE 5-2

Mechanical Thrombectomy Devices

Device

Aspiration Devices
- Export® Catheter (Medtronic Corporation, Minneapolis, MN)
- Pronto® Extraction Catheter (Vascular Solutions, Inc, Minneapolis, MN)

Hemodynamic Recirculation Devices
- Angiojet® (Possis Medical, Minneapolis, MN)
- Hydrolyser® (Cordis Corporation, Miami, FL)
- Oasis® (Boston Scientific, Natick, MA)

Rotational Devices
- HELIX® Clot Buster Thrombectomy device (ev3 Inc, Plymouth, MN)

Ultrasonic Devices
- Resolution® Ultrasonic Endovascular Ablation System (OmniSonics Medical Technologies, Inc, Wilmington, MA
- Acolysis® (Vascular Solutions, Inc, Minneapolis, MN)

Miscellaneous Group
- X-SIZER® Catheter (ev3 Inc, Plymouth, MN)
- Trellis® Thrombectomy System (Bacchus Vascular, Santa Clara, CA)

for the treatment of arterial thrombus. Table 5-2 shows a listing of these devices.

Simple Aspiration Catheters

The simplest thrombectomy devices are catheters with a large distal port for application of suction. Currently there are two aspiration catheters available for use in the coronary and peripheral circulations: the Export® Catheter and the Pronto® Extraction Catheter (Fig. 5-1). Both of these catheters have a monorail design, and are delivered over a 0.014″ guidewire. The suction lumen is large (Fig. 5-1), and extends from the tip of the catheter to the hub, where a syringe is attached for aspiration.

These catheters work most effectively when there is no flow in the artery. In the presence of flow, the catheter aspirates blood instead of thrombus. For maximum efficacy, the catheter is placed in the midst of a thrombus and suction is applied as the catheter is gradually withdrawn over the monorail. These steps are typically repeated several times. If the catheter gets clogged, the catheter should be removed outside of the

body and flushed. In small vessels (i.e., up to 4 mm to 5 mm) these catheters seem to work well. When the thrombus burden is large, other mechanical devices are generally required to remove the remaining thrombus. These catheters may be used as a pretreatment, in some cases, prior to using more bulky devices for thrombectomy (see below), in an effort to minimize distal embolization at the time of insertion of the latter devices.

Hydrodynamic Aspiration Devices

This group of devices exploits the use of high-speed saline jets to create a Venturi effect at the catheter tip, which results in lysis and aspiration of thrombus. Saline is injected though a narrow injection lumen toward the catheter tip. Using a variety of designs, the jet(s) is (are) then directed backwards, toward the proximal portion of the catheter. A low pressure zone is thus created around these high speed jets, which has the effect of fragmenting and aspirating the thrombus

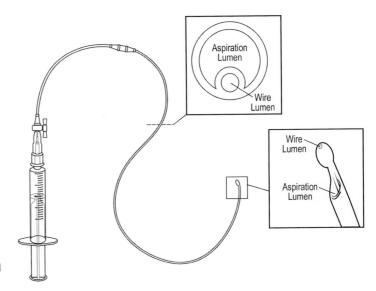

FIGURE 5-1 ● Schematic illustration of Pronto® aspiration catheter with a magnified cross-sectional view and magnified view of the catheter tip.

through the hole(s) that are present in the catheter tip. A large export lumen then carries the aspirated thrombus toward a collection area. Various designs of the fluid delivery, pressure generation, and suction provide specific advantages and disadvantages to these systems. The specific design features of the three representatives of this class of thrombectomy device are outlined in the following section.

AngioJet

The AngioJet® has three components: a drive unit that monitors the performance of the system, and a pump set that is responsible for delivery and removal of equal volumes of fluid from the final component of the system, the catheter. The drive unit and pump set are housed in a large console whose platform accommodates an array of catheters that have been developed for use in vessels of different caliber (Table 5-3).

It is important to be aware of the appropriate wire and guide/sheath compatibilities of the various devices. The Xpeedior® and AVX® catheters are specifically marketed for use in the peripheral circulation. They are each delivered over an 0.035″ wire, and their outer diameters mandate the use of an 8-Fr guide or 6-Fr sheath. They differ only in the catheter length (i.e., 50 cm versus 120 cm). In smaller vessels in the periphery, it is appropriate to use the XVG® and XMI® catheters, which are specifically marketed for use in saphenous vein grafts and native coronary arteries, respectively.

All catheters share the same basic technology. At the tip of the catheter, the fluid that is delivered into the catheter by the pump is directed

TABLE 5-3

AngioJet® Catheters

Catheter	XMI	XMI-Rx	XVG	Xpeedior	AVX
Minimal vessel diameter	≥2 mm	≥2 mm	≥3 mm	≥3 mm	≥3 mm
Optimal vessel range	2–5 mm	2–5 mm	3–8 mm	4–12 mm	4–12 mm
Working length	135 cm	135 cm	140 cm	120 cm	50 cm
Wire	OTW 0.014″	Monorail 0.014″	OTW 0.014″	OTW 0.035″	OTW 0.035″
Guide	6 F	6 F	7 F	8 F	8 F
Sheath	4 F	4 F	5 F	6 F	6 F

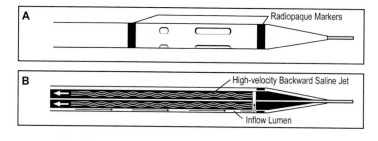

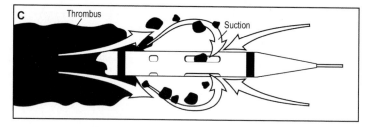

FIGURE 5-2 ● Schematic illustration of the distal portion of the Angiojet® catheter. **A:** Intact distal portion of the catheter showing the site of the radiopaque markers and entry holes. **B:** Cross-sectional view through the distal portion of the catheter, showing the location and backward direction of the high-speed saline jets. **C:** Activation of the saline jets results in aspiration of thrombus through the holes in the distal portion of the catheter.

backwards toward the operator from the tip in six high-velocity jets (Fig. 5-2). These jets create a low pressure zone at the catheter tip, producing a vacuum that draws thrombus through holes located between the two radiopaque markers in the distal portion of the catheter. Once captured in the hole, the thrombus is fragmented by the saline jets and returned to the pump set. Calculations of pressure at the tip of the Angiojet catheter show it to be an almost perfect vacuum (i.e., negative 760 mmHg). If one considers that the normal pressure inside an artery is approximately 100 mmHg, one may begin to appreciate the pressure difference (i.e., 860 mmHg) that drives thrombotic debris through the openings at the catheter tip (5).

Prior to insertion in the patient, the catheter is flushed outside the body, by activating the pump (using a pedal), for a duration of approximately 20 seconds, while keeping the catheter tip under water. There is continued debate over the best strategy for the initial activation of the device in the patient; some operators activate the pump when advancing the catheter into the thrombus, while others activate while withdrawing the catheter from the thrombus. The manufacturer recommends the latter approach. Following the initial activation, the pump is activated during both advancement and withdrawal of the catheter. This is repeated several times until the bulk of the thrombus burden is removed, as determined by angiography.

There are a number of potential complications associated with the use of the Angiojet device. The large size of the catheter may cause distal embolization while traversing the thrombus. Some operators employ an adjunctive distal-emboli prevention device to minimize the risk of this complication (Fig. 5-3). Significant vessel dissection may also occur following Angiojet use. This is more commonly seen with the larger catheter sizes, and emphasizes the need to use the appropriately sized catheter, based on vessel size.

Hydrolyser System

The Hydrolyser® device is marketed for use in the treatment of thrombus in hemodialysis fistulas and acute arterial thrombosis below the inguinal ligament, in either native arteries or synthetic grafts. This device is available in 6 Fr and 7 Fr sizes, whose specifications are summarized in Table 5-4.

The device functions as follows (Fig. 5-4): heparinized saline is injected through a narrow injection lumen, using a conventional power injector. The recommended maximum flow and pressure settings on the power injector are 5 mL per second and 750 psi, respectively. A total of 100 mL to 150 mL of saline is typically injected during passage of the catheter through the thrombus. At the catheter tip, the injection lumen makes a 180° loop and terminates just distal to an oval side hole located 4 mm proximal to

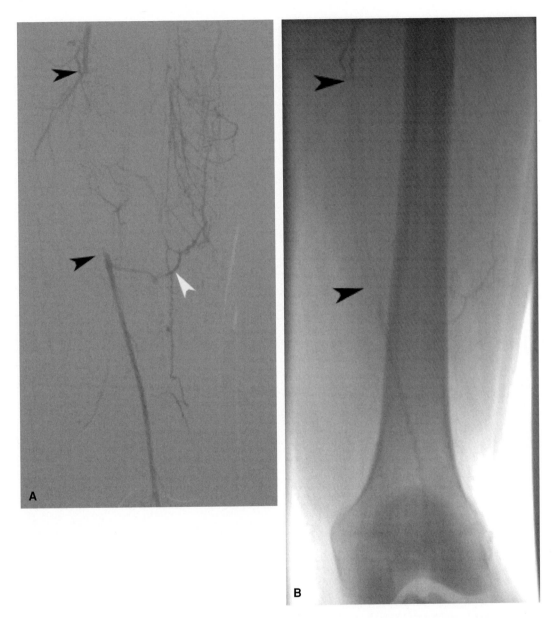

FIGURE 5-3 ● **Example of thrombotic occlusion of left superficial femoral artery (SFA) treated with Angiojet® device.** Two months previously, this 57 year-old female had a 7.0 mm × 100 mm Dynalink® stent placed for the treatment of a 7-cm distal SFA occlusion. She presented with 4-day history of left lower extremity pain. **A:** Baseline digital subtraction angiography (DSA) demonstrating occlusion of the distal SFA. Black arrowheads indicate margins of occlusion. Collateral channel indicated by white arrowhead. **B:** Baseline angiography demonstrating the thrombotic occlusion that extends the length of the stent. Stent margins are indicated by arrowheads, and correspond to the length of occlusion. (*Continued*)

the distal smooth tip. The proximally directed jet of saline creates a pressure reduction at the site of the oval hole, which aspirates and fragments thrombus from around the catheter into a larger exhaust lumen that empties into a collection bag. With a guidewire in place, the device performs isovolumetrically. The eccentric location of the hole in this device is a potential disadvantage in that the suction vortex created is less than 360°. This raises the potential for asymmetric suction on the vessel wall, increasing the risk for vessel trauma.

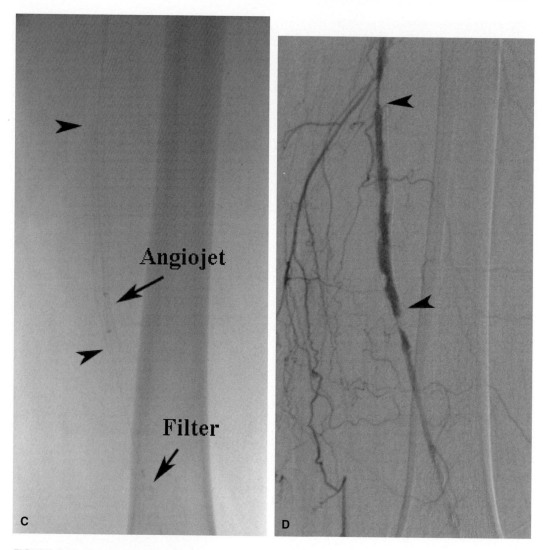

FIGURE 5-3 ● (*Continued*) **C:** The lesion was crossed with a FilterWire® embolic protection device, and the filter was deployed in the popliteal artery. Several passes of an Angiojet catheter were performed to debulk the thrombus. Black arrowheads indicate the stent margin. **D:** Angiography following thrombectomy with Angiojet. Note that significant thrombus remains adherent to the vessel wall and stent. Black arrowheads indicate stent margin. Adjunctive angioplasty using 6.0 mm × 40 mm OptaPro® balloon was performed along the length of the stent, as well as proximally and distally to the stent, after which 7.0 mm × 20 mm Precise® stents were placed proximal and distal to the previous stent. **E:** and **F:** Final angiographic appearance of the proximal and distal stent, respectively. There remains some residual thrombus in the proximal portion of the stent (*black arrowheads*).

Oasis System

The Oasis® thrombectomy catheter (i.e., formerly known as the Shredding Embolectomy Thrombectomy (SET) catheter) is the third member of the hydrodynamic aspiration device group. The device is a triple lumen catheter with an outer diameter of 6 Fr, and working lengths of 65 cm and 100 cm. The guidewire lumen accepts a 0.018″ guidewire. A smaller injection lumen communicates with a J-tipped, stainless-steel

channel at the tip of the catheter that directs the saline jet into the larger exhaust lumen (Fig. 5-5).

This creates the low-pressure zone at the tip for aspiration of thrombus into the exhaust lumen. Unlike the Angiojet and Hydrolyser devices, this system does not perform isovolumetrically. In one study, the ratio of injected saline to aspirated fluid was 0.6. This introduces the risk of procedure-related anemia with this device.

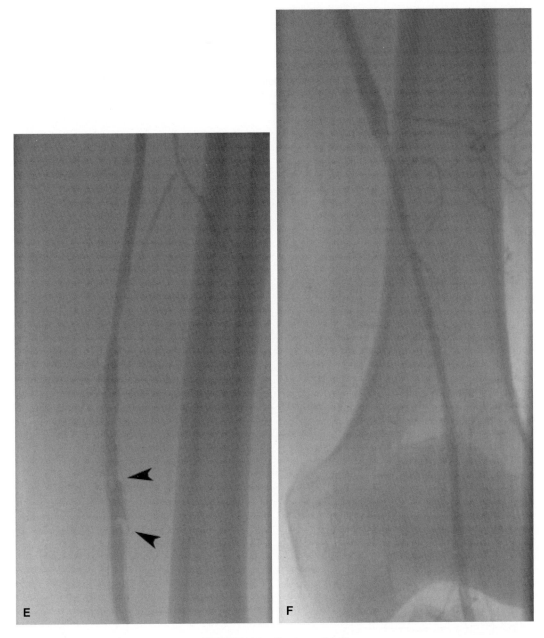

FIGURE 5-3 ● *(Continued)*

Complications with Hydrodynamic Aspiration Devices

Macroembolization

All of these devices are relatively bulky and are potential causes of distal macroembolization during manipulation of the catheters in thrombus-laden vessels. While hemodialysis fistulas usually tolerate this downstream embolization into the large capacitance venous system, this event is typically poorly tolerated in the peripheral arterial circulation (6).

Vessel Trauma

In theory, these devices exert their effect without making contact with the vessel wall. However, in practice, the negative suction effect created at the tip of these catheters has the potential to draw

TABLE 5-4

Specifications of Hydrolyser® Device

Descriptor	6 Fr Triple-lumen Device	7 Fr Double-lumen Device
Guide/Sheath compatibility	8 Fr Guide 6 Fr Sheath	9 Fr Guide 7 Fr Sheath
Wire compatibility	OTW 0.018″	OTW 0.025″
Device length (cm)	65, 100	65, 100
Design	Triple lumen • Injection lumen • Exhaust lumen • Guidewire lumen	Double lumen • Injection lumen • Exhaust lumen shared with guidewire through hemostatic device
Vessel treatment size	3 mm to 6 mm	5 mm to 9 mm

the vessel wall into the openings in the catheter tip. Angiographically, it is rare to observe evidence of vessel trauma (i.e., frank vessel dissection), but angioscopic and histologic studies commonly demonstrate evidence of endothelial denudation (7). The asymmetry in the opening of the Hydrolyser device may increase the risk of this complication compared to that associated with the Angiojet or Oasis devices. Reducing the flow rate of the saline solution is likely to reduce the risk of this complication.

Hemolysis and Anemia

Hemolysis resulting in anemia may occur during the mechanical disruption of red blood cells in the path of the high-velocity saline jets. Long activation runs of these devices, together with larger amounts of applied saline increase the risk of this complication. One of the effects of hemolysis is the release of adenosine, which may cause significant heart block in some patients. This is very commonly seen during coronary artery intervention, but has been observed in peripheral arterial and venous interventions also. The Oasis device may create a dilutional anemia, since the volume of injected saline exceeds that retrieved through the export lumen.

Fragmentation Devices

This group of thrombectomy devices exerts its actions by mechanically fragmenting the thrombus, and then dispersing the dissolved thrombus. In theory, these devices are more likely to be associated with distal embolization, since there

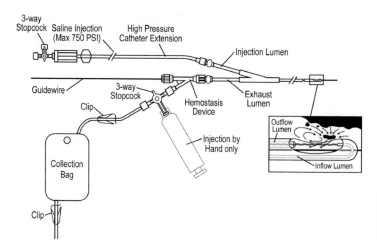

FIGURE 5-4 ● **7 Fr, dual-lumen Hydrolyser® thrombectomy system.** Inset shows magnified view of the tip of the catheter.

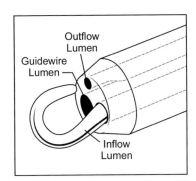

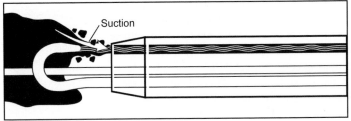

FIGURE 5-5 ● Oasis® thrombectomy catheter. Upper figure shows 3D depiction of the distal portion of the catheter. Lower figure shows cross-sectional view of the distal portion of the catheter.

is no attempt to aspirate the thrombus from the vessel.

HELIX Clot Buster Thrombectomy Device

The HELIX® Clot Buster Thrombectomy Device (formerly known as Amplatz Thrombectomy Device) was the first member of this group of thrombectomy devices. The device has a 7-Fr outer lumen and is delivered, without the use of a guidewire, to the desired location within the vessel (i.e., has no guidewire lumen). It is available in catheter lengths of 75 cm and 120 cm.

A compressed gas-driven turbine (i.e., using air or nitrogen) activates a drive shaft running the length of the catheter. This causes rotation of an encapsulated impeller housed at the distal end of the device, at approximately 100,000 rpm. The miniature impeller creates a recirculating vortex that draws thrombus to the catheter tip, where it is macerated into microscopic fragments and dispersed into the bloodstream. A Turbo Wash™ Hydraulic fluid is injected through the catheter to facilitate removal of adherent mural thrombus, without allowing contact between the device and vessel wall.

Ultrasound-Induced Thrombolysis

The use of ultrasound for purposes other than diagnostic imaging has evolved considerably over

the last decade. Two devices have now been developed that exploit the tissue effects of low-frequency (i.e., 20 kHz to 40 kHz), high-energy ultrasound waves. In liquid media such as blood, these energy waves create tiny microvacuums by a process known as cavitation. When these bubbles contract, they release a focused shock wave of acoustic energy that may cause the disintegration of surrounding tissue, such as thrombus, into microemboli of subcapillary size, while sparing the normal tissue of the vessel wall. The effect is therefore to achieve thrombus lysis without causing macroembolization. Two devices have been developed that are based on this principle.

Resolution 360 Ultrasonic Wire

The Resolution 360® Ultrasonic Wire is an investigational device designed for the rapid ablation of thrombus in both grafts and native vessels. The system consists of an ultrasonic generator that puts out low-power ultrasonic energy (i.e., 2 watts), a hand piece that converts this energy into acoustic energy, and a disposable titanium wire that releases the acoustic energy circumferentially (i.e., a full 360°) around its active length and promotes thrombus lysis. The advantage of this system over older devices that have sought to exploit this technology is the length of the active segment of wire, which dramatically increases its ability to treat a larger thrombus burden. In the current designs of the system, the wire is envisioned to have an active length of up to 30 cm, and comes in lengths varying from 40 cm to 140 cm. The goal is to use this wire as an interventional wire on which other devices may be delivered.

Acolysis

Although the principle of the Acolysis® ultrasound thrombolysis system is similar to that of the Resolution 360 Ultrasonic Wire system, they differ in the design used to transmit the ultrasonic energy to the thrombus. The Acolysis system consists of a 125-cm long, 4.5 Fr catheter that is delivered using a monorail delivery system, over conventional 0.014″ wires. Connected to the proximal end of the catheter is a piezoelectric transducer that generates low-frequency ultrasonic energy (i.e., 41.9 kHz). This energy is transmitted to a flexible wire segment (i.e., 18-cm long) at the end of the catheter, in the form of longitudinal vibrations, which cause disruption of thrombus in this segment of vessel.

This device is currently available only in non-US markets and is in the clinical planning stages in the United States. Despite early, encouraging case series, recent randomized data using this system during saphenous vein graft interventions proved disappointing (8). There was an increased incidence of adverse angiographic and clinical events in the Acolysis group. This setting of the saphenous vein graft use is somewhat distinct from the treatment of frank thrombus in peripheral arteries, and further data in the latter setting are eagerly awaited.

Miscellaneous Group

A number of newer devices have been developed that do not fit neatly into any specific category of thrombectomy device.

X–Sizer Catheter System

The X-Sizer® Catheter is a novel device that functions as both a fragmentation and aspiration device (9,10). It has recently received approval for use in native coronary arteries and saphenous vein grafts in the United States, and will likely find application in the treatment of thrombus in smaller peripheral vessels. The specifications of

TABLE 5-5

Specifications of X-Sizer® Devices

Descriptor	1.5-mm Device	2.0-mm Device
Diameter of Helix cutter	1.5 mm	2.0 mm
Outer catheter diameter	4.5 Fr	5.5 Fr
Guide/Sheath compatibility	7 Fr Guide 5 Fr sheath	8 Fr Guide 6 Fr Sheath
Guidewire compatibility	0.014″ OTW	0.014″ OTW
Catheter length	135 cm	135 cm

the two available types of this catheter system are summarized in Table 5-5.

The device contains a hand-held control unit that houses a battery-powered motor. When activated, a motor-driven drive shaft runs the length of the catheter and rotates (i.e., 2,100 rpm) a stainless steel helical cutter, which extends approximately 1 mm beyond a protective housing at the catheter tip (Fig. 5-6). The rotating helix entrains and macerates the thrombus and allows its aspiration through the vacuum port. The vacuum mechanism, which generates a negative pressure of approximately 700 mmHg, is activated simultaneously with the helical cutter by the motor unit.

Trellis Thrombectomy System

The Trellis® catheter is a further example of a novel device for the treatment of arterial thrombus. Using a unique design and technology, it allows both localized mechanical lysis and pharmacologic fibrinolysis of thrombus in the arterial circulation. Currently, the FDA has only approved the device for the administration of fibrinolytic agents.

The device contains a 6 Fr, multi-lumen catheter. Near the distal end of the catheter, there are two compliant balloons with infusion holes located in between (Fig. 5-7).

When inflated, the compliant balloons isolate a treatment zone that effectively maintains the concentration of the infused fluid. Depending on

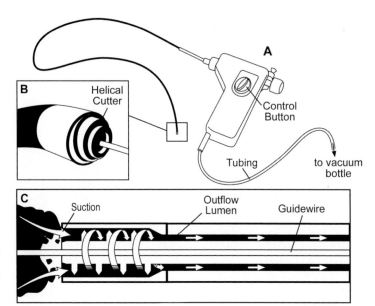

FIGURE 5-6 ● X-sizer® **thrombectomy system. A:** Low magnification view of entire system. **B:** High magnification view of the helical cutter at the tip of the catheter. **C:** High magnification view of the helical cutter at the tip of the catheter in cross-section.

the length of thrombus to be treated, catheters with a 10-cm or 20-cm distance between the balloons may be chosen. The device also has a central through-lumen that is compatible with a 0.035″ guidewire, to allow delivery of the device. The mechanical thrombectomy component of the system requires that the guidewire be exchanged for the dispersion wire component, which is a shape-set nitinol cable. Once placed, the shape-set region of the dispersion wire resides between the two balloons of the catheter. The dispersion wire is connected to an integral drive unit that oscillates the dispersion wire within the isolated region, to further disperse the infused fluid and mechanically lyse the thrombus.

CLINICAL OUTCOMES WITH MECHANICAL THROMBECTOMY FOR ACUTE PERIPHERAL ARTERIAL OCCLUSIVE DISEASE

There is a paucity of clinical data comparing the effectiveness of the various forms of mechanical thrombectomy, and an absence of randomized data comparing mechanical thrombectomy with surgical or pharmacologic therapies. The result

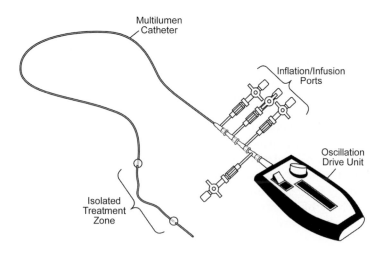

FIGURE 5-7 ● Trellis® thrombectomy catheter showing major components of system.

is that an assessment made of the efficacy of the various methods of mechanical thrombectomy is currently based largely on case reports, and single and multicenter registry experiences with these devices, without any comparison control group (summarized in Table 5-6).

The largest amount of data is available for the AngioJet system. Initial thrombus extraction rates have ranged from 52 to 95%. Most of the studies have used adjunctive therapy, including thrombolytic agents, balloon angioplasty, and stenting, to achieve adequate reperfusion. When mechanical therapy with the Angiojet is used in isolation, the results are only moderately good.

In a study reported from the Cleveland Clinic involving 83 patients, the initial success rate was 61% with the AngioJet as stand-alone therapy. Adjunctive thrombolytic therapy was used in 50 patients, the majority for angiographic evidence of distal small vessel occlusion (i.e., beyond the reach of the device). Müller-Hülsbeck et al reported the use of the AngioJet thrombectomy catheter in 112 patients with occluded arterial or bypass grafts. Overall angiographic success (i.e., greater than 75% thrombus removal) was seen in 88.4% of patients and adjunctive thrombolytic therapy was required in 29% of these patients. Mild elevation in plasma free hemoglobin was noted for 24 hours postprocedure, with no adverse clinical sequelae. Immediate amputations were required in two patients and the 2-year amputation-free survival rate was 75%.

Rilinger et al reported the largest experience in the use of the Helix Clot Buster thrombectomy system for acute peripheral arterial ischemia. A majority of the patients had an embolic occlusion (n = 32) with a mean duration of ischemia of 2 days. Complete thrombus extraction with the device, as stand-alone therapy, was seen in 75% of the patients, which is impressive. No clinically relevant distal embolization was reported in this series. There were no in-hospital deaths, adjunctive thrombolytic therapy was used in eight patients, and two patients required early amputation. Of particular concern however, was the reported inability to remove the device percutaneously in 7.5% of patients. In a smaller study involving 14 patients, a similar initial success of 71% was reported with 6-month patency rate of 43%.

Clinical information for acute leg ischemia with the Hydrolyser catheter has been limited. In two clinical trials the initial success rate was high at 82% and 83%, respectively. Reekers et al reported higher success rates for procedures performed on grafts (88%) compared to those performed on native vessels (73%). They noted a mean catheter activation time of only 3 minutes, and the avoidance of thrombolytic drugs in 58% of patients. Angiographic evidence of embolization was noted in seven patients of which six underwent successful management with percutaneous aspiration or thrombolysis; the remaining patient required an amputation.

Although data for the Trellis infusion catheter system for local fibrinolytic therapy have been encouraging, the data on the mechanical catheter are relatively sparse (20,21).

LESSONS LEARNED

A number of lessons have been learned from the experience with mechanical thrombectomy devices (MTDs). First, mechanical thrombectomy does not eliminate the need for pharmacologic thrombolysis or surgical therapies. When distal small vessel occlusion is present, the current generations of MTDs are too bulky to allow treatment at these sites. Second, MTDs are less successful when treating older adherent thrombus; in these cases, pharmacologic thrombolysis has an advantage. These considerations likely explain the high use of adjunctive thrombolysis in almost all series using MTDs to treat acute peripheral arterial occlusive disease (range 10 to 66%). Finally, MTDs do not treat the culprit lesion underlying the cause of acute vessel occlusion. This requires the use of adjunctive endovascular or surgical therapies, to prevent recurrences.

Despite these shortcomings, mechanical thrombectomy does have a number of distinct advantages in the treatment of arterial thrombosis. It rapidly debulks thrombus, and therefore minimizes the duration of tissue ischemia in the area supplied by that arterial segment. There is clearly an advantage of using mechanical thrombectomy in patients who are either high-risk for open surgery, or who have contraindications to pharmacologic thrombolysis. In patients with a

TABLE 5-6

Literature on the Use of the Mechanical Catheters for Limb-threatening Ischemia

Study	Device	Trial Design	N	Native Vessel (%)	Adjunctive Lysis (%)	Complications (%)				Primary Patency (%)
						Emboli	Bleeding	Amputation	Death	
Wagner 1997 (11)	Angiojet	Prospective Multicenter	50	78	30	6	2	8	0	30 d: 76 1 y: 69
Silva 1998 (5)	Angiojet	Prospective	21	62	–	9	10	5	14	6 mo: 89
Müller-Hülsbeck 2000 (12)	Angiojet	Prospective	112	86	18	10	N/A	2	7	6 mo: 68 2 y: 60 3 y: 58
Kasirajan 2001 (13)	Angiojet	Retrospective	86	63	58	2	11	12	9	3 mo: 90 6 mo: 79
Hopfner 1999 (14)	Oasis	Prospective	51	86	10	5	N/A	18	8	1 mo: 64 6 mo: 54
Reekers 1996 (15)	Hydrolyser	Prospective	28	39	39	18	0	11	0	1 mo: 50
Henry, 1998 (16)	Hydrolyser	Prospective	41	68	24	2.4	N/A	0	0	1 mo: 73
Tadavarthy 1994 (17)	Amplatz	Retrospective	14	14	28	14	14	0	0	6 mo: 43
Rilinger 1997 (18)	Amplatz	Prospective	40	100	22	0	2.5	5	0	N/A
Görich 1998 (19)	Amplatz	Retrospective	18	100	66	N/A	6	6	N/A	N/A

(adapted from Kasirajan et al. (6))

relative contraindication to thrombolysis, mechanical thrombectomy may enhance the effectiveness of pharmacologic thrombolysis by exposing a greater surface area of thrombus to the agent. The dose and duration of pharmacologic therapy may therefore be minimized, reducing the risk of bleeding.

SUMMARY OF STRATEGY FOR TREATMENT OF ACUTE PERIPHERAL OCCLUSIVE DISEASE

With the limited data comparing mechanical versus pharmacologic therapy, the selection of a particular therapy is dependent largely on the characteristics of the thrombotic occlusion (e.g., location, thrombus burden, age of thrombus), the feasibility of mechanical therapy, the risk of bleeding with thrombolytic therapy, and the operative risk assessment of the patient. Mechanical therapy may be attempted first if the vessel can be successfully crossed with a guide wire. Even for local thrombolytic therapy this is an essential step. If the lesion can not be crossed with a guide wire (which is rare), then surgical treatment is necessary. If the thrombus can not be adequately removed despite mechanical thrombectomy, local thrombolytic treatment may be attempted. Thrombolytic therapy may also be helpful with distal embolization in some cases. Combination of glycoprotein IIbIIIa inhibitors and fibrinolytic medications has shown some promise in this situation.

REFERENCES

1. Fogarty TJ, Cranley JJ, Krause RJ, et al. A method for extraction of arterial emboli and thrombi. *Surg Gynecol Obstet.* 1963;116:241–244.
2. Sniderman KW, Bodner L, Saddekni S, et al. Percutaneous embolectomy by transcatheter aspiration. Work in progress. *Radiology.* 1984;150:357–361.
3. Starck EE, McDermott JC, Crummy AB, et al. Percutaneous aspiration thromboembolectomy. *Radiology.* 1985;156:61–66.
4. Bush RL, Lin PH, Lumsden AB. Management of thrombosed dialysis access: thrombectomy versus thrombolysis. *Semin Vasc Surg.* 2004;17:32–39.
5. Silva JA, Ramee SR, Collins TJ, et al. Rheolytic thrombectomy in the treatment of acute limb-threatening ischemia: immediate results and six-month follow-up of the multicenter AngioJet registry. Possis Peripheral AngioJet Study AngioJet Investigators. *Cathet Cardiovasc Diagn.* 1998;45:386–393.
6. Kasirajan K, Haskal ZJ, Ouriel K. The use of mechanical thrombectomy devices in the management of acute peripheral arterial occlusive disease. *J Vasc Interv Radiol.* 2001;12:405–411.
7. Vesely TM, Hovsepian DM, Darcy MD, et al. Angioscopic observations after percutaneous thrombectomy of thrombosed hemodialysis grafts. *J Vasc Interv Radiol.* 2000;11:971–977.
8. Singh M, Rosenschein U, Ho KK, et al. Treatment of saphenous vein bypass grafts with ultrasound thrombolysis: a randomized study (ATLAS). *Circulation.* 2003;107:2331–2336.
9. Stone GW, Cox DA, Low R, et al. Safety and efficacy of a novel device for treatment of thrombotic and atherosclerotic lesions in native coronary arteries and saphenous vein grafts: results from the multicenter X-Sizer for treatment of thrombus and atherosclerosis in coronary applications trial (X-TRACT) study. *Catheter Cardiovasc Interv.* 2003;58:419–427.
10. Kornowski R, Ayzenberg O, Halon DA, et al. Preliminary experiences using X-sizer catheter for mechanical thrombectomy of thrombus-containing lesions during acute coronary syndromes. *Catheter Cardiovasc Interv.* 2003;58:443–448.
11. Wagner HJ, Muller-Hulsbeck S, Pitton MB, et al. Rapid thrombectomy with a hydrodynamic catheter: results from a prospective, multicenter trial. *Radiology.* 1997;205:675–681.
12. Muller-Hulsbeck S, Kalinowski M, Heller M, et al. Rheolytic hydrodynamic thrombectomy for percutaneous treatment of acutely occluded infra-aortic native arteries and bypass grafts: midterm follow-up results. *Invest Radiol.* 2000;35:131–140.
13. Kasirajan K, Gray B, Beavers FP, et al. Rheolytic thrombectomy in the management of acute and subacute limb-threatening ischemia. *J Vasc Interv Radiol.* 2001;12:413–421.
14. Hopfner W, Vicol C, Bohndorf K, et al. Shredding embolectomy thrombectomy catheter for treatment of acute lower-limb ischemia. *Ann Vasc Surg.* 1999;13:426–435.
15. Reekers JA, Kromhout JG, Spithoven HG, et al. Arterial thrombosis below the inguinal ligament: percutaneous treatment with a thrombosuction catheter. *Radiology.* 1996;198:49–53.
16. Henry M, Amor M, Henry I, et al. The Hydrolyser thrombectomy catheter: a single-center experience. *J Endovasc Surg.* 1998;5:24–31.
17. Tadavarthy SM, Murray PD, Inampudi S, et al. Mechanical thrombectomy with the Amplatz device: human experience. *J Vasc Interv Radiol.* 1994;5:715–724.
18. Rilinger N, Gorich J, Scharrer-Pamler R, et al. Mechanical thrombectomy of embolic occlusion in both the profunda femoris and superficial femoral arteries in critical limb ischaemia. *Br J Radiol.* 1997;70:80–84.
19. Gorich J, Rilinger N, Sokiranski R, et al. Mechanical thrombolysis of acute occlusion of both the superficial and the deep femoral arteries using a thrombectomy device. *AJR Am J Roentgenol.* 1998;170:1177–1180.
20. Sarac TP, Hilleman D, Arko FR, et al. Clinical and economic evaluation of the trellis thrombectomy device for arterial occlusions: preliminary analysis. *J Vasc Surg.* 2004;39:556–559.
21. Kasirajan K, Ramaiah VG, Diethrich EB. The Trellis Thrombectomy System in the treatment of acute limb ischemia. *J Endovasc Ther.* 2003;10:317–321.

CHAPTER 6

Carotid Intervention

Ivan P. Casserly and Jay S. Yadav

In 1905, Chiari reported that embolization of thrombotic material formed on the surface of atherosclerotic plaque in the carotid sinus was a cause of apoplexy (i.e., sudden impairment of neurologic function, stroke). Further published work by Miller Fisher in the 1950s solidified the association between carotid artery disease and stroke and led to the development of carotid endarterectomy (CEA) as a treatment option for patients with carotid artery disease. It took nearly 50 years before large, randomized, clinical trials demonstrated that this therapy improved outcomes for symptomatic patients with moderate-to-severe carotid stenosis, and asymptomatic patients with severe carotid stenosis. Based on these data, CEA established itself as the gold standard for carotid revascularization.

Coincident with the development of endovascular therapies at other vascular sites, a small number of investigators began to perform angioplasty of the carotid artery in the early 1980s (1). These investigators faced a number of unique challenges. The hazard of distal embolization and resultant stroke, at the time of endovascular intervention, limited the ability to offer this therapy to surgically eligible patients, where cross-clamping of the carotid distally provides protection against embolization. By the early 1990s, it was clear that percutaneous carotid intervention would not become a viable therapy without addressing this limitation. A variety of emboli-protection devices (EPDs) were developed that served to limit or prevent distal embolization.

Unfortunately, it has taken nearly a decade to get FDA approval for these devices.

As in other vascular territories, the use of stents in the carotid artery gained acceptance in the mid-1990s, as operators sought to achieve a predictable angiographic result, treat procedural complications such as abrupt closure and dissection, eliminate vessel recoil, and reduce the risk of restenosis. However, conventional balloon-expandable stents in the carotid location proved suboptimal for two reasons: (1) conventional balloon-expandable stents were too rigid and resulted in kinking of the internal carotid artery in the length between the stent and the petrous portion of the artery, particularly in tortuous vessels (Fig. 6-1), and (2) balloon-expandable stents were associated with a high incidence of loss of apposition between the stent and vessel wall.

These considerations led to the development of nitinol self-expanding stents that have performed well in the carotid location and are now receiving FDA approval for use in the carotid location.

In addition to the technical issues related to the procedure, percutaneous carotid intervention has had to overcome a number of political hurdles. Among providers in the surgical community, there has been an understandable reluctance to abandon the old gold standard of CEA for the treatment of carotid disease. Among endovascular specialists, there have been significant turf wars about who should be allowed to perform these procedures. The national non-coverage policy for carotid intervention, determined by the Center for Medicare and Medicaid

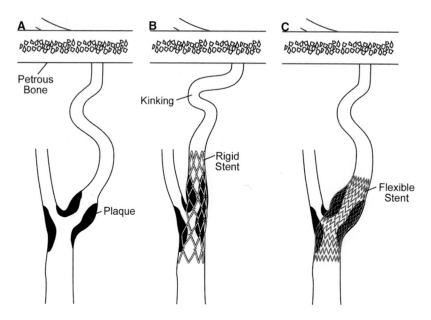

FIGURE 6-1 ● Schematic illustrating the effect of rigid stainless-steel, balloon-expandable **(panel B)** and self-expanding nitinol stents **(panel C),** in the carotid location. Nitinol stents conform to the tortuosity in the carotid artery, minimizing any kinking, distally.

Services (prior to FDA approval), also hampered the early dissemination of this technique.

Having met the major technical challenges of the procedure and slowly addressed the political issues, proponents of percutaneous carotid intervention have made it a reality. A major shift away from CEA is imminent and is supported by an increasing body of evidence. This chapter will summarize the evidence for carotid artery stenting, and provide a comprehensive description of the technical aspects of the technique, and the periprocedural management of these patients.

ANATOMIC CONSIDERATIONS

The right common carotid artery (CCA) arises in remarkably constant fashion from the bifurcation of the innominate artery (Fig. 6-2). It may rarely arise as a separate branch off the aortic arch, or in conjunction with the left CCA (i.e., common carotid trunk) (Fig. 6-3).

In contrast, the origin of the left CCA is variable. In approximately 75% of cases, it arises as the second great vessel off the aortic arch, in a plane posterior to the innominate artery (Fig. 6-2). In the remaining cases, the left CCA

shares its origin off the aortic arch with the innominate artery (i.e., approximately 10 to 15%), or arises from the innominate artery (i.e., bovine origin, approximately 10%) (Fig. 6-4).

At the level of the upper border of the thyroid cartilage, each CCA bifurcates into an external

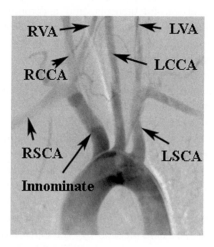

FIGURE 6-2 ● Normal anatomy of the aortic arch and great vessels. LCCA, left common carotid artery; RCCA, right common carotid artery; LVA, left vertebral artery; RVA, right vertebral artery; LSCA, left subclavian artery; RSCA, right subclavian artery.

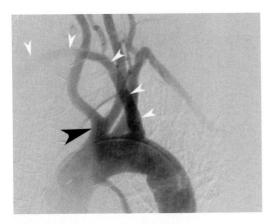

FIGURE 6-3 ● Arch aortogram from patient with common carotid trunk (black arrowhead) and anomalous origin of the right subclavian artery, distal to the origin of the left subclavian artery (white arrowheads).

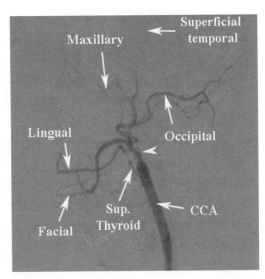

FIGURE 6-5 ● **Anatomy of the external carotid artery.** Angiogram of the common carotid artery (CCA) shows occlusion of the internal carotid artery (white arrowhead) facilitating identification of the branches of the external carotid artery.

and internal branch. During diagnostic angiography, the angle of the mandible serves as a useful landmark for the carotid bifurcation, although significant variation in the level of the carotid bifurcation is common. The external carotid artery (ECA) is easily recognized, owing to its numer-

ous branches to the face, scalp, and thyroid. A basic understanding of the anatomy of the ECA is important because this vessel and its branches are often wired during carotid intervention (see below). Anterior branches arise in the following order: the superior thyroid, lingual, and facial. The occipital branch arises posteriorly, at the level of the facial artery. The ECA terminates by giving off the internal maxillary branch that is directed anteriorly, and the superficial temporal branch that runs along the path of the ECA toward the temporal-scalp region (Fig. 6-5).

Under normal conditions, the internal carotid artery (ICA) contains a bulbous dilation at its origin, referred to as the carotid sinus. The adventitia in this region contains the mechanoreceptors responsible for blood pressure regulation. In its proximal portion, the ICA lies posterior and medial to the ECA. These relationships may be appreciated in the lateral and posteroanterior (PA) projections by angiography, respectively.

By convention, the ICA is divided into four sections (Fig. 6-6):

1. the *pre-petrous* or *cervical portion*. This defines the segment of vessel between the CCA bifurcation and the petrous bone, and contains no arterial branches. Most carotid

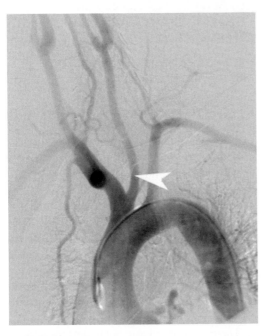

FIGURE 6-4 ● Arch aortogram with bovine origin of the left common carotid artery off the innominate artery (arrowhead).

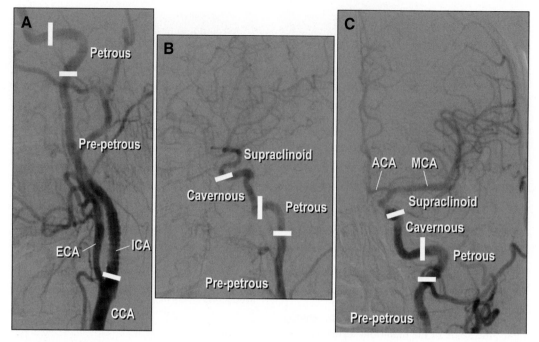

FIGURE 6-6 ● **Anatomy of the internal carotid artery (ICA). A:** LAO oblique view showing the proximal portion of the left ICA. **B:** Lateral view of distal portion of the left ICA. **C:** Posteroanterior (PA) cranial view of the distal left ICA and its cerebral branches. ICA, internal carotid artery; ECA, external carotid artery; CCA, common carotid artery; MCA, middle cerebral artery; ACA, anterior cerebral artery.

intervention involves treatment of atherosclerosis of the ostium and proximal portion of this segment of vessel;

2. the *petrous portion.* This refers to the L-shaped section of vessel (i.e., rotated 90°) that courses through the petrous bone;

3. the *cavernous portion,* which courses through the cavernous sinus; and

4. the *supraclinoid portion,* which gives off the important ophthalmic, posterior communicating, and anterior choroidal branches, and terminates in the middle and anterior cerebral arteries.

The ophthalmic artery supplies the ipsilateral retina and optic nerve and is an important route for collateral flow between the ICA and ECA (via maxillary branches). Similarly, the posterior communicating branch links the ICA with the posterior cerebral artery, providing an important collateral link between the anterior and posterior cerebral circulations. The area of the brain supplied by the anterior- and middle-cerebral arteries is termed the *carotid territory.*

CURRENT INDICATIONS FOR CONTEMPORARY CAROTID INTERVENTION

High-Risk Patients—Symptomatic and Asymptomatic

Having established the technique of carotid intervention using self-expanding carotid artery stents and embolic protection devices, investigators sought to establish the evidence base for contemporary carotid intervention by initially focusing on a group of patients at high-risk for poor outcomes of CEA. The surgical literature had identified the characteristics of this high-risk group (listed in Table 6-1), which included both anatomic and clinical variables. Patients with these characteristics were systematically excluded from the large randomized CEA trials, leading to clinical uncertainty regarding the efficacy of CEA in this group.

There were two basic study designs used to examine outcomes in high-risk patients. The majority of studies were prospective, single-center, multi-center, or corporate-sponsored registry

TABLE 6-1

Criteria Used to Define High-Risk in Carotid Artery Stent Studies

High-Risk Criteria

Clinical

Age >80 years

Congestive heart failure (class III/IV)

Known severe left ventricular dysfunction, LV EF <30%

Open heart surgery needed within six weeks

Recent MI (>24 hrs. and <4 weeks)

Unstable angina (CCS class III/IV)

Severe pulmonary disease

Contralateral laryngeal nerve palsy

Anatomic

Previous CEA with recurrent stenosis

High cervical ICA lesions or CCA lesions below the clavicle

Contralateral carotid occlusion

Radiation therapy to neck

Prior radical neck surgery

Severe tandem lesions

ICA, internal carotid artery; CCA, common carotid artery; LV EF, left ventricular ejection fraction; MI, myocardial infarction; CEA, carotid endarterectomy.

studies evaluating the outcome of consecutively treated patients (Table 6-2) (2). Enrollment in these studies required that the patients have one or more high-risk anatomic or clinical characteristics, and have a carotid stenosis of at least 80% in asymptomatic patients or at least 50% in symptomatic patients. A single, randomized trial (SAPPHIRE, Stenting and Angioplasty with Protection in Patients at High Risk for Endarterectomy) was also performed. The enrollment criteria for this study were similar to that for the high-risk registries except in one important respect: the carotid lesion had to be equally amenable to revascularization by surgical or percutaneous methods (3,4). Therefore, the overall risk of the cohort in this trial was likely somewhat less than in registry-type studies, where such a requirement did not exist. A carotid-artery stent registry component was prospectively incorporated within the SAPPHIRE trial that enrolled patients who were deemed ineligible for CEA by the vascular surgeon investigator. Because of this

requirement, it is likely that the risk of this group exceeded that in other high-risk registries. These considerations are important in interpreting the data from the randomized and registry arms of the SAPPHIRE trial, and in comparing outcomes from high-risk registries with the results obtained in this trial.

Given its randomized design, the randomized arm of the SAPPHIRE trial provides the most robust data supporting the role of CAS with emboli protection in high-risk patients (Table 6-3).

At 30-day and 1-year follow-up examination, there was a trend toward a reduction in the incidence of stroke, or death, and a significant reduction in the incidence of myocardial infarction in patients from the stent arm. Target-lesion revascularization and cranial-nerve palsies were also significantly reduced in the stent arm population. Overall, the data support the conclusion that CAS with embolic protection is at least of equivalent safety with CEA, in high-risk patients. Further corroborating evidence for this conclusion is provided by the outcomes from other high-risk registries, using a variety of stents and embolic protection devices, and the registry arm of the SAPPHIRE trial. These studies show a remarkable consistency in the frequency of the composite endpoint of death/stroke/MI at 30 days that is similar to that reported in the randomized cohort of the SAPPHIRE trial (Fig. 6-7).

Based on the results of the SAPPHIRE trial and the ARCHER registry, the FDA Circulatory Systems Devices Panel has voted for approval of CAS using the Precise® or Acculink® nitinol stent in conjunction with the Angioguard XP® or Accunet® filter, respectively, for the treatment of symptomatic and asymptomatic patients with at least 50% and at least 80% carotid stenosis, respectively. These devices will have become available to qualified operators for routine clinical use, for the approved indications, by the middle of 2005. Several other carotid stent/filter combinations will be seeking the same approval, and are expected to become available in the next 1 to 2 years.

Low-Risk Symptomatic Patients

Carotid intervention remains investigational in patients other than those at high-risk for CEA. The CAVATAS trial (Carotid and Vertebral

TABLE 6-2

Summary of 'High-Risk' Carotid Artery Stenting with Embolic Protection Device Registries

Study	Sponsor	Sample Size	Stent	Embolic Protection Device	Status
SAPPHIRE (CAS registry)	Cordis	409	Precise®	Angioguard®	30-day and 1-year outcomes presented
ARCHER 2, 3	Guidant	ARCHER 2—278 ARCHER 3—145	Acculink® (OTW & Rx)	Accunet®	30-day outcome ARCHER 3 and 1-year outcome of ARCHER 2 presented
SECURITY	Abbott Vascular Devices	320	MedNova® Xact®	MedNova NeuroShield®/EmboShield®	30-day outcomes presented
BEACH	Boston Scientific	480	Wallstent®	FilterWire® EX and EZ	Enrollment completed
CABERNET	EndoTex	380	NexStent®	FilterWire® EX	30-day outcomes presented
MAVERIC Int'l	Medtronic	51	Exponent®	Interceptor®	CE mark approved
MAVERIC II	Medtronic	Phase I—99 Phase II—399	Exponent	GuardWire®	30-day outcomes presented
PASCAL	Medtronic	115	Exponent	Any CE Mark-approved device	Enrollment completed
CREATE	ev3	400	Protegé®	Spider®	Enrollment completed

CAS, carotid artery stent; OTW, over-the-wire; Rx, monorail; SAPPHIRE, Stenting and Angioplasty with Protection in Patients at High Risk for Endarterectomy. (Adapted from Endovascular Today, September 2003, p 83.)

TABLE 6-3

30-day and 1-year Outcomes (Based on Actual Treatment Analysis) in the SAPPHIRE Trial

	Randomized Trial	
	CAS	CEA
30-day Outcome		
Death	0.6	2.0
Stroke	3.1	3.3
MI	1.9	6.6
Death/Stroke/MI	4.4	9.9
1-year Outcome		
Death	7.0	12.9
Stroke	5.8	7.7
MI	2.5	8.1
30-day Death/stroke/MI + death and ipsilateral stroke between 31 days and 1 year.	12.0	20.1

CAS, carotid artery stenting; CEA, carotid endarterectomy; MI, myocardial infarction; MACE, major adverse cardiac event. (Adapted from Table 3. N Engl J Med 2004, 351, 1–9.)

Artery Transluminal Angioplasty Study) did randomize low-risk, largely symptomatic patients with carotid disease, to carotid intervention or CEA. However, in the endovascular arm, embolic protection devices were not used, and stenting was performed in only 25% of patients. Although the results of this trial were favorable for carotid angioplasty, the use of an antiquated endovascu-lar strategy raises significant doubts regarding the current applicability of the findings (5). Table 6-4 summarizes the ongoing clinical trials randomizing low-risk symptomatic patients (i.e., *without* high-risk criteria) to either CEA or contemporary carotid intervention (6–10).

A cut-off criterion of at least 50% stenosis by angiography (NASCET criteria) is being used in most studies. The carotid interventional technique will involve carotid-artery stenting in all studies, and the use of an embolic protection device is either mandatory or strongly encouraged. Unfortunately, the enrollment in these studies has been extremely slow, and will likely be further jeopardized by low-risk, carotid-artery stent registries that are currently being planned. Completion of enrollment and follow-up monitoring of these studies, together with FDA approval (i.e., assuming the data support carotid artery stenting) may take a further 3 to 5 years.

Low-Risk Asymptomatic Patients

Low-risk, asymptomatic patients with CAD have not been included in carotid intervention studies to date. This is likely related to the low frequency of events in this group, when treated medically. Randomized and case-controlled studies of CEA versus CAS are planned for this patient population. Based on the results of the asymptomatic European (ACST) and North American (ACAS) studies, there is likely some potential benefit for carotid intervention in this group, provided complication rates can be kept to a low level.

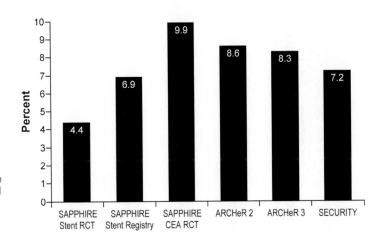

FIGURE 6-7 ● Incidence of death/stroke/myocardial infarction at 30 days from 'high-risk' carotid stent registries and randomized portion of SAPPHIRE trial. RCT, randomized controlled trial.

TABLE 6-4

Summary of 'Low-Risk' Carotid Artery Stent Trials in Progress

Trial	Sample Size	Sites of Enrollment	Funding	Clinical Enrollment Criteria	Lesion Enrollment Criteria	Endovascular Strategy	Primary Endpoints	Status of Trial
ICSS (CAVATAS-2)	1500	Europe Australia Canada	Stroke Association Sanofi Synthelabo European Commission	TIA/Stroke within 12 months	>50% by NASCET method or noninvasive equivalent	CAS ± EPD	• 30-day death/stroke/ MI • 3 year death/disabling stroke	Expect to complete enrollment by 2007
EVA-3S	900	France	National Research Organization	TIA/Stroke within 4 months	>60% by NASCET or noninvasive equivalent	CAS + EPD	• 30-day death/stroke • 30-day death/stroke + ipsilateral stroke at 2–4 years.	300 enrolled April 2004
SPACE	1,900	Germany Austria Switzerland	Federal Ministry of Education and Research German Research Foundation Industry Funding	TIA/Stroke within 6 months	>50% by NASCET or 70% by Doppler	CAS ± EPD	• 30-day death/ipsilateral stroke • 2-year death/ipsilateral stroke	667 enrolled Feb 2004
CREST	2,500	North America Europe	National Institute of Neurological Disorders and Stroke—National Institute of Health Guidant Coroporation	Symptomatic	>50% by NASCET	CAS + EPD*	• 30-day death/stroke/MI ipsilateral stroke after 30 days	Currently enrolling

ICSS, International Carotid Stenting Study; SPACE, Stent-Supported Percutaneous Angioplasty of the Carotid Artery versus Endarterectomy Trial; CREST, Carotid Revascularization Endarterectomy versus Stent Trial; EVA-3S, Endarterectomy Versus Angioplasty in patients with Symptomatic Severe carotid Stenosis; CAS, Carotid artery stenting; EPD, embolic protection device; MI, myocardial infarction; TIA, transient ischemic attack.

*Acculink® stent and Accunet® EPD.

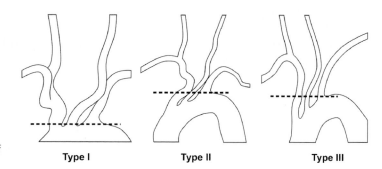

FIGURE 6-8 ● Illustration of aortic arch types.

Type I   **Type II**   **Type III**

Diagnostic Carotid Angiography

Prior to performing a diagnostic carotid angiography, one should first make an assessment of the anatomy of the aortic arch. Noninvasive studies such as computed tomography (CT) or magnetic resonance angiography (MRA) that provide a 3D assessment of the arch are ideal for this purpose. Conventional aortic arch angiography provides a 2D assessment of the arch that often underestimates the degree of tortuosity in the innominate and common carotid arteries. Rotational angiography of the aortic arch, if available, is preferable.

The information that needs to be gleaned from the aortic arch assessment includes: (1) the aortic arch type (Fig. 6-8), (2) the presence of any variant anatomy in the origins of the great vessels off the aortic arch, and (3) the presence of atherosclerotic disease or tortuosity in the proximal portions of the great vessels.

These factors strongly influence the choice of diagnostic catheter (Fig. 6-9) and the interventional strategy selected.

For all patients with Type I, and most patients with Type II, aortic arch anatomy, our practice is to use a JR4 diagnostic catheter for carotid angiography. The exception to this rule involves patients with a bovine origin of the left CCA, where a Vitek® catheter is often required, regardless of the aortic arch type. In patients with Type III aortic arches, a Vitek catheter is usually required, especially for engagement of the innominate artery. Only rarely is a Simmons® catheter required. Selective angiography of the left CCA and bifurcation is performed with the diagnostic catheter at the origin of the vessel, although in some cases the catheter may need to be advanced over an angled glide wire toward the midportion of the vessel. For right CCA angiography, the innominate artery is first engaged with the diagnostic catheter. Typically, a roadmap angiogram of the innominate artery is performed in the RAO projection, which splays the origins of the right subclavian artery and right CCA. A stiff-angled glidewire is advanced into the right CCA and the catheter is advanced over the wire to the midportion of the vessel.

In most patients, ipsilateral oblique (30° to 45°) and left lateral views of the CCA of interest are adequate to define the anatomy of the carotid bifurcation. Additional views (e.g., straight AP, contralateral oblique, or adding cranial or caudal angulation to standardized views) may be required to define a lesion of interest, especially in situations where significant tortuosity distorts the normal geometric relationship between the ICA and ECA. The anatomic features that require assessment during angiography of the carotid bifurcation, and the potential influence of these features on the interventional strategy or technique employed, are summarized in Table 6-5.

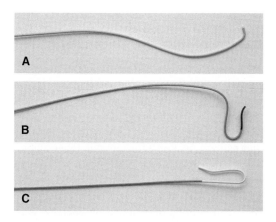

A

B

C

FIGURE 6-9 ● **Diagnostic catheters used during carotid-artery angiography. A:** JR 4. **B:** Vitek. **C:** Simmons 1.

TABLE 6-5

Influence of Assessments Made During Diagnostic Carotid Angiography on Carotid Interventional Procedures

Angiographic Assessment	Impact on Interventional Procedure
Assess Lesion Characteristics	
Precise location of the lesion, with definition of the proximal and distal extent of lesion	Influences planned location for stent placement and stent length
	Influences strategy for delivery of guide/sheath to distal CCA
Approximate length of lesion	Stent length
Complex lesion ulceration	Predict difficulty of crossing lesion with filter device
Severity of stenosis	Predict difficulty of crossing lesion with filter device
	Predict need for predilation of lesion prior to filter delivery
Calcification	Predict ability to achieve good stent expansion
Diameter of CCA and ICA	Influences choice of stent diameter and filter diameter
Assess the entire pre-petrous portion of the ICA	Influences the choice of landing zone for the filter device
Tortuosity distal to the lesion and proximal to the landing zone for filter	Favors use of guide to provide support
	Predict degree of difficulty in delivering filter
Patency of external carotid artery	Influences strategy for delivery of guide/sheath to distal CCA

Additionally, a baseline angiography of the anterior cerebral circulation is routinely performed prior to any planned carotid intervention. This serves as a reference against which the postprocedural cerebral angiogram may be compared, thus facilitating the prompt diagnosis of distal embolization related to the procedure. Additionally, the presence of associated, significant intracranial or distal extracranial atherosclerotic-artery disease, or other vascular pathology that might influence management, will be uncovered. A shallow PA cranial view (i.e., with enough cranial angulation to position the petrous bone at the base of the orbit) and left lateral views are the standard projections used by most operators. To obtain good quality cerebral angiograms, the diagnostic catheter ideally should be placed in the distal CCA. For this reason, we typically delay cerebral angiography on the side of the carotid intervention until there is placement of the sheath or guide in the distal CCA.

CAROTID INTERVENTION

Pharmacology

In the practice of the authors, all patients receive aspirin and clopidogrel for at least 3 days, prior to carotid artery stenting. In the absence of contraindication, a small bolus of heparin (i.e., 2,000 units to 3,000 units) is administered prior to diagnostic carotid angiography, and this is supplemented during the intervention to achieve an ACT of 275 to 300 seconds. In patients with a contraindication to heparin, carotid-artery stenting may be performed using the direct thrombin inhibitor, bivalirudin. However, there currently are insufficient data documenting the safety of bivalirudin for *routine* use during CAS.

Delivery of Sheath or Guide to CCA

With rare exception, carotid intervention is performed using femoral arterial access. Having achieved access, the first task is the successful delivery of a sheath or guide to the distal CCA. With currently available stent-delivery systems and balloon-dilation catheters, the inner diameter of an 8-Fr guide or 6-Fr sheath is required to allow easy delivery of required devices. Although the particular choice of the use of a guide or sheath is often determined by operator bias, there are objective advantages and disadvantages to either, which are summarized in Table 6-6.

Given the familiarity with guide catheters from coronary intervention, and an experience

TABLE 6-6

Advantages and Disadvantages of Guide and Sheath-Based Approaches to Carotid Artery Stenting Procedures

	Guide	Sheath
Advantages	• Torque control of tip allows orientation of guide with respect to the ICA • Provides superior support • More resistant to kinking in tortuous vessels or Type III arches • Easier to deliver to CCA in presence of ECA occlusion	• 6-Fr sheath adequate for carotid intervention minimizing arteriotomy size, risk of limb ischemia in patients with PVD • Smooth transition between dilator and sheath advantageous in patients with diseased CCA • Easier to deliver through CCA tortuosity
Disadvantages	• 8-Fr guide required for carotid intervention • Transition from diagnostic catheter to guide less optimal than with sheath and dilator	• Provides less support than guide • More likely to be displaced distally into CCA during intervention • No torque capability

that guides provide for greater flexibility during carotid intervention, our practice is to use a guide catheter in most cases. Guides should certainly be considered in situations where added support is required (e.g., significant tortuosity distal to ICA lesion, critical ICA stenosis). Sheaths should be favored in patients with severe peripheral vascular disease owing to the smaller arteriotomy required. They should also be considered in patients with CCA disease because the smaller outer diameter of the 6-Fr sheath, compared with an 8-Fr guide, and the smooth transition between the dilator and sheath catheter.

Standard Guide Technique

Our guide of choice is the H-1 guide (Fig. 6-10). The standard technique for delivery is (Fig. 6-11) as follows: a long (i.e., 125 cm) diagnostic catheter is advanced through a Tuohy-Borst type adaptor at the hub of the guide, such that its tip extends beyond the tip of the guide (Fig. 6-12). One should use the diagnostic catheter that successfully engaged the carotid of interest during the diagnostic angiogram (see above). Over a soft-tipped 0.035″ wire, the catheter-guide combination is delivered into the thoracic aorta. The diagnostic catheter is engaged into the ostium of the innominate or

left CCA. It is important to keep the tip of the guide approximately 6 cm to 7 cm proximal to the tip of the catheter, to enable manipulation of the catheter tip. A roadmap of the CCA is then performed at low magnification, in a view that allows clear visualization of the ICA and ECA.

Using this roadmap, a stiff-angled glide wire is then advanced through the diagnostic catheter into the ECA. In situations where the ECA has

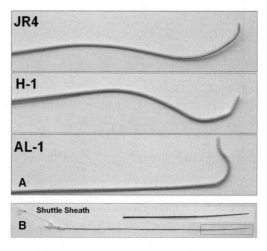

FIGURE 6-10 ● Picture of guide catheters **(A)** and shuttle sheath **(B)** used during carotid intervention.

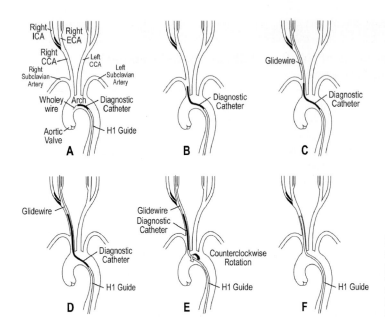

FIGURE 6-11 ● Schematic of technique used to deliver a guide to the distal common carotid artery and ICA. See text for details. ICA, internal carotid artery; ECA, external carotid artery; CCA, common carotid artery.

severe proximal disease or is occluded, or the distal CCA has significant disease, the stiff-angled glide wire should instead be positioned in the distal CCA, proximal to any disease. At this point, the diagnostic catheter is slowly advanced over the wire to the distal CCA or ECA (when patent and not significantly diseased). The guide is then carefully advanced, using slow counterclockwise rotation over the catheter-wire combination, to the distal CCA. Finally, the catheter-

wire combination is carefully removed under fluoroscopic guidance.

Modifications to the Standard Guide Technique

Modifications to the above technique will be required in a number of situations, most notably in patients with more difficult aortic arch types: a bovine origin of the left CCA, tortuosity of the innominate or CCA, and an ECA that is unavailable

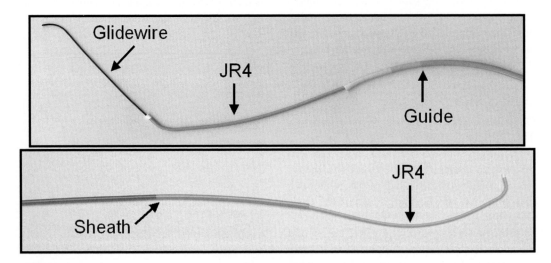

FIGURE 6-12 ● Illustration of diagnostic catheter advanced through the guide catheter and shuttle sheath, for the telescoping technique used to deliver the sheath or guide to the common carotid artery during carotid intervention. See text for details.

for use. The following section describes the most common modifications to the technique outlined above, which are divided into grades I–III in increasing order of complexity and risk.

Grade I Modification

In patients with Type III arches or severe CCA tortuosity, the support provided by the combination of the diagnostic catheter and glidewire may be inadequate to allow delivery of the guide catheter. In this situation, with the diagnostic catheter in the ECA or distal CCA, the glidewire is exchanged for a stiff Amplatz® wire with a 6-cm soft tip, and the guide advanced over the catheter-stiff Amplatz wire combination. Following delivery of the guide, the process of removal of the catheter-wire combination is carefully observed under fluoroscopy, and accomplished with slight backward tension on the guide, owing to the tendency of the guide to prolapse forward.

Grade II Modification

In patients with the complex anatomy types outlined above, the diagnostic catheter will occasionally provide inadequate support, in itself, to allow delivery of the stiff-angled glide wire into the ECA or distal CCA. In this circumstance, one may have to engage the innominate or left CCA, directly, with the guide catheter. Great care with this maneuver is required because there is an increased risk of guide-related trauma. Although an H-1 guide may occasionally be successful, in the authors' experience, typically, an AL1 guide is required in this situation (Fig. 6-10). The terminal tip of the AL1 guide is removed using a metal wire introduced into the catheter tip, and a blow heater to mold the tip. With the AL1 or H-1 guide at the origin of the innominate or left CCA, the ECA or distal CCA is wired. If the ECA is available, it is worth spending the time to advance the wire far distally into one of the major branches of the ECA (e.g., occipital) for enhanced support. The diagnostic catheter is then advanced as far as possible. At this point, it is best to exchange the glidewire for a stiff-Amplatz wire (i.e., generally, with a 6-cm soft tip) in anticipation of the extra support required to deliver the guide to the distal CCA. If an H-1 guide has been used, it may be advanced safely over the catheter-stiff wire combination. How-

ever, this maneuver should never be attempted with the AL1 guide. Owing to the shape of this guide, the risk of trauma to the CCA during such an attempt is prohibitively high. Therefore, with the catheter and stiff Amplatz wire in the ECA or distal CCA, the AL1 guide should be exchanged for an H-1 guide, which is subsequently advanced to the distal CCA.

Grade III Modification

Very rarely, the anatomic considerations outlined above may make it impossible to deliver a guide catheter into the distal CCA. If that situation exists, it may be elected to abandon the procedure or to attempt to perform the procedure with the guide (i.e., typically an AL1) positioned in the origin of the CCA or innominate artery (Fig. 6-13).

Clearly, only the most experienced operators are qualified to make this judgment and attempt such procedures. If the procedure is attempted, an extra-support 0.014″ wire (e.g., Ironman®)

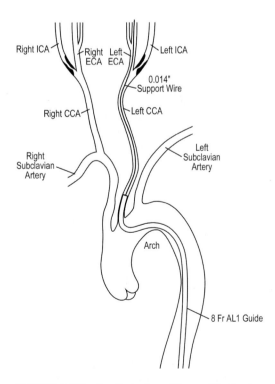

FIGURE 6-13 ● Illustration of the modification to the standard-guide technique in patients with Type III arches that do not allow delivery of a guide to the common carotid artery. See text for details.

advanced into the ECA provides the added support to facilitate delivery of equipment to the carotid bifurcation. Alternatively, if one increases the size to a 9-Fr guide, a 0.035" wire may be advanced into the ECA, for superior support. Great care needs to be exercised during these procedures, as any maneuver that tends to back the guide away from the ostium of the great vessel (e.g., stent delivery) will also tend to drag the filter or distal balloon-occlusion device proximally, potentially across the bifurcation lesion. For this reason, one should try to use a low-magnification view during critical maneuvers, keeping the guide and embolic protection device in view.

Standard Sheath Technique

The standard technique for delivery of a sheath to the distal CCA is similar to that described for guides and is as follows: (1) the dilator is removed from the 90-cm sheath; (2) a 125-cm long, diagnostic catheter is then advanced through the sheath; and is used selectively to engage the innominate or left CCA; (3) using the methodology described above, a stiff-angled glide wire is advanced through the diagnostic catheter into the ECA or distal CCA; and (4) the diagnostic catheter is then advanced over the glidewire to the ECA or distal CCA. At this point, there are two possible approaches:

1. the sheath may be directly advanced over the glidewire-catheter combination. This is the most economic approach but suffers from the potential hazard of uplifting plaque, due to the potential space between the diagnostic catheter and sheath. This approach should therefore be avoided in patients with angiographic evidence of CCA atherosclerosis.
2. the glidewire may be exchanged for a stiff Amplatz wire (6-cm soft tip), the diagnostic catheter is removed, and the sheath with its dilator is advanced over the stiff Amplatz wire into the distal CCA.

The latter is the more standard approach and is recommended for patients with more complex arterial anatomy, where extra support is required to deliver the sheath. It is important to be aware that the sheath dilator is not radiopaque and extends approximately 3 cm beyond the tip of the sheath. Fluoroscopically, its position may be in-

ferred from the straightening effect the dilator tip has on the wire. It is recommended that the tip of the dilator not extend beyond the distal target for the sheath. Thus, when the tip of the sheath reaches the mid-CCA, the dilator is detached from the sheath, and the sheath is advanced, independently, over the dilator for the last 3 cm of its course in the distal CCA.

Based on this discussion, it should be clear that the use of a guide, compared to a sheath, allows for a much greater variety of strategies toward achieving the goal of delivery to the distal CCA. This is not an issue in patients with straight-forward vascular anatomy, but becomes a very real consideration in patients with more complicated anatomy. The recommendation is that all operators should become facile with both techniques.

Emboli Protection Devices

Having secured delivery of a sheath or guide to the distal CCA, the next task during carotid intervention is to place an embolic protection device, to prevent or limit distal embolization during the angioplasty and stenting portion of the procedure. A variety of emboli protection devices are available, and are summarized in the following section.

Filter-Type EPDs

Filter-type EPDs are the most popular and user-friendly of the carotid EPDs and have the largest body of data to support their use in carotid intervention (Table 6-7, Fig. 6-14).

In design, these devices most commonly contain a polyurethane membrane with pores of fixed size—ranging from 80μm to 140μm between devices—which is supported by a nitinol frame. The filter is integrated with a 0.014" guidewire with a 3-cm to 4-cm malleable floppy tip. During the carotid intervention, the filter is delivered in a collapsed form across the carotid lesion on the attached guidewire. Ideally, the filter is positioned and deployed in the cervical portion of the ICA, just proximal to the petrous section of the vessel, where the ICA typically is straight and free of disease (Fig. 6-15).

Tortuosity or disease in the cervical portion of the ICA may require an alternate placement, but the filter must always be positioned at least

TABLE 6-7

Summary of Filter-Type Embolic Protection Devices Used During Carotid Intervention

Filter	Manufacturer	Diameters	Pore Size	Filter and Guidewire Integrated	Filter Type
Interceptor®	Medtronic, Minneapolis, MN	4.5, 5.5, 6.5	100 μm	Yes	Supported
Rubicon®	Rubicon Medical Corp., Salt Lake, Utah	4, 5, 6	100 μm	Yes	Supported
FilterWire® EX FilterWire® EZ	Boston Scientific, Natick, MA	3.5–5.5	80 μm 110 μm	Yes	Unsupported
Angioguard® XP Angioguard® RX	Cordis, Warren, NJ	4, 5, 6, 7, 8	100 μm	Yes	Supported
NeuroShield®/ EmboShield®	Abbott Laboratories, Abbott Park, IL	3, 4, 5, 6	140 μm	No	Supported
Spider®	ev3, Plymouth, MN	3, 4, 5, 6, 7	50–200 μm	Yes	Supported
Accunet® OTW Accunet® RX	Guidant, Indianapolis, IN	4.5, 5.5, 6.5, 7.5	120 μm	Yes	Supported

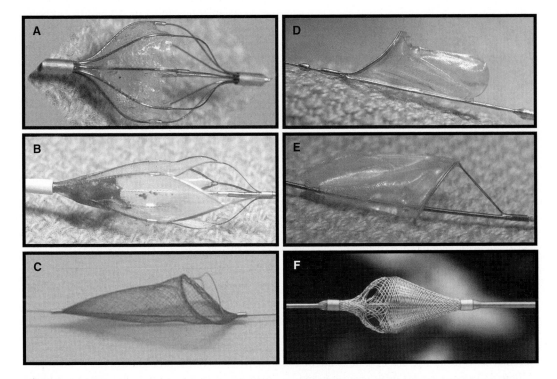

FIGURE 6-14 ● **Examples of filter-type embolic protection devices used during carotid intervention.** **A:** Angioguard® XP (Cordis, Warren, NJ). **B:** Accunet® (Guidant Corporation, Santa Clara, CA). **C:** Spider® (ev3, Plymouth, MN). **D:** FilterWire EX® (Boston Scientific, Natick, MA). **E:** FilterWire EZ® (Boston Scientific, Natick, MA). **F:** Interceptor® (Medtronic, Minneapolis, MN).

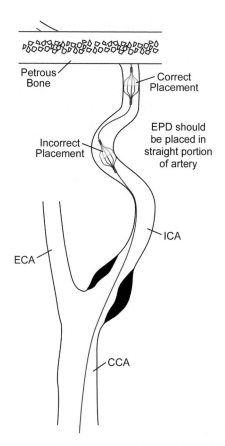

Petrous
Bone

Correct
Placement

EPD should
be placed in
straight portion
of artery

Incorrect
Placement

ICA

ECA

CCA

FIGURE 6-15 ● Schematic of internal carotid artery demonstrating correct placement of filter-type embolic protection device.

approximately 2 cm distal to the bifurcation lesion, to allow delivery of the interventional equipment.

Delivery of the filter through tortuosity distal to the ICA lesion is sometimes impossible (Fig. 6-16). There are defined maneuvers that may be used to overcome this problem, but should only be employed by experienced operators. Initially, a soft-tipped, 0.014″, low-support wire (e.g., Balance Trek®) is advanced through the lesion and positioned in the petrous portion of the ICA. Occasionally, this wire may provide a sufficient straightening effect on the cervical ICA to allow delivery of the filter. If this fails, a coronary over-the-wire balloon is then advanced over this wire to its tip, and a further attempt at filter delivery is made, using the wire-and-balloon combination to provide support and a straightening effect. If this fails, the final maneuver is to exchange the low-support wire for a soft-

tipped, heavy-support wire (e.g., Ironman). This wire will usually provide sufficient support and straightening effect, alone, without the balloon. Excessive straightening of the cervical ICA may be problematic, as it may produce severe kinking of the vessel that both interferes with antegrade flow and makes delivery of the filter more difficult. Once the filter has been successfully delivered, it is important to remember to bring the support wire proximal to the filter, so that it does not compromise the apposition of the filter with the wall of the vessel.

The major advantage of filter-type EPDs is that they allow continued antegrade flow during carotid intervention, an important consideration for patients with compromised collateral flow to the ipsilateral carotid territory (e.g., patients with contralateral carotid disease or occlusion). Although the crossing profile of these EPDs is slightly greater than distal balloon-occlusion devices, in the authors' experience, predilation of the carotid lesion to facilitate delivery of the filter is required in less than 5% of cases. Finally, it is important to emphasize that filter-type EPDs serve as embolic-limitation devices that prevent embolization of particles greater than approximately 80 μm to 100μm in diameter, while allowing particles of smaller diameter to pass through.

Distal Occlusion Balloon EPDs

This is the second most popular type of EPD used in carotid intervention and was the first EPD used during a carotid intervention (circa 1998). There is currently only one example of this EPD type available: the GuardWire®. In essence, this device contains a compliant balloon that is inflated and deflated through a hollow, nitinol hypotube, located in a 0.014″ angioplasty-style wire. The GuardWire is advanced in its deflated state across the carotid lesion. A marker indicating the position of the balloon is placed in the same location in the prepetrous portion of the cervical ICA, as would a filter-type device. The balloon is then inflated, producing complete cessation of antegrade flow. Following the angioplasty and stenting portions of the procedure, a monorail-export catheter is used to aspirate the column of blood proximal to the filter, thus removing any debris that may have embolized from the carotid plaque. The balloon is then deflated and the GuardWire

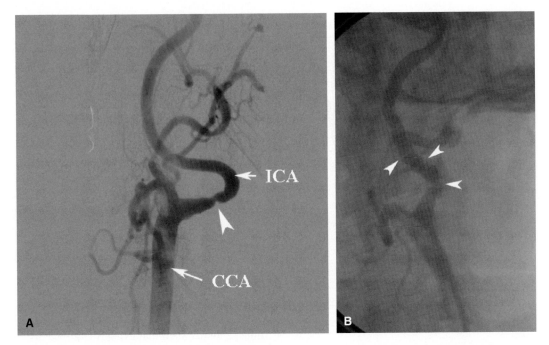

FIGURE 6-16 ● **A:** Common carotid-artery angiogram from a patient with severe tortuosity distal to a focal internal carotid artery lesion (arrowhead) that would not allow delivery of the filter device. **B:** Angiogram following placement of a stiff Ironman® wire in the internal carotid artery, demonstrating the straightening effect on the artery. Also note the kinking (arrowheads) in the artery created by the wire.

removed. The GuardWire has a lower crossing profile, compared to filter-type EPDs. In theory, this type of EPD should serve as a true embolic prevention device, by removing all embolized debris regardless of particle size. In practice, the device functions more as an embolic-limitation device. Its major limitation is that complete cessation of antegrade ICA flow may be poorly tolerated in patients with compromised collateral flow to the anterior cerebral circulation.

Proximal-Occlusion Devices

Proximal-occlusion devices are the most recent group of EPDs developed for carotid intervention. Two examples of such devices currently exist: The Parodi® Anti-embolism System and MO.MA® system (Fig. 6-17).

These devices function by generating retrograde flow in the ICA, which theoretically should protect the brain from distal embolization during the intervention. This is achieved by inflating compliant balloons in the distal CCA and ECA, which interrupts antegrade carotid flow, and allows retrograde flow along the ICA from the circle of Willis. The lumen of the catheter whose tip is in the CCA, and distal to the occlusive balloon, is connected through a blood-return system to the femoral vein. This provides a gradient for flow between the ICA and the femoral vein, ensuring continued retrograde ICA flow.

These devices are cumbersome and technically challenging to use, and are unlikely to rival the filter-type EPDs in selection for use. In their current iteration, the catheter sizes are larger than for other types of EPDs. In addition, they require an adequate collateral circulation in the Circle of Willis to ensure retrograde flow along the ICA. These devices may find particular use for patients in whom tortuosity or disease distal to the carotid-bifurcation lesion prevents the use of other EPDs. It should be stressed that the use of proximal-occlusion type EPDs is, currently, strictly investigational.

Angioplasty and Stenting (Fig. 6-18)

Balloon Predilation

Following placement of the EPD, it may be necessary to dilate the carotid bifurcation lesion in approximately 75% of cases, prior to stenting.

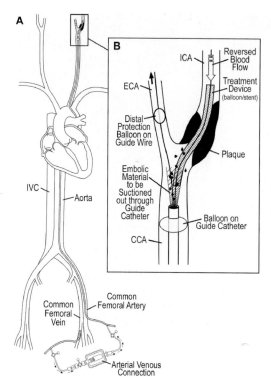

FIGURE 6-17 ● **Illustration of proximal balloon-occlusion type embolic protection device.** Occlusion of the common (CCA) and external carotid (ECA) arteries blocks antegrade flow in the internal carotid artery (ICA). The connection between the catheter placed in the CCA and the common femoral vein creates a gradient for retrograde flow along the ICA, providing embolic protection during the procedure.

The primary purpose of predilation is to ensure the subsequent delivery of the stent. In general, the greater the degree of lesion calcification and severity of stenosis, the more likely that predilation will be necessary, to allow successful stent delivery. Predilation also serves several useful secondary functions: (1) it provides a rough assessment of the length of the lesion, and diameters of the ICA and CCA, which influences the choice of stent; (2) the hemodynamic response to predilation provides some insight into the likely hemodynamic consequences of stent deployment and postdilation, enabling the operator to take appropriate prophylactic measures (e.g., the administration of intravenous atropine or more aggressive fluid management); and finally (3) the ease with which balloon predilation achieves its nominal diameter gives some assessment of the rigidity of the plaque.

Predilation is generally performed using a 4.0-mm diameter coronary balloon (e.g., Maverick®). Balloon lengths for predilation are also conservative, with a targeted balloon: lesion length of approximately 1:1. The balloon is inflated to nominal pressure for 10 to 15 seconds.

Stent Deployment

Following predilation, carotid-bifurcation lesions are stented using a variety of self-expanding nitinol stents. These stents are available in cylindrical and tapered shapes (Fig. 6-19).

The lengths and diameters typically employed in the carotid location vary from 20 mm to 40 mm and from 5 mm to 10 mm, respectively. In addition to the lesion length and vessel diameter, the most important determinant of stent length and diameter is lesion location (Fig. 6-20).

The majority of carotid-bifurcation lesions involve the ostium of the ICA, and in such situations, a longer stent that extends from the distal CCA into the ICA should be chosen. In this circumstance, assuming a cylindrical stent is the only stent available, the stent diameter chosen should match the estimated diameter of the distal CCA. With tapered stents, which are ideally suited for this purpose, the larger diameter of the taper should match the CCA diameter, and the smaller diameter of the taper should match the ICA diameter.

For lesions that are truly confined to the ICA, a cylindrical stent confined to the ICA is entirely appropriate, and the stent diameter may match the ICA diameter. It should be stressed that self-expanding stents appose the arterial wall less well than balloon-expandable stents. For this reason, the authors generally add 1 mm to the estimated vessel diameter size, to arrive at the stent diameter to be used.

Stent placement using balloon-expandable stents is less precise than with balloon-expandable stents. There is often a tendency for self-expanding stents to move forward during deployment. Pulling back on the stent to the correct position, prior to deployment, will minimize this phenomenon. In addition, the initial phase of deployment should be done slowly and carefully, as one may continue to adjust the stent position up until the deployment of the first few stent cells. One should be aware that once any of the cells are deployed, the stent should not be pushed forward,

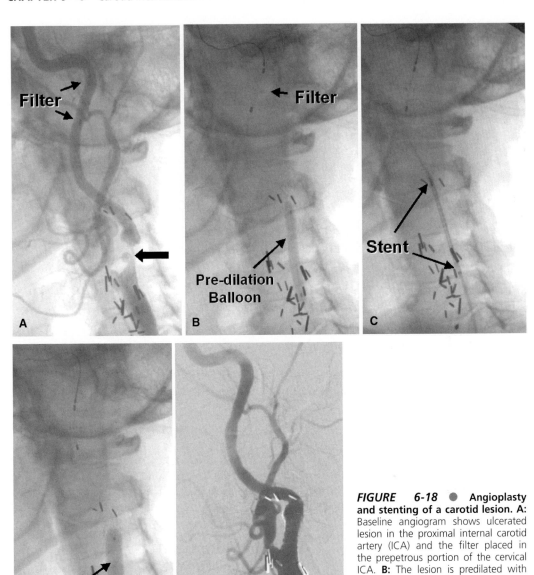

FIGURE 6-18 ● **Angioplasty and stenting of a carotid lesion. A:** Baseline angiogram shows ulcerated lesion in the proximal internal carotid artery (ICA) and the filter placed in the prepetrous portion of the cervical ICA. **B:** The lesion is predilated with a 4.0 × 30-mm balloon. **C:** An 8.0 × 30-mm stent is placed across the lesion, extending into the common carotid artery. **D:** Postdilation with a 5.5. × 30-mm balloon. **E:** Final angiogram following removal of filter.

but typically may be pulled backwards, provided only a few cells have been deployed. When positioning the stent, one should avoid allowing the proximal margin of the stent to straddle the distal CCA, as this may complicate retrieval of filter-type EPDs by impeding delivery of the retrieval sheath (Fig. 6-21). It may also impede delivery of the export catheter when using a distal balloon-occlusion EPD.

Postdilation

Most operators dilate the stent following deployment, using 5.0-mm to 6.0-mm diameter balloons (e.g., Viatrec®) inflated to nominal pressure for 10 to 15 seconds. Generally, the balloon length should be shorter than the stent length, to minimize the risk of dissection caused by angioplasty beyond the limits of the stent. In contrast to coronary intervention, mild residual stenosis (i.e.,

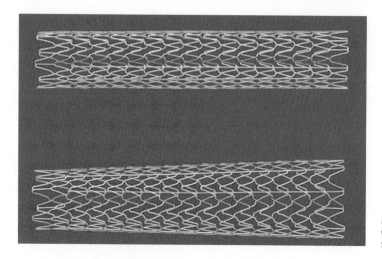

FIGURE 6-19 ● Cylindrical (upper) and tapered (lower) nitinol self-expanding carotid stents.

up to 20%) is generally tolerated during carotid stenting, owing to the low risk of restenosis.

In heavily calcified lesions that do not expand well in response to stenting, resulting in a larger residual stenosis, one needs to be wary against overaggressive postdilation of the stent. This may produce a tear in the media or adventitia of the vessel, which typically results in a contained-vessel perforation. The authors advocate a conservative approach to balloon postdilation in symptomatic patients and patients with soft plaque; the reasoning is that aggressive postdilation in these situations increases the likelihood of excessive extrusion of plaque elements, which increases the risk for distal embolization. In these situations, if an adequate angiographic

result is achieved with stenting alone, one may elect to avoid postdilation altogether.

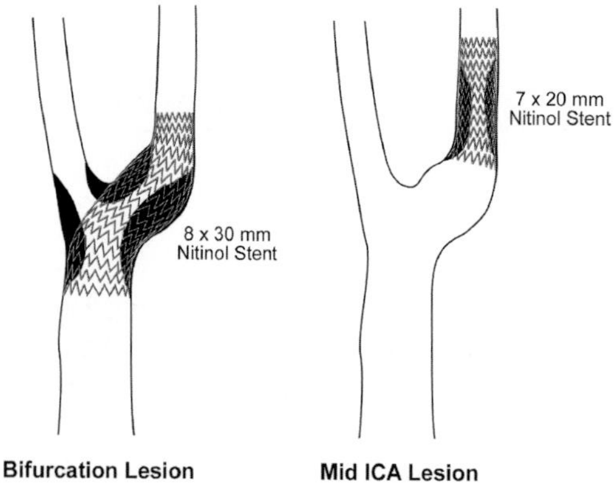

Removal of EPD and Final Angiography

Following the angioplasty and stenting portion of the procedure, the EPD is removed. Careful angiography of the lesion site and ipsilateral anterior-cerebral circulation is performed. The authors also suggest performing angiography of the ipsilateral CCA, to document the absence of trauma to the CCA from delivery of the sheath or guide.

MANAGEMENT OF COMPLICATIONS OF CAROTID INTERVENTION

Hemodynamic Complications

Hypotension and Bradycardia

Angioplasty and stenting in the region of the carotid sinus results in stretching of mechanoreceptors at this location. This generates afferent impulses in the glossopharyngeal nerve (i.e., CN IX) that activate the vasomotor center in the medulla. The efferent output from this area activates the vagus nerve (i.e., CN X) and reticulospinal tract, resulting in peripheral vasodilation, and a reduction in heart rate and contractility of the heart (Fig. 6-22).

This mechanism underlies the combination of transient hypotension and bradycardia that is

7 x 20 mm Nitinol Stent

8 x 30 mm Nitinol Stent

Bifurcation Lesion   Mid ICA Lesion

FIGURE 6-20 ● Schematic of internal carotid artery, demonstrating appropriate stent placement, sizing, and length, based on lesion location.

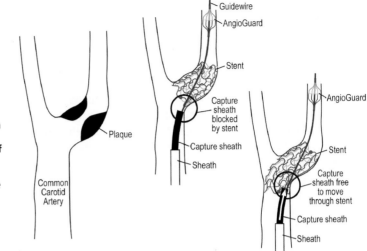

FIGURE 6-21 ● **Illustration of the problem created by placing a stent at the ostium of the internal carotid artery.** The stent struts, inferiorly, may interfere with advancement of the filter retrieval sheath **(middle panel).** By placing the proximal portion of the stent in the distal common carotid artery, this problem is overcome **(right panel).**

frequently observed (i.e., approximately 40%) during CAS and during the postprocedural period (11–15). It also explains why hypotension and bradycardia are most commonly seen during the treatment of bifurcation lesions involving the ICA ostium, as opposed to procedures on isolated ICA lesions. The effect is seen for seconds to minutes following predilation, stent placement, and postdilation. Since postdilation typically produces the maximal stretch on the carotid sinus, the maximal effect is usually seen at this point in time. More modest effects may be seen up to 24 to 48 hours following the procedure.

Some operators routinely administer atropine prior to the angioplasty and stenting portion of the procedure, in an effort to prevent procedure-related hypotension and bradycardia. In the au-

thors' experience, this is unnecessary. Indeed, routine administration of atropine may increase procedure-related morbidity, since in elderly patients, atropine is associated with significant side effects, including urinary retention, confusion, and severe dry mouth. In patients with critical coronary artery disease, the tachycardia induced by atropine may precipitate coronary ischemia. It is preferable to administer prophylactic atropine only in select situations, including: (1) in patients with exaggerated hypotensive or bradycardia response to predilation or stent deployment, and (2) in patients with critical aortic stenosis. In the latter situation, even brief episodes of hypotension and bradycardia may be poorly tolerated and result in hemodynamic collapse. Using this approach,

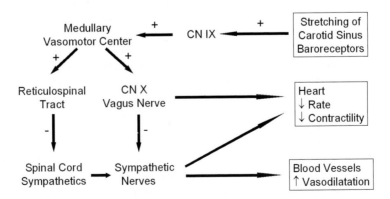

FIGURE 6-22 ● Diagrammatic representation of the effect of activation of mechanoreceptors in the carotid sinus, during carotid intervention.

atropine is administered in approximately 5% of the cases seen by the authors.

Procedure-related hypotension is certainly mitigated by aggressive, preprocedural hydration. All patients commence receiving intravenous fluids 2 to 3 hours prior to the procedure, which are continued during the procedure (i.e., at approximately 200 mL per hour). Intraprocedurally, the first line of therapy for hypotension is similarly aggressive intravenous hydration. If the patient becomes symptomatic, or if severe asymptomatic hypotension develops (i.e., systolic blood pressure [SBP] lower than 75 mmHg), intravenous dopamine is commenced (i.e., at the rate of 5μcg/Kg) and titrated to achieve a SBP higher than 90 mmHg, or to alleviate symptoms.

Hypotension in the postprocedural period should always be carefully evaluated. Typically, hypotension caused by stretch from the carotid stent will first manifest during the procedure and persist into the postprocedural period. It is important to remember to withhold all blood pressure medications, and aggressively hydrate the patient with intravenous fluids. For asymptomatic patients with severe hypotension, we use oral pseudoephedrine, 60-mg tablet every 4 hours. If the patient becomes symptomatic, intravenous dopamine should be given and titrated to achieve an asymptomatic status. When administering these sympathomimetic agents, one should be aware of the risk of inducing coronary ischemia, since 50 to 60% of patients with carotid artery disease will have significant coronary artery disease. Bradycardia postintervention rarely, if ever, requires intervention, other than to modify the dose of AV-nodal antagonist agents.

Hypertension

Hypertension is a frequent finding during, and following, carotid artery stenting. Most commonly, it reflects a persistence of the patients' baseline condition (14). Although acute hypertension caused by carotid endarterectomy has been described, and attributed to transient dysfunction of adventitial baroreceptors at the endarterectomy site (16), there is no report of evidence that this phenomenon occurs with carotid intervention.

The importance of periprocedural hypertension is emphasized by the strong association between hypertension and hyperperfusion to the ipsilateral cerebral hemisphere (17). This complication was first described in patients undergoing carotid endarterectomy. Mechanistically, it is explained as follows: (a) the presence of a critical carotid stenosis compromises cerebral blood flow; (b) compensatory dilation of the cerebral vessels occurs in an attempt to maintain the baseline flow;(18) (c) chronic dilation of the vessels results in a loss of their normal vasomotor response (i.e., their ability to vasoconstrict and limit cerebral flow); and (d) the sudden removal of carotid stenosis by carotid-artery stenting restores carotid flow, and in the presence of dilation of the cerebral vessels, there is hyperperfusion to the brain.

Retrospective registry data suggest an incidence of hyperperfusion following carotid artery stenting of between 1% and 5% (17). Based on the carotid endarterectomy experience and limited carotid-intervention data, it appears that hypertension in conjunction with the treatment of a critical, ipsilateral carotid stenosis (i.e., of greater than 90%), and the presence of a contralateral stenosis (i.e., of more than 80%), or occlusion, predicts the group at highest risk for this complication (19). Clinically, patients complain of a headache that lateralizes to the side of the intervention. The headache has a throbbing quality and may be located in the facial, temporal, or retro-orbital regions. Nausea, vomiting, focal neurologic deficits, or seizures often accompany the headache.

The absence of abnormal findings on CT of the head, and increased flow velocities in the ipsilateral middle cerebral artery, as assessed by transcranial Doppler, provide supportive evidence for the diagnosis of hyperperfusion (20). Prompt diagnosis and emergent management are the keys to a successful outcome from this complication. Aggressive treatment with intravenous antihypertensive medication is mandatory. In the authors' practice, the preferred agents are beta-blockers (beta antagonists), owing to the risk of associated coronary artery disease in 'high-risk' patients and the neutral effect of beta-blockers on cerebral blood flow. Intravenous nitroglycerin is also used, although the development of a 'nitrate headache' may confuse the clinical picture, occasionally.

Following the acute control of hypertension, aggressive reinstitution of the patient's baseline oral, antihypertensive regimen is also important. If neurologic symptoms are prominent, typically, the patient's routine postprocedural aspirin and clopidogrel therapy are held until the neurologic symptoms resolve and the blood pressure is controlled. This is because the most feared complication of the hyperperfusion syndrome is cerebral hemorrhage (17,21–24). This diagnosis carries a very high mortality rate (i.e., approximately 30 to 80%), and among those who survive, 20 to 40% have significant residual neurologic dysfunction (25). In the single institution registry of 450 carotid interventions administered by the authors, intracranial hemorrhage occurred in three of the five patients with hyperperfusion syndrome (i.e., 0.67%). Although this frequency is low, the morbidity and mortality associated with the condition underscores the importance of meticulous attention to hypertension management, and the necessity for early recognition and appropriate management of hyperperfusion syndrome.

Stroke

Stroke is the major feared complication of carotid artery stenting. In the high-risk carotid-stent registries to date, the 30-day incidence of stroke with CAS is approximately 3%, (26,27) which compares favorably to the rate of 3.3% in the CEA arm of the SAPPHIRE trial (3). One may not use the stroke rates reported from the CEA trials of the 1990s for comparison, however, as the patient populations were different. It is encouraging that the majority of strokes following CAS are classified as minor (i.e., resolution within 30 days, or NIH Stroke Scale 3 or less).

Distal embolization of extruded atherosclerotic debris, during angioplasty and CAS, is a universal finding in carotid intervention and is clearly the dominant mechanism of procedure-related stroke. However, it is important to be aware of other potential etiologies, most notably, the manipulation of wires, catheters, and guides in the aortic arch and common carotid artery. These manipulations are not protected by an EPD. Distal embolization of debris, at the time of these manipulations, should certainly be implicated as the likely mechanism in patients who experience strokes outside of the territory of the treated carotid artery (i.e., posterior or contralateral anterior circulation stroke) (28). This phe-

nomenon also explains why even an EPD that functions perfectly may not be expected to reduce the risk of stroke during CAS to zero.

If a neurologic deficit occurs during the carotid procedure, cerebral angiography should be performed, as further management is largely dictated by these angiographic findings. In the presence of a normal angiogram, the clinical outcome in these patients is predictably excellent, and they should be managed conservatively. If a large artery (i.e., 2-mm to 2.5-mm diameter, or greater) occlusion that is the result of distal embolization is identified, it is reasonable for a suitably qualified interventionalist to attempt recanalization, using a combination of mechanical (i.e., angioplasty) and pharmacologic (i.e., thrombolytic, glycoprotein IIb/IIIa) therapies (Fig. 6-23).

Unfortunately, there are no guidelines for the dosing of thrombolytics or glycoprotein IIb/IIIa agents in this situation. Empirically, we have administered a dose of 0.125 mg/kg of abciximab, alone or in combination with 5 mg to 20 mg of tissue plasminogen activator (tPA), given

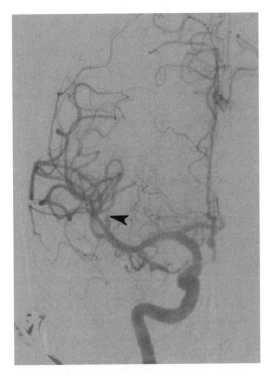

FIGURE 6-23 ● Example of distal embolization to a major branch of the M-2 segment of the right middle-cerebral artery (arrowhead) in a patient, following carotid stenting.

intra-arterially in divided doses at the site of the occlusion. Unfortunately, the efficacy of these maneuvers is unpredictable, which is likely explained by the fact that these emboli are composed of atheromatous debris and generally do not respond to conventional intervention techniques (29). Occlusions of smaller branch vessels (i.e., those of less than 2-mm diameter) are probably best managed noninvasively. If the patient has a significant neurologic deficit, a bolus and infusion of an intravenous glycoprotein IIb/IIIa inhibitor through a peripheral IV system may be administered in an effort to minimize the infarct size.

Strokes beyond the immediate periprocedural period (i.e., but within the first 2 weeks following carotid intervention) are rare, and are typically minor in severity (5). The mechanism of these strokes is unclear. Manipulation of atheroma in the aortic arch or CCA may result in delayed embolization of plaque elements or of platelet thrombi that form on the surface the traumatized atheroma. The stent surface may also serve as a focus for platelet thrombi formation and embolization, and delayed extrusion of plaque elements through the interstices of the stent may also occur. If a patient presents with a delayed stroke following carotid intervention, the first priority should be to rule out an intracranial hemorrhage. In the absence of hemorrhage, management is typically conservative.

Adverse Cardiac Events

The frequency of myocardial infarction in high-risk patients in the 30 days following CAS is ~2% in most series (27,30). Of these, the majority are non-Q wave in type. In the randomized cohort of the SAPPHIRE trial, the 30-day incidence of myocardial infarction in the stent arm was 1.9%, compared to 6.6% in the CEA arm. This difference was statistically significant and suggests a major advantage of CAS over CEA in patients with significant coronary artery disease (30).

Despite these data, caution is recommended in the use of CAS in the subset of patients with critical coronary or cardiac disease awaiting open-heart surgery. This is an extremely high-risk patient subset, with a significant risk of mortality during the typical 3- to 4-week waiting period between CAS and open-heart surgery. Previously,

the authors' strategy in this group was to perform carotid intervention using stents. The patient received a minimum of 4 weeks of antiplatelet therapy with aspirin and clopidogrel, followed approximately 5 to 7 days later by open-heart surgery. Using this strategy, the anecdotal experience had been an excess of cardiac mortality in this patient cohort during this waiting period. As a result, the strategy has been revised significantly. Now, the use of stents during the carotid intervention is avoided, and carotid angioplasty is performed alone, using cutting balloons to minimize the risk of dissection.

The goal of therapy is to achieve normal carotid flow, and a moderate residual stenosis is tolerated. Antiplatelet therapy consists of aspirin and one of the short-acting, small-molecule, intravenous GP IIb/IIIa inhibitors. Following the procedure, the patient proceeds within the next 1 to 2 days to open-heart surgery, stopping the glycoprotein IIb/IIIa inhibitor 4 to 6 hours prior to surgery. Postoperatively, the patient receives aspirin therapy, and clopidogrel is added within 48 hours. At 6 to 8 weeks, a carotid ultrasound is performed, and if needed a carotid stent may be placed in an elective procedure, using routine antiplatelet and anticoagulant pharmacotherapy.

Slow-Flow

Delayed antegrade flow in the ICA is frequently observed during CAS procedures using filter-type EPDs, and is referred to as slow-flow. This phenomenon is likely explained by excessive distal embolization of plaque elements that block the pores of the filter and thus interfere with antegrade flow through the filter (Fig. 6-24).

The phenomenon is most commonly observed following postdilation of the stent (i.e., approximately 75%) and stent deployment (i.e., about 25%). Angiographically, the spectrum of slow-flow may vary from mild delay to complete cessation of antegrade flow.

In an analysis of some 420 patients from the carotid intervention registry at our institution, slow-flow occurred in approximately 10% of patients. Symptomatic status (i.e., stroke or transient ischemic attack within the last 6 months), increased patient age, and larger stent sizes were independently associated with this event. Comparing patients who experienced slow-flow

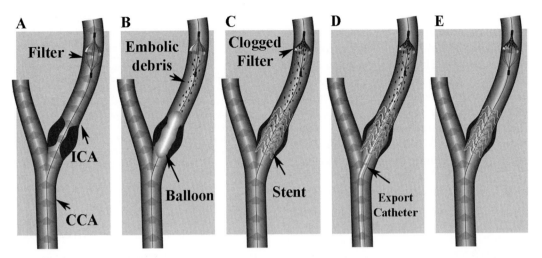

FIGURE 6-24 ● **Schematic of proposed mechanism of slow-flow and rationale for aspiration. A:** Carotid bifurcation lesion with filter placed distally. **B:** and **C:** Balloon angioplasty and stenting results in embolization of debris from atherosclerotic plaque, toward filter, causing occlusion of filter pores and accumulation of debris in column of blood proximal to the filter. **D:** and **E:** Aspiration proximal to filter removes debris from column of blood without affecting debris causing occlusion of filter.

to those with normal flow, there was a significantly increased risk of periprocedural stroke in the slow-flow group (i.e., 9.5% versus 1.7%), although the majority of these were minor. The mechanism of this increased stroke risk is debatable. The belief is that it results from the accumulation of embolized debris in the column of blood, proximal to the filter, under the conditions of slow-flow (i.e., when the filter pores are blocked). For this reason, it is generally recommended to aspirate the column of blood proximal to the filter when slow-flow is observed. This is achieved using the export catheter of the Percusurge® system. The export catheter is advanced over the filter wire to the level of the filter. It is then withdrawn toward the stent and approximately 20cc of blood is aspirated. This process is repeated three to four times. This aspiration does not affect the angiographic appearance of flow since the filter remains obstructed with debris. Failure to aspirate however, exposes the patient to a potentially large burden of embolized debris at the time of filter retrieval. Filter retrieval universally restores normal antegrade flow.

Post-Procedural Care and Follow-Up Monitoring

At our center, patients are admitted overnight, to a step-down telemetry care unit and typically, are discharged the following day. The major management issue following intervention is blood pressure. Nursing and medical staff should be keenly aware of the importance of this fact, and respond appropriately to both hypotension and hypertension. Particular attention should be paid to the reintroduction and titration of blood pressure medications. This process requires a significant investment of time, involving making arrangements for twice-daily blood pressure measurements and daily contact between the patient and health-care professional until a stable blood pressure state has been reached. A stable state is usually reached about 1 week following the procedure, but for some patients, it may take longer.

Secondary risk-factor modification is also mandatory. All patients should receive life-long aspirin therapy unless contraindicated, and clopidogrel therapy is recommended for a minimum of 4 weeks following the procedure. There are currently no data to support more prolonged use of clopidogrel in patients with carotid disease, but future trials (e.g., CHARISMA) may help answer this question. It is also reasonable to treat all patients with a statin drug.

Long-term follow-up evaluation of patients involves monitoring for evidence of restenosis or progression of disease in the contralateral carotid artery. Fortunately, CAS is associated with a low rate of restenosis (i.e., 2 to 5%). The target-lesion revascularization rate at 1 year in the CAS arm of the randomized SAPPHIRE cohort was 0.7%. Ipsilateral stroke or TIA beyond the initial 2 weeks following CAS are extremely rare. These data certainly underscore the long-term durability and efficacy of the procedure. There is no consensus regarding the management of severe restenosis following CAS. The risk of stroke from restenosis is poorly defined, but is suggested to be low (31). The authors adopt an aggressive approach to the treatment of high-grade restenosis (i.e., greater than 80%). In the past, angioplasty and brachytherapy using γ radiation was the most commonly employed treatment strategy (30). Unfortunately, γ-brachytherapy systems for vascular treatment are no longer available. In the absence of this therapy, angioplasty alone, with peripheral cutting balloons is a reasonable percutaneous option.

CONCLUSIONS

Carotid intervention using carotid stents and EPDs is finally a reality, and over the next decade is likely to replace CEA as the revascularization strategy-of-choice for management of all patients with CAD. The technique has many technical challenges, and requires a thorough knowledge of the anatomy, vascular biology, and pathology of the cerebrovascular system. In addition, these procedures are associated with a number of well recognized complications that require careful management by a multidisciplinary team of endovascular specialists, cardiologists, internists, and neurologists.

REFERENCES

1. Brown MM. Carotid artery stenting—evolution of a technique to rival carotid endarterectomy. *Am J Med.* 2004;116:273–275.
2. Ouriel K, Yadav JS. The role of stents in patients with carotid disease. *Rev Cardiovasc Med.* 2003;4:61–67.
3. Yadav JS. Stenting and angioplasty with protection in patients at high risk for endarterectomy: 30-day results. In: *The American Heart Association Scientific Sessions.* Chicago, IL;2002.
4. Yadav JS. Stenting and angioplasty with protection in patients at high risk for endarterectomy: 1-year results. In: *Transcatheter Cardiovascular Therapeutics Meeting.* Washington DC;2003.
5. Endovascular versus surgical treatment in patients with carotid stenosis in the Carotid and Vertebral Artery Transluminal Angioplasty Study (CAVATAS): a randomised trial. *Lancet.* 2001;357:1729–1737.
6. Featherstone RL, Brown MM, Coward LJ. International carotid stenting study: protocol for a randomised clinical trial comparing carotid stenting with endarterectomy in symptomatic carotid artery stenosis. *Cerebrovasc Dis.* 2004;18:69–74.
7. Endarterectomy vs. Angioplasty in Patients with Symptomatic Severe Carotid Stenosis (EVA-3S) Trial. *Cerebrovasc Dis.* 2004;18:62–65.
8. Ringleb PA, Kunze A, Allenberg JR, et al. The Stent-Supported Percutaneous Angioplasty of the Carotid Artery vs. Endarterectomy Trial. *Cerebrovasc Dis.* 2004; 18:66–68.
9. Hobson RW II. Update on the Carotid Revascularization Endarterectomy versus Stent Trial (CREST) protocol. *J Am Coll Surg.* 2002;194:S9–S14.
10. Hobson RW II. Rationale and status of randomized controlled clinical trials in carotid artery stenting. *Semin Vasc Surg.* 2003;16:311–316.
11. Bush RL, Lin PH, Bianco CC, et al. Reevaluation of temporary transvenous cardiac pacemaker usage during carotid angioplasty and stenting: a safe and valuable adjunct. *Vasc Endovascular Surg.* 2004;38:229–235.
12. Mlekusch W, Schillinger M, Sabeti S, et al. Hypotension and bradycardia after elective carotid stenting: frequency and risk factors. *J Endovasc Ther.* 2003;10:851–859; discussion 860–861.
13. Mendelsohn FO, Weissman NJ, Lederman RJ, et al. Acute hemodynamic changes during carotid artery stenting. *Am J Cardiol.* 1998;82:1077–1081.
14. Qureshi AI, Luft AR, Sharma M, et al. Frequency and determinants of postprocedural hemodynamic instability after carotid angioplasty and stenting. *Stroke.* 1999;30:2086–2093.
15. Leisch F, Kerschner K, Hofmann R, et al. Carotid sinus reactions during carotid artery stenting: predictors, incidence, and influence on clinical outcome. *Catheter Cardiovasc Interv.* 2003;58:516–523.
16. Bove EL, Fry WJ, Gross WS, et al. Hypotension and hypertension as consequences of baroreceptor dysfunction following carotid endarterectomy. *Surgery.* 1979;85:633–637.
17. Abou-Chebl A, Yadav JS, Reginelli JP, et al. Intracranial hemorrhage and hyperperfusion syndrome following carotid artery stenting: risk factors, prevention, and treatment. *J Am Coll Cardiol.* 2004;43:1596–1601.
18. Sundt TM, Jr., Sharbrough FW, Piepgras DG, et al. Correlation of cerebral blood flow and electroencephalographic changes during carotid endarterectomy: with results of surgery and hemodynamics of cerebral ischemia. *Mayo Clin Proc.* 1981;56:533–543.
19. Sbarigia E, Speziale F, Giannoni MF, et al. Postcarotid endarterectomy hyperperfusion syndrome: preliminary observations for identifying at risk patients by transcranial Doppler sonography and the acetazolamide test. *Eur J Vasc Surg.* 1993;7:252–256.
20. Jansen C, Sprengers AM, Moll FL, et al. Prediction of intracerebral haemorrhage after carotid endarterectomy by clinical criteria and intraoperative transcranial Doppler monitoring: results of 233 operations. *Eur J Vasc Surg.* 1994;8:220–225.
21. McCabe DJ, Brown MM, Clifton A. Fatal cerebral reperfusion hemorrhage after carotid stenting. *Stroke.* 1999;30:2483–2486.
22. Morrish W, Grahovac S, Douen A, et al. Intracranial hemorrhage after stenting and angioplasty of

extracranial carotid stenosis. *AJNR Am J Neuroradiol.* 2000;21:1911–1916.

23. Al-Mubarak N, Roubin GS, Vitek JJ, et al. Subarachnoidal hemorrhage following carotid stenting with the distal-balloon protection. *Catheter Cardiovasc Interv.* 2001;54:521–523.

24. Caplan LR, Skillman J, Ojemann R, et al. Intracerebral hemorrhage following carotid endarterectomy: a hypertensive complication? *Stroke.* 1978;9:457–460.

25. Cheung RT, Eliasziw M, Meldrum HE, et al. Risk, types, and severity of intracranial hemorrhage in patients with symptomatic carotid artery stenosis. *Stroke.* 2003;34:1847–1851.

26. Wholey MH, Al-Mubarek N. Updated review of the global carotid artery stent registry. *Catheter Cardiovasc Interv.* 2003;60:259–266.

27. Reimers B, Schluter M, Castriota F, et al. Routine use of cerebral protection during carotid artery stenting: results of a multicenter registry of 753 patients. *Am J Med.* 2004;116:217–222.

28. Schluter M, Tubler T, Steffens JC, et al. Focal ischemia of the brain after neuroprotected carotid artery stenting. *J Am Coll Cardiol.* 2003;42:1007–1013.

29. Wholey MH, Tan WA, Toursarkissian B, et al. Management of neurological complications of carotid artery stenting. *J Endovasc Ther.* 2001;8:341–353.

30. Yadav JS. Stenting and angioplasty with protection in patients at high risk for endarterectomy. In: *The American Heart Association Meeting.* Chicago, Illinois, USA;2002.

31. Ansel GM. Treatment of carotid stent restenosis. *Catheter Cardiovasc Interv.* 2003;58:93–94.

CHAPTER 7

Vertebral Artery Disease

Debabrata Mukherjee and Ken Rosenfeld

O ur knowledge about ischemia of the posterior cerebral circulation is more rudimentary, compared with that of anterior cerebral circulation ischemia. With improved technology, allowing imaging of the brain and vascular lesions causing vertebrobasilar ischemia (VBI), this gap has closed and many misconceptions have been challenged. Based on data from a well-characterized group of patients with signs and symptoms of posterior circulation ischemia (n = 407), the causes of VBI have been defined (1). Embolism is the dominant mechanism, accounting for approximately 40% of cases. Emboli may arise from the heart (usually thrombus), aorta (usually atheroma), or proximal vessel thrombus (predominantly the vertebral artery).

Large artery disease, predominantly involving the vertebral artery, is the second most common mechanism accounting for approximately 32% of cases, with ischemia being produced on a hemodynamic basis or by occlusion of important penetrating or circumferential branches arising from the diseased vessel. The remaining cases are caused by a variety of conditions such as dissection, fibromuscular dysplasia, migraine, and rare arteriopathies that often involve the vertebral artery. These data highlight the importance of vertebral artery disease in causing posterior cerebral circulation ischemia, a phenomenon that has previously been under-appreciated in clinical practice.

Atherosclerosis is the dominant pathology seen in the vertebral artery and has a predilection for the origin and proximal section of the extracranial portion of the vessel (i.e., termed the V1 segment) and the intracranial portion of the vessel. The focus of this chapter will be on the interventional management of patients with proximal extracranial vertebral artery (ECVA) disease. Management of intracranial artery disease is discussed in Chapter 9A. Although it has generally been considered that ECVA disease has a more benign outcome compared to intracranial vertebral artery disease, significant occlusive disease of the proximal vertebral artery was present in 20% of patients who presented with VBI at a tertiary referral center, and was felt to represent the primary cause of ischemia in 9% of patients (2).

ANATOMY

The vertebral artery typically arises from the supero-posterior aspect of the first part of the subclavian artery, and is usually the first branch of this vessel. In approximately 5% of patients, the left vertebral artery arises directly from the aortic arch, between the origin of the left common carotid and left subclavian arteries (Fig. 7-1).

Other rare anomalies have been described including: origin directly from the aortic arch distal to the left subclavian artery, origin distal to the thyrocervical branch of the subclavian artery, origin of the right vertebral from the right common carotid artery, and duplication of the vertebral artery that may occur at any level of the artery (3).

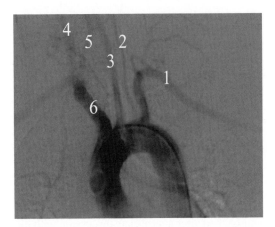

FIGURE 7-1 ● **Left vertebral artery arising directly from the aortic arch.** 1. Left subclavian; 2. Left vertebral; 3. Left common carotid; 4. Right common carotid; 5. Right vertebral; 6. Innominate.

The vertebral arteries converge beyond the base of the skull and form the basilar artery at the base of the pons. The vertebral artery is arbitrarily divided into four anatomic parts [Fig. 7-2]

- V1 - The origin to the point at which it enters the transverse foramina of either the fifth or sixth cervical vertebra
- V2 - Course within the intervertebral foramina until exiting behind the atlas (i.e., C2)
- V3 - The extracranial segment between the transverse process of the C2 and the base of the skull, as it enters the foramen magnum
- V4 - Final intracranial part begins as it pierces the dura and arachnoid mater, at the base of the skull, and ends as it meets its opposite vertebral artery to form the midline basilar artery at the level of the medullopontine junction

The intracranial part gives off major anterior and posterior spinal arteries to the medulla and spinal cord, minute penetrating vessels to the medulla and the largest branch—the posterior inferior cerebellar artery (PICA)—which supplies a portion of the dorsal medulla and cerebellum. One of the vertebral arteries is often larger (i.e., left more frequently than right) and provides most of the blood supply to the posterior circulation (i.e., dominant artery). Stenosis of the dominant artery is more likely to cause symptoms.

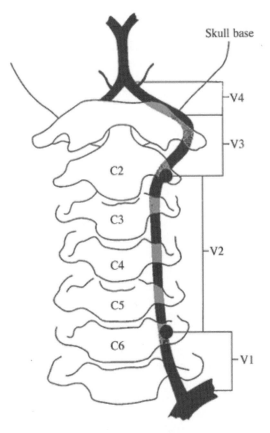

FIGURE 7-2 ● Schematic of the four parts of the vertebral artery. Adapted from Cloud et al. (15).

CLINICAL PRESENTATION OF EXTRACRANIAL VERTEBRAL ARTERY DISEASE

Extracranial vertebral artery (ECVA) disease causing hemodynamic compromise typically produces dizziness accompanied by other signs of hind-brain ischemia (e.g., diplopia, hemiparesis, bilateral leg weakness, numbness) consistent with global ischemia of the posterior circulation (4). The non-specific nature of a number of these symptoms, particular in an elderly population, has contributed to the failure to associate vertebral artery disease and VBI.

Embolization from proximal vertebral atherosclerosis produces a variety of syndromes based on the site of distal embolization. The typical sites of embolization include the PICA, superior cerebellar artery (SCA), and posterior cerebral artery. Obstruction of circumferential arteries (e.g., PICA, SCA) results in typical lateral syndromes that affect cerebellar function, sensation, and lateral cranial nerves. In contrast, the clinical presentation following obstruction of midline perforator branches is highly variable. In general, midline syndromes tend to affect the pyramidal system, consciousness, and midline cranial nerves.

PATIENT SELECTION

Considerable controversy surrounds the indications for endovascular intervention for occlusive disease of the ECVA. The reasons for this have been well described and are multiple (5). Relatively inexpensive, noninvasive testing with ultrasonography has been unreliable in this location, requiring the use of routine angiography and magnetic resonance angiography (MRA) to help make a reliable diagnosis. The absence of an effective and safe surgical therapy for the treatment of proximal ECVA disease has engendered a nihilistic approach to patient management, with medical therapy being offered rather than performing apparently futile diagnostic tests. These factors have contributed to a knowledge gap, with respect to vertebral artery disease and the potential for revascularization to alter the natural history of the disease.

Endovascular approaches to proximal ECVA disease have transformed approaches to therapy. In contrast to surgical revascularization, where surgical accessibility is particularly demanding and likely contributes to the very high morbidity and mortality rates for these procedures (i.e., approximately 20%) (6), endovascular access is straightforward, and the techniques of angioplasty and stenting are readily applied to the treatment of proximal ECVA stenoses. Although endovascular ECVA revascularization has been practiced at multiple centers for over 2 decades, the techniques continue to evolve, and currently available data are still derived from relatively small registries. Therefore, appropriate decisions regarding patient management remain hampered by a lack of data.

Despite these limitations, it is generally accepted that intervention is indicated in patients with symptomatic vertebral artery stenosis who fail, or who are intolerant of medical therapy. Intervention in patients with symptomatic disease without a trial of medical therapy is also prob-

ably justified, in view of the outcomes reported from observational studies. Decisions regarding intervention in asymptomatic patients are more uncertain. A thorough review of the clinical history and angiographic findings by a neurologist, together with the interventionist, is recommended. Factors that will influence the decision include: the severity of the stenosis, angiographic appearance of the stenosis (i.e., friability, presence of ulceration), the adequacy of collateral flow, and the age of the patient. A severe, ulcerated stenosis without good collateral flow, in a relatively young, asymptomatic patient may be approached after appropriate discussion with the patient.

ACCESS

The choice of an appropriate arterial access site is crucial to performing safe and successful angiography, and intervention of the vertebral artery. Access is typically obtained using the retrograde common femoral artery (CFA) approach. Ipsilateral brachial artery access is considered in individuals with bilateral, severe, iliac artery stenosis or distal aortic occlusions. Brachial access may also be indicated in patients with severe tortuosity or stenosis of the proximal subclavian artery, or Type III aortic arch anatomy. If brachial or radial artery access is used, 3000 U to 5000 U of unfractionated heparin should be injected immediately following sheath insertion, to minimize the risk of thrombosis. Specifically, in the case of radial artery access, an additional 50 mcg to 100 mcg of intra-arterial nitroglycerin, or 100 mcg to 200 mcg of verapamil may be administered to minimize the risk of spasm.

DIAGNOSTIC ANGIOGRAPHY

Arch Aortogram

An arch aortogram should be performed prior to attempts at selective cannulation of the vertebral arteries. This is performed in the LAO 30° to 45° projection, to assess the origin of the great vessels and delineate the tortuosity of the arch (Fig. 7-3).

Typical arch anatomy with separate origin of the brachiocephalic, left carotid, and left subclavian arteries is seen in more than 70% of cases.

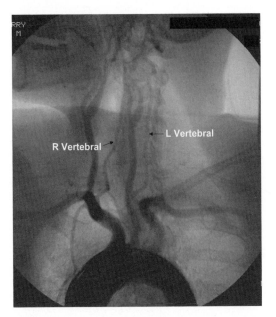

FIGURE 7-3 ● Arch aortogram in left anterior oblique 30° projection visualizing both vertebral arteries.

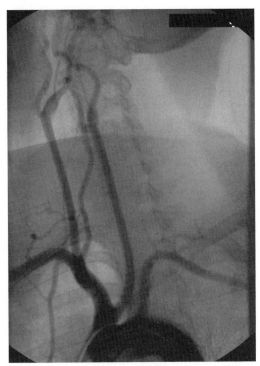

FIGURE 7-4 ● A bovine arch, which defines the origin of the left common carotid artery from the brachiocephalic trunk.

A shared origin of the brachiocephalic trunk and left common carotid artery is seen in 15% of cases, while a bovine arch (i.e., origin of the left common carotid artery from the brachiocephalic trunk) is seen in 8 to 10% of cases (Fig. 7-4).

With increasing age, hypertension, and atherosclerotic changes in the aorta, the arch sinks deeper into the thoracic cavity and draws the origin of the great vessels along with it. An aortogram helps define the type and tortuosity of the aortic arch, identify any anomalies of the vertebral artery origin, and helps the operator choose the appropriate diagnostic catheter for the case.

Selective Vertebral Artery Angiography

One should start with a catheter appropriate to the degree of angulation or tortuosity of the arch, rather than repeatedly scraping the arch with an inappropriate catheter that increases the risk of stroke and other procedural complications. Most vertebral arteries may be cannulated with a Judkins® Right (JR4) catheter. It is however, inappropriate to try to cannulate the great vessels with a JR4 catheter in an individual with a severely angulated and tortuous aortic arch.

A Vitek® (COOK Inc., Bloomington, IN) or a Headhunter® (Meditech, Watertown, MA) catheter should be the initial catheter of choice in individuals with a moderately tortuous arch and a Simmons® 1 or 2 catheters (Angiodynamics, Queensbury, NY) should be chosen for cannulating great vessels in an individual with a severely tortuous arch. Since even small emboli may have devastating consequences in this territory, the use of gentle and meticulous technique is imperative. The authors' practice is to perform nonselective vertebral artery angiography, with the catheter tip close to the origin of the vertebral artery but not engaged in the ostium. This is particularly important where proximal V1-segment disease is suspected. An inflated blood pressure cuff on the ipsilateral arm will help maximize visualization of the vertebral artery during nonselective angiography.

The ostia of the vertebral arteries are typically visualized in the contralateral oblique projection, although some variation should be expected. The remainder of the V1 segment, and the V2 and V3 segments, are visualized using

INTERVENTION

Anticoagulation/Antithrombotics

All patients should have received aspirin (i.e., 325 mg daily) and clopidogrel (i.e., 300 mg to 600 mg loading dose, followed by 75 mg daily) for at least 2 days prior to the procedure. A baseline, activated clotting time (ACT) is obtained prior to the interventional procedure. The patient then receives a weight-adjusted bolus of unfractionated heparin of 60 U/kg body weight, to ensure a value greater than twice baseline ACT, or longer than 250 seconds. The role of glycoprotein IIb/IIIa inhibitors during vertebral artery intervention is not well defined and therefore, currently, is not recommended.

Guide/Sheath

Either a long sheath or a preshaped guide may be used for vertebral artery interventions. For brachial access, the 6 Fr sheath (i.e., 35 cm to 55 cm length) is a good choice as it minimizes the risk of occlusion of the brachial artery and allows delivery of appropriately sized balloons and stents. A long, 80-cm 6-Fr shuttle sheath may be an option when using the retrograde CFA approach, in patients with severe PVD or ostial subclavian-artery disease. Preferably, guides should be 8 Fr (e.g., JR4, H1, or Multipurpose), although with newer stents, 7-Fr systems may also be used.

When using a guide, the telescoping technique employed for carotid intervention may be employed to facilitate safe delivery of the guide in the region of the vertebral artery ostium (Fig. 7-7).

With this technique, a long 125-cm diagnostic catheter (e.g., JR4) is telescoped through the guide and used to engage the ostium of the subclavian/innominate artery. A wire (e.g., Wholey® or stiff-angled glidewire) is then advanced into the axillary artery, and the diagnostic catheter is advanced over the wire, into the distal subclavian artery. The guide is then advanced over the wire-catheter combination into the proximal subclavian artery, near the vertebral artery origin. A useful option is to leave an 0.035″ Wholey wire in place in the axillary or brachial artery, to stabilize the guide during the intervention. This may be particularly useful in patients with marked

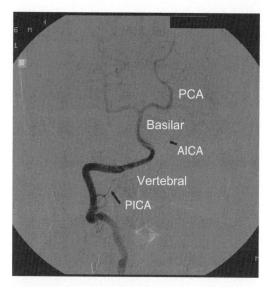

FIGURE 7-5 ● Digital subtraction angiogram of the right vertebral artery in the postero-anterior (PA) projection. AICA, anterior inferior cerebellar artery; PICA, anterior inferior cerebellar artery.

postero-anterior (PA) and lateral views. Alternatively, a single ipsilateral oblique view may suffice. The intracranial posterior circulation is best visualized in steep (i.e., approximately 40°) PA cranial (i.e., Townes view) (Fig. 7-5) and cross-table views (Fig. 7-6).

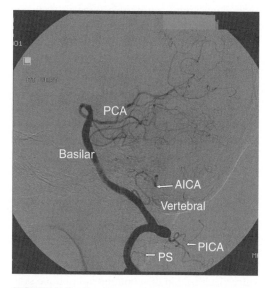

FIGURE 7-6 ● Digital subtraction angiogram of the right vertebral artery in the lateral projection. AICA, anterior inferior cerebellar artery; PICA, anterior inferior cerebellar artery; PS, posterior spinal artery.

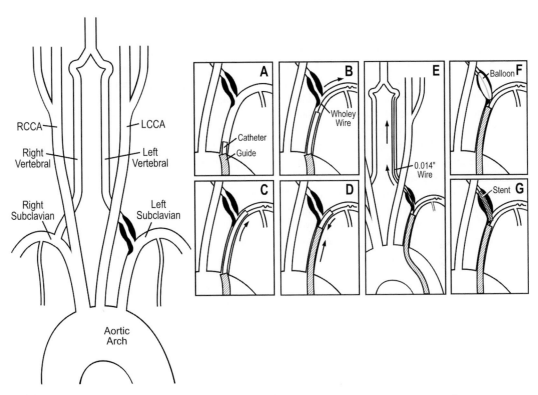

FIGURE 7-7 ● Schematic of vertebral artery intervention from the femoral approach. LCCA, Left Common Carotid Artery; RCCA, Right Common Carotid Artery.

proximal tortuosity of the subclavian or innominate arteries.

When using a sheath, one may similarly telescope the long, 125-cm diagnostic catheter through the sheath, engage the subclavian with the catheter, advance the 0.035″ wire (Wholey or angled glidewire) distally as before, and advance the diagnostic catheter into the axillary artery. At this point, the authors typically exchange the 0.035″ wire for a stiff wire (e.g., stiff Amplatz wire), remove the diagnostic catheter, and advance the sheath with its dilator, such that the sheath is positioned proximally to the vertebral artery. The sheath tip is placed very close to the ostium of the vertebral artery, without actually intubating it.

Wires

Once the ACT is longer than 250 seconds, the lesion is traversed with a 0.014″ exchange length wire (i.e., BMW® wire, Guidant Corporation). Hydrophilic wires should generally be avoided, to minimize the risk of dissection or perforation,

which could have devastating consequences in this area. Some vertebral arteries are very tortuous and a hydrophilic wire may be necessary, initially, to wire the vessel (e.g., Whisper®, Pilot® 50, Guidant Corporation). These may then be exchanged using an over the wire balloon for a more friendly wire like the BMW or Balance® Trek (Guidant Corporation).

It should be noted that in patients with severe vertebral artery tortuosity and even in some patients in which tortuosity is not initially obvious, there is a propensity for pseudostenoses to develop following wire placement, which may compromise vertebral flow. The operator should always check flow following wire placement. If diminished flow is present, one needs to exchange for a softer, nonhydrophilic wire, or one may have to use a hydrophilic wire for the entire procedure.

PTA vs PTA-Plus-Stent

The normal size of the proximal vertebral artery is typically between 3.0 mm to 6.0 mm.

Predilation with a balloon serves two functions: it allows subsequent passage of a balloon-mounted stent, and it also allows an objective assessment of the length and diameter of the vessel. Generally, angioplasty balloon sizing is conservative in an effort to minimize the risk of dissection: typically we use a coronary balloon (Maverick®, Boston Scientific) that is approximately two-thirds of the initially estimated diameter of the vessel. Stenting of ostial lesions is performed usually with an appropriately sized (i.e., 3.5-mm to 6.0-mm diameter] balloon-mounted stent (Figs. 7-7 and 7.8). The choice of stent for vertebral ostial lesions represents a balance between the need for radial strength, and the likelihood of creating distal kinking of the artery after stenting in a tortuous vessel.

Coronary stents are attractive because of their flexibility, but they lack the radial strength of peripheral balloon-expandable stents (e.g., Herculink, Genesis). Therefore, in nontortuous vessels, the stiffer peripheral balloon-expandable stents are preferred, whereas in tortuous vessels, coronary stents represent an adequate compromise (7,8). Before deployment, angiograms are performed in orthogonal projections to determine appropriate placement of the stent. It is of paramount importance that the stent cover the ostium of ostial lesions. This will usually necessitate that 1 mm to 2 mm of stent will be free in the subclavian artery (Figs. 7-8, 7-9). The overhang is typically asymmetric because of the angulation of the vertebral artery, off the subclavian artery.

Nonostial lesions are uncommon but technically more straightforward than ostial lesions. Appropriate treatment of these lesions in the vertebral arteries is still uncertain, but stenting is assumed to be the optimal management strategy by preventing elastic recoil and reducing the risk of restenosis (9). The choice of stent is determined by the location, with balloon-expandable stents being used in the fixed extracranial V2, and self-expanding stents in the V3 segment,

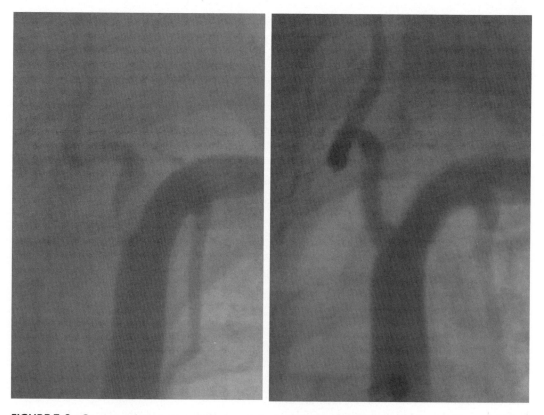

FIGURE 7-8 ● Successful balloon angioplasty and stenting of the proximal left vertebral artery that produced complete resolution of symptoms in a 73-year-old male with drop attacks.

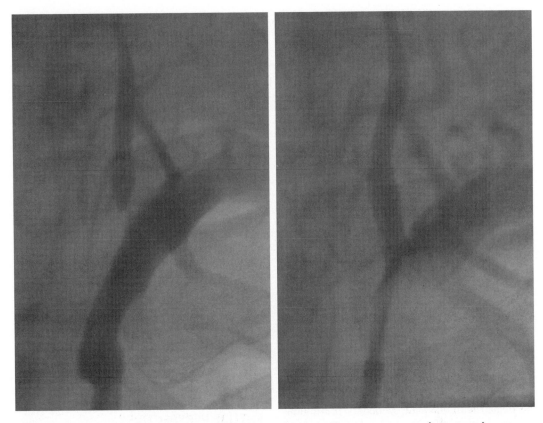

FIGURE 7-9 ● Successful balloon angioplasty associated with significant improvement of symptoms from a severe ostial left vertebral artery stenosis in a 76-year-old female with diplopia and gait disturbances.

which has significant tortuosity and is subject to torsion. Radial force is less of an issue in the nonostial location, and either coronary or peripheral balloon-expandable or self-expandable stents may be used.

Distal Embolic Protection

The use of emboli-protection devices during vertebral artery intervention is uncommon. The practice is to reserve their use to cases in which the angiographic appearance of the lesion suggests there is an increased risk of embolization (i.e., bulky, hazy lesions), and in which the diameter of the V2 segment is large enough to accommodate the currently available filter device (i.e., greater than 4 mm). Since the FilterWire® (Boston Scientific) is the only currently FDA-approved filter, this is the current embolic protection device of choice. In the near future, the Angioguard® filter (Cordis) is likely to be approved and may be a viable alternative. The Percusurge® (Medtronic) occlusive device has a lower crossing profile than either of these filters and may be used for severe stenoses in which occlusion of ipsilateral vertebral flow does not produce symptoms.

Potential Complications

Potential major complications include posterior circulation distribution strokes and transient ischemic attacks (TIAs). These events are generally embolic, and occur in approximately 1% of interventions. Most other complications are related to access site issues (e.g., in patients with brachial access) and include hematomas, pseudoaneurysms and arteriovenous fistulas.

POSTPROCEDURAL CARE

Patients are generally observed overnight following the procedure, with frequent neurologic checks. Hypertension should be treated, to

TABLE 7-1

Studies of Vertebral Artery Stenting

	n	Technical Success	Procedural Complications	Improvement in Symptoms	Mean Follow-up (Months)	Late Stroke	Restenosis
Mukherjee et al (14)	12	100%	none	12/12	6.4	0	1/12
Malek et al (13)	13	100%	1 TIA	11/13	20.7	0	N/A
Jenkins et al (17)	32	100%	1 TIA	31/32	10.6	0	1/32
Chastain et al (8)	50	98%	None	48/50	25	1	5/50

TIA, Transient ischemic attack; N/A, not available.

minimize the risk of reperfusion hemorrhage, and hypotension should also be avoided. The optimum blood pressure range is 110 mmHg to 130 mmHg systolic, over 70 mmHg to 85 mmHg diastolic. Patients are discharged on lifelong aspirin therapy and clopidogrel, 75 mg daily, for 1 to 12 months. Long-term appropriate follow-up monitoring is extremely important in detecting potential recurrence of symptoms and restenosis. It is also imperative that these patients be treated with adequate secondary prevention agents, such as beta-blockers, statins, and angiotensin converting enzyme (ACE) inhibitors, which in turn translates into improved clinical outcomes (10).

OUTCOME

In patients with significant stenosis involving the vertebral or basilar artery territories, transluminal angioplasty may be of significant benefit in alleviating symptoms and improving blood flow to the posterior cerebral circulation. However, adequate dilation of the origin of the vertebral artery with balloon angioplasty, alone, has resulted in high restenosis rates of 10% in one series (11) and up to 75% in another series (12). Arterial spasm and dissection may occur in some instances, with subsequent hemodynamic compromise (5,9). These data have encouraged the use of stents for vertebral artery lesions.

Several case series of patients treated with vertebral artery stenting have been reported (Table 7-1) (8,13–15).

The data show that stent placement for symptomatic stenosis involving the vertebral artery is safe and effective for alleviating symptoms of vertebrobasilar ischemia, with good long-term results. Overall technical success is greater than 90%, with less than 1% risk of procedural complications including stroke. Late stroke is uncommon (i.e., less than 1%) and restenosis is seen in 8 to 10% of patients. The use of drug-eluting stents may further reduce restenosis rates in the future.

FUTURE PERSPECTIVES

Future advances using MR technology to delineate plaque composition/characteristics may help better define the indications for intervention, particularly in asymptomatic patients. Randomized trials with, and without, the use of filter devices will better define the risks and benefits of intervention compared to medical therapy. As mentioned before, drug-eluting stents may further improve long-term outcomes in patients undergoing vertebral artery intervention by reducing restenosis. Continued innovation and refinement of endovascular devices and techniques, together with optimization of pharmacologic regimens, will improve technical success rates, reduce complications, and broaden the applications of endovascular therapy for cerebrovascular diseases.

REFERENCES

1. Caplan L. Posterior circulation ischemia: then, now, and tomorrow. The Thomas Willis Lecture-2000. *Stroke.* 2000;31(8):2011–2023.
2. Wityk RJ, Chang HM, Rosengart A, et al. Proximal extracranial vertebral artery disease in the New England

Medical Center Posterior Circulation Registry. *Arch Neurol.* 1998;55(4):470–478.

3. Koenigsberg RA, Pereira L, Nair B, et al. Unusual vertebral artery origins: examples and related pathology. *Catheter Cardiovasc Interv.* 2003;59(2):244–250.

4. Caplan LR. Vertebrobasilar disease. *Adv Neurol.* 2003;92:131–140.

5. Rocha-Singh K. Vertebral artery stenting: ready for prime time? *Catheter Cardiovasc Interv.* 2001;54(1): 6–7.

6. Phatouros CC, Higashida RT, Malek AM, et al. Endovascular treatment of noncarotid extracranial cerebrovascular disease. *Neurosurg Clin N Am.* 2000;11(2):331–350.

7. Jain SP, Ramee SR, White CJ. Treatment of atherosclerotic vertebral artery disease by endoluminal stenting: Results from a multicenter registry. *J Am Coll Cardiol.* 2000;35:86A.

8. Chastain HD II, Campbell MS, Iyer S, et al. Extracranial vertebral artery stent placement: in-hospital and follow-up results. *J Neurosurg.* 1999;91(4):547–552.

9. Piotin M, Spelle L, Martin JB, et al. Percutaneous transluminal angioplasty and stenting of the proximal vertebral artery for symptomatic stenosis. *AJNR Am J Neuroradiol.* 2000;21(4):727–731.

10. Mukherjee D, Lingam P, Chetcuti et al. Missed opportunities to treat atherosclerosis in patients undergoing peripheral vascular interventions: insights from the University of Michigan Peripheral Vascular disease quality improvement initiative (PVD-Q1[2]). *Circulation.* 2002;106:1909–1912.

11. Higashida RT, Tsai FY, Halbach VV, et al. Transluminal angioplasty for atherosclerotic disease of the vertebral and basilar arteries. *J Neurosurg.* 1993;78(2): 192–198.

12. Crawley F, Brown MM. Percutaneous transluminal angioplasty and stenting for vertebral artery stenosis. *Cochrane Database Syst Rev.* 2000(2):CD000516.

13. Malek AM, Higashida RT, Phatouros CC, et al. Treatment of posterior circulation ischemia with extracranial percutaneous balloon angioplasty and stent placement. *Stroke.* 1999;30(10):2073–2085.

14. Mukherjee D, Roffi M, Kapadia SR, et al. Percutaneous intervention for symptomatic vertebral artery stenosis using coronary stents. *J Invasive Cardiol.* 2001;13(5):363–366.

15. Jenkins JS, White CJ, Ramee SR, et al. Vertebral insufficiency: when to intervene and how? *Curr Interv Cardiol Rep.* 2000;2(2):91–94.

16. Cloud GC, Markus HS. Diagnosis and management of vertebral artery stenosis. *QJM.* 2003;96(1):27–54.

17. Jenkins JS, White CJ, Ramee SR, et al. Vertebral artery stenting. *Catheter Cardiovasc Interv.* 2001;54(1):1–5.

CHAPTER 8

Subclavian, Brachiocephalic, and Upper Extremity

Leslie Cho, Ivan P. Casserly, and Mark H. Wholey

Brachiocephalic or subclavian artery obstruction accounts for about 15% of symptomatic, extracranial, cerebrovascular disease. Rapid advances in technology and evolution in technique over the last decade have resulted in percutaneous revascularization techniques supplanting surgery as the therapy of choice for the treatment of these lesions. Owing to the predilection of atherosclerosis for these sites, and the relative sparing of more distal upper extremity vessels, brachiocephalic and subclavian-artery intervention comprise the majority of upper-extremity endovascular procedures and will form the major focus of this chapter. Additional, less common vascular pathologies encountered during angiography of the upper-extremity arterial circulation will also be highlighted.

ANATOMY (1,2)

The subclavian arteries originate from the bifurcation of the brachiocephalic artery on the right, and directly from the aortic arch as the third, and final, of the great vessels on the left (Fig. 8-1A).

In approximately 0.5% of patients, the right subclavian artery arises anomalously, as the terminal vessel from the descending thoracic aorta, and courses toward its normal distribution to the right upper extremity (Fig. 8-1B).

Rarely, the right subclavian artery and right common carotid arteries have a separate origin from the arch (Fig. 8-1C).

Additional variations in arch anatomy that are important during upper extremity angiography include: common origin of the innominate and left common carotid artery from the arch (about 15%) (Fig. 8-1D), and bovine origin of the left common carotid artery from the innominate artery (about 10%) (Fig. 8-1E).

In healthy young individuals, the great vessels arise from the horizontal portion of the arch. With increasing age and atherosclerotic disease, this portion of the arch descends into the thoracic cavity together with the origin of the great vessels, such that they appear to arise from the ascending portion of the arch (Figs. 8-1F and 8-1G).

The most important branches of the subclavian artery arise from the first segment of the artery (i.e., medial to the scalenus anterior muscle) (Fig. 8-2A). The vertebral and internal mammary artery branches of the subclavian artery are remarkably constant in their origin and course, arising as the first and second branches respectively. These branches supply the posterior cerebral circulation and the anterior chest wall, respectively. In 1 to 5% of patients, the left vertebral artery had a direct origin from the aortic arch, typically between the origins of the left common-carotid artery and the left subclavian artery (Fig. 8-2B).

In contrast, the thyrocervical trunk, which arises as the third branch, demonstrates significant variation in both the pattern and size of its various branches (i.e., inferior thyroid, suprascapular, ascending cervical, transverse cervical).

At the lateral margin of the first rib, the subclavian artery becomes the axillary artery. At the anatomic neck of the humerus, the axillary artery changes name to become the brachial artery (Fig. 8-2C).

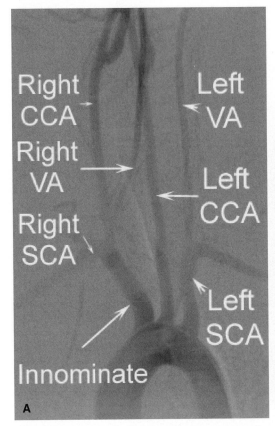
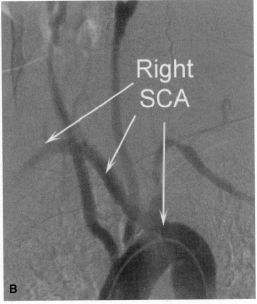

FIGURE 8-1 ● Normal and variant anatomy of the aortic arch. **A: Arch aortogram in LAO projection demonstrating normal angiographic anatomy.** CCA common carotid artery, VA vertebral artery, SCA subclavian artery **B:** Anomalous origin of right subclavian artery (SCA) as terminal great vessel off aortic arch. (*continued*)

In the arm, the brachial artery supplies the deep brachial branch that runs posteriorly, relatively minor compared to its counterpart in the thigh, and the superior and inferior ulnar collateral arteries that supply collateral flow to the elbow region. Opposite the neck of the radius, the brachial artery then divides into the radial and ulnar arteries (Fig. 8-2D).

The ulnar artery is usually the larger of the terminal branches of the brachial artery. Just distal to its origin, it gives off the anterior and posterior ulnar recurrent arteries that supply collateral flow to the elbow, and then gives off its major branch, the common interosseous. Thereafter, the ulnar artery descends on the medial side of the forearm. The radial artery supplies a radial recurrent branch to the elbow, and descends on the lateral side of the forearm. In some cases, the radial artery may originate high from the axillary or upper-brachial artery. This is an impor-

tant anatomic variant, as it may cause significant confusion during diagnostic angiography if its presence is not appreciated.

The arterial anatomy of the hand is extremely variable, and deviations from the classic patterns are common (Figs. 8-2E and 8-2F).

The ulnar artery supplies the superficial palmar arch and the radial artery supplies the deep palmar arch. In 10% of the population, the anterior interosseous or median artery persists and supplies the deep-palmar arch. Typically, the superficial arch is dominant and lies distal to the deep arch. The princeps pollicis and radialis indicis arteries arise from the radial artery and supply the thumb and index finger. The superficial-palmar arch gives off three or four common palmar digital arteries, and the deep arch gives off the palmar metacarpal arteries. At the bases of the proximal phalanges, adjacent metacarpal vessels from each arch join and then immediately

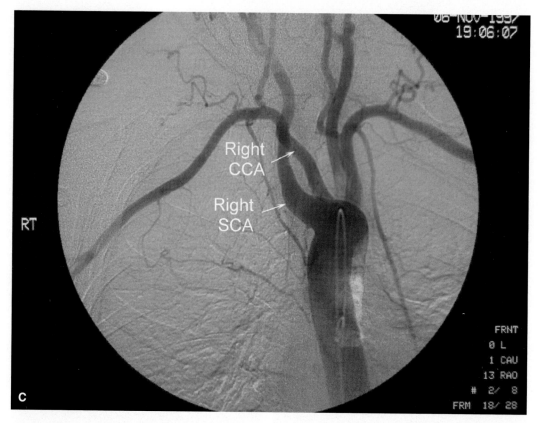

FIGURE 8-1 ● **C:** Separate origin of right subclavian (SCA) and common carotid (CCA) arteries from aortic arch demonstrated in aortogram in RAO projection **D:** Common origin of innominate and left common carotid artery (CCA) from aortic arch **E:** Bovine origin of left common carotid artery (CCA) from innominate artery **F:** Type II aortic arch **G:** Type III aortic arch.

divide into proper digital arteries, which supply apposing surfaces of the fingers.

BRACHIOCEPHALIC AND SUBCLAVIAN ARTERY INTERVENTION

Patient Selection

As in all endovascular procedures, careful patient selection is absolutely crucial to the success of the intervention (Table 8-1).

With some exceptions, intervention is generally reserved for patients with symptomatic subclavian or brachiocephalic stenoses. It is worth emphasizing that most patients with angiographic evidence of subclavian or brachiocephalic artery stenosis are asymptomatic. When symptoms are present, they may be attributable to ischemia of the upper extremity that is typically

precipitated by upper extremity activity. Alternatively, symptoms may be attributable to 'steal' of blood flow from the posterior cerebral circulation toward the upper extremity, via retrograde flow along the ipsilateral vertebral artery, caused by significant proximal brachiocephalic/subclavian stenosis or obstruction (Fig. 8-3) (3,4). When symptomatic (i.e., subclavian steal syndrome), patients present with symptoms of posterior circulation ischemia including: nausea, dizziness, diplopia, nystagmus, ataxia, and visual symptoms. Again, it is worth emphasizing that the presence of retrograde flow along the vertebral artery is most commonly asymptomatic, and is referred to as the 'subclavian steal phenomenon'.

In patients with prior bypass surgery involving 'in situ' right, or left internal mammary artery grafts, coronary 'steal' may also occur as a result of retrograde flow along the graft from the coronary circulation toward the distal subclavian

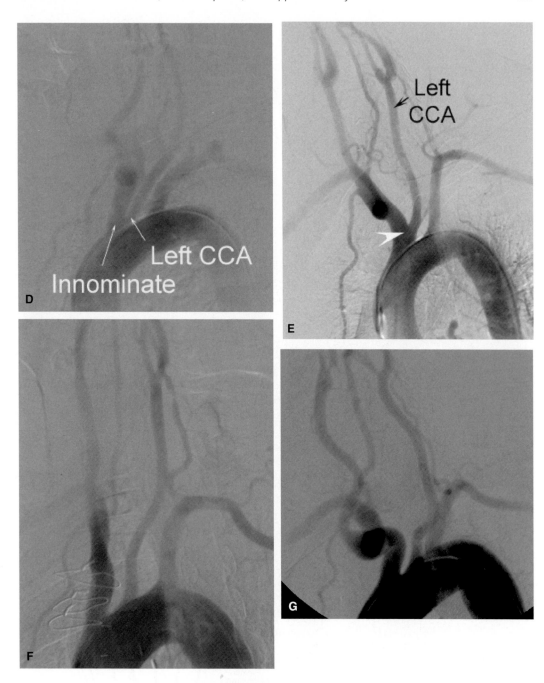

FIGURE 8-1 ● *(Continued)*

artery, precipitating coronary ischemia (Fig. 8-4) (5).

Typically, these 'steal' syndromes are worsened by upper extremity activity. Specific to brachiocephalic artery lesions, ischemia in the distribution of the right internal carotid artery may be the presenting symptom, on the basis of atherothrombotic embolization from the lesion, or hemodynamic compromise of flow. In asymptomatic patients, subclavian or brachiocephalic artery intervention may be performed to protect the inflow to a variety of surgical grafts including: axillo-axillary, axillo-femoral, subclavian-carotid, and IMA-coronary.

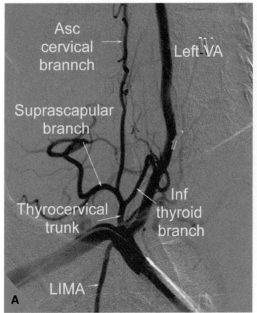

A

Asc cervical brannch
Left-VA
Suprascapular branch
Thyrocervical trunk
Inf thyroid branch
LIMA

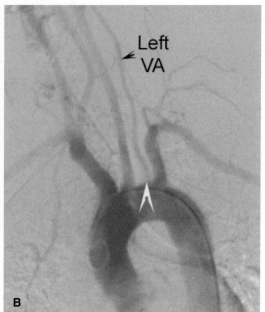

B

Left VA

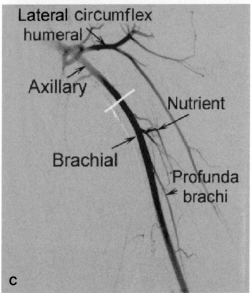

C

Lateral circumflex humeral
Axillary
Nutrient
Brachial
Profunda brachi

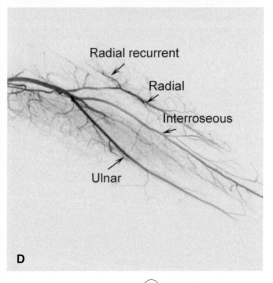

D

Radial recurrent
Radial
Interroseous
Ulnar

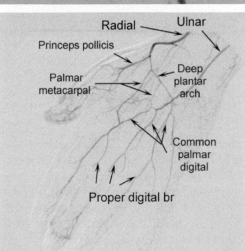

E

Radial
Ulnar
Princeps pollicis
Palmar metacarpal
Deep plantar arch
Common palmar digital
Proper digital br

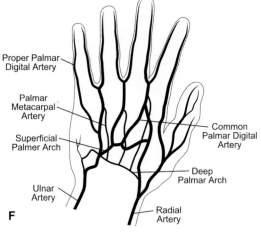

F

Proper Palmar Digital Artery
Palmar Metacarpal Artery
Superficial Palmar Arch
Ulnar Artery
Common Palmar Digital Artery
Deep Palmar Arch
Radial Artery

TABLE 8-1

Indications for Subclavian Artery or Innominate Artery Revascularization

Vertebral Basilar Insufficiency

Symptomatic subclavian steal syndrome
Disabling upper extremity claudication
Preservation of flow to in-situ LIMA or RIMA grafts
Preservation of inflow to axillary graft or dialysis conduit
Embolization to the fingers from subclavian disease

The dominant contraindication to subclavian/brachiocephalic percutaneous intervention is the presence of fresh thrombus. Embolization to the vertebral artery or right internal carotid artery during subclavian and brachiocephalic artery intervention is an important complication in this circumstance. There are significant technical challenges to the use of emboli protection devices (EPDs) for these procedures that further add to the risk in this setting. Therefore, with thrombotic lesions, the authors recommend either thrombolysis, or 2 to 4 weeks of anticoagulation, prior to proceeding with intervention. If the lesion must be dealt with immediately, use of a glycoprotein IIb/IIIa inhibitor, in addition to emboli protection is recommended.

Upper Extremity Angiography (2,6)

Aortogram

The major indications for upper extremity angiography are listed in Table 8-2.

Prior to selective angiography of the upper extremity, it is prudent to always perform an arch aortogram (40° LAO projection). Our practice is to use a multi-sidehole pigtail catheter (Fig. 8-5 [a]) for this purpose.

The arch aortogram facilitates the detection of important anomalies, as outlined above, and anatomic features (e.g., tortuosity of brachiocephalic or proximal subclavian artery, Type III aortic arch) that influence the choice of equipment used to perform angiography and intervention, and increase the technical complexity of these procedures. An RAO view is rarely helpful, except in circumstances where there is significant overlap of vessels in the LAO view. Ideally, rotational angiography would be the gold standard, allowing a complete 3-D assessment of the arch and the origins of the great vessels.

When selective angiography of the entire upper extremity is required, it is advisable to adopt a systematic, step-wise approach, starting proximally and working distally. This approach facilitates the prompt detection of anomalies, such as the high origin of either the radial or ulnar artery from the brachial artery (i.e., 15 to 20%), or the origin of the radial artery from the axillary artery (i.e., 1 to 3%). Failure to adopt this approach may result in an erroneous diagnosis of vessel occlusion. Iodixanol, an iso-osmolar nonionic contrast agent, is the preferred contrast medium for use in upper-extremity angiography because of its excellent tolerability. By using hand injections of 5 mL to 10 mL of contrast agent with digital subtraction angiography (DSA), adequate visualization of all major vessels is achieved.

Subclavian and Brachiocephalic Artery Angiography

Selective engagement of the brachiocephalic artery and left subclavian artery may generally be achieved using a JR4 diagnostic catheter (Fig. 8-5[b]). For patients with unfolding of the aortic arch (i.e., Type III arches), alternative catheters may be required (e.g., Vitek®, Simmons® catheter, Cobra®, Headhunter-1®) (Fig. 8-5[c–e]). The appropriate use of these

---

FIGURE 8-2 ● Angiographic anatomy of upper extremity. **A:** Angiography of right subclavian artery (PA) demonstrating origin and course of the major branches from the first segment of the vessel **B:** Arch aortogram demonstrating anomalous origin of left vertebral artery from typical location on aortic arch **C:** Angiography of left axillary and brachial artery **D:** Angiography of distal left brachial artery and ulnar and radial branches **E:** Angiography of right hand from patient with small vessel vasculitis involving the proper digital branches **F:** Stylistic diagram of typical anatomy of the blood vessels in the hand. VA, vertebral artery; Inf, inferior; Asc, ascending; LIMA, left internal mammary artery.

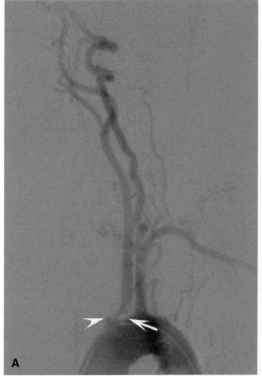

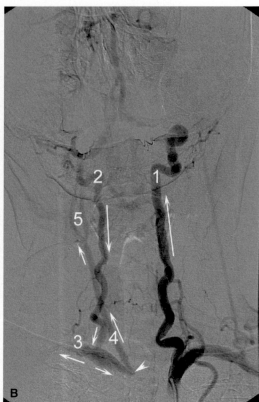

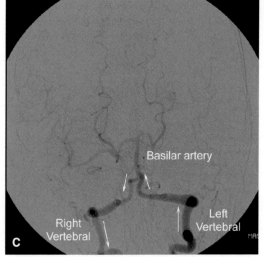

FIGURE 8-3 ● Demonstration of subclavian artery steal from vertebrobasilar circulation in a patient with innominate artery occlusion. **A:** Arch aortogram demonstrating innominate artery occlusion (*arrowhead*) and ostial left common carotid artery stenosis (*arrow*) **B:** Left subclavian artery angiography demonstrating antegrade flow along left vertebral artery (1), and retrograde flow along right vertebral artery (2), toward the right subclavian artery (3), and right common carotid artery (CCA) (4). Arrows indicate the direction of flow. (5) Right CCA bifurcation **C:** Selective angiography of left vertebral artery showing that flow from the left to right vertebral artery occurs at the level of the origin of the basilar artery. Arrows indicate the direction of flow.

catheters is important. In the case of the Vitek catheter, the practice is to advance the catheter to the descending-thoracic aorta, direct the tip posteriorly, and then advance the catheter over the arch. This will result in the tip of the catheter engaging the origin of the great vessels sequentially.

Safe removal of the Vitek catheter is accomplished by advancing the catheter into the ascending aorta, passing a long wire through the catheter beyond the tip to straighten the curve, and then removing the catheter and wire in unison. This technique minimizes trauma to the arch from the catheter tip. Owing to the larger primary curve of the Simmons catheter, it is more challenging to use because of the difficulty in reshaping the catheter in the aortic arch. The practice is to

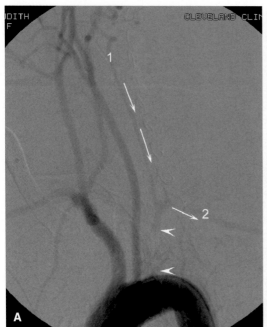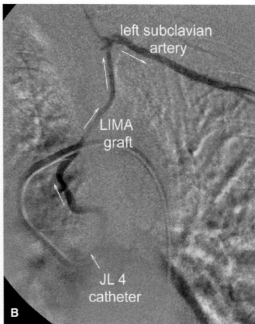

FIGURE 8-4 ● Demonstration of subclavian artery steal from coronary circulation in patient with left subclavian artery occlusion and prior left internal mammary artery (LIMA) graft to left anterior descending artery graft **A:** Arch aortogram demonstrating left subclavian artery occlusion. Arrows indicate the direction of flow, arrowheads delineate the proximal and distal extent of the left subclavian artery occlusion, 1. left vertebral artery, 2. left subclavian artery **B:** Selective angiography of left main coronary artery showing retrograde flow along left internal mammary artery graft toward the left subclavian artery. Arrows indicate the direction of flow.

reshape the catheter in the ascending aorta, advance a soft-tipped wire beyond the tip of the catheter, and then withdraw the catheter into the origin of the great vessels. A similar removal technique for the Simmons catheter is employed, as described, for the Vitek catheter.

TABLE 8-2

Indications for Upper Extremity Angiography

Acute Upper Extremity Ischemia

Extreme arm claudication
Blue digit syndrome
Severe digital ischemia
Blunt trauma with signs of vascular injury
Penetrating trauma with signs of vascular injury

Following selective engagement of the left subclavian artery and brachiocephalic artery, angiography is performed in orthogonal oblique projections. The bifurcation of the brachiocephalic artery and origin of the right subclavian artery is well delineated in the RAO projection. The origins of the right vertebral artery and right internal mammary artery (RIMA) are usually best visualized in the LAO projection. For the left subclavian artery, the origins of the left vertebral artery and left internal mammary artery (LIMA) are usually best visualized in the RAO projection. Subclavian artery angiography is performed with the patient's arm adducted at the patients side (i.e., neutral position). In the specific circumstance when thoracic outlet syndrome causing arterial compression is suspected, angiography is performed in the posteroanterior (PA) projection with the arm in neutral position, and repeated with the shoulder in full abduction, external rotation, and retroversion (i.e., the throwing position).

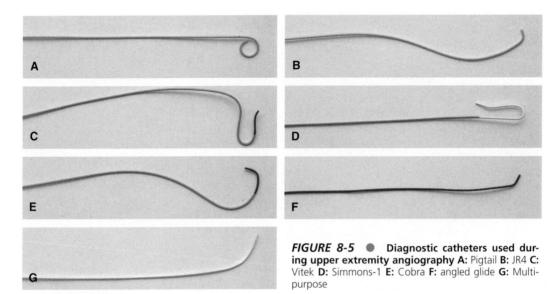

FIGURE 8-5 ● Diagnostic catheters used during upper extremity angiography **A:** Pigtail **B:** JR4 **C:** Vitek **D:** Simmons-1 **E:** Cobra **F:** angled glide **G:** Multipurpose

Axillary and Brachial Artery Angiography

Selective angiography of the axillary or brachial arteries requires delivery of the diagnostic catheter into the distal subclavian artery, beyond the brachiocephalic/left subclavian artery ostium. Following the initial engagement of the respective ostia with the diagnostic catheter, a long (i.e., 300 cm) soft-tipped, 0.035″ wire (e.g., Wholey/Magic Torque®) is advanced into the brachial artery, using the DSA road-mapping function, and then the diagnostic catheter is advanced over this wire. This is a straight forward maneuver when the diagnostic catheter is a JR4 or angled glide catheter. When a Vitek or Simmons catheter is required to engage the respective ostia, an alternative strategy is usually required. In this circumstance, a soft-tipped wire, or stiff-angled glide wire, is advanced into the brachial artery, and the Vitek or Simmons catheter is then exchanged for a 'friendly' diagnostic catheter (e.g., angled glide catheter or multipurpose catheter) (Fig. 8-5[f–g]). The angled glide wire is very steerable but care is required so as not to cause vessel dissection. Additionally, catheter exchanges over this wire are difficult. Axillary artery angiography is performed with the arm in the neutral position or slightly abducted, whereas brachial artery angiography is performed with the arm abducted, and the forearm placed supine on an arm board.

Forearm and Hand Angiography

Adequate angiography of the forearm and hand requires that the diagnostic catheter be advanced to the level of the mid-distal brachial artery, over an appropriate wire (e.g., angled glidewire, Wholey). Liberal administration of vasodilators (e.g., nitroglycerin, calcium channel antagonists) is recommended, because of the propensity of the brachial artery to spasm, and vasodilators may also improve visualization of the digital vessels.

Appropriate positioning of the forearm and hand are important. The forearm and hand must be placed supine on an arm board; the fingers of the hand are splayed, and the thumb is abducted. It is advisable to tape the digits and thumb in this position to minimize motion artifacts. Some operators will wrap the hands with warm cloths to promote vasodilatation and improve visualization of the digital vessels. Angiography is usually performed in the PA projection, although angulated views sometimes may be helpful. For example, during forearm angiography, an ipsilateral-oblique projection may help separate the course of the ulnar, interosseous, and radial arteries.

Interventional Technique

Although subclavian and brachiocephalic artery interventions are often pooled together, brachiocephalic artery intervention presents a number of unique, technical challenges that are not encountered in subclavian artery intervention. Therefore, a description of the technique for subclavian artery intervention is first described, and building on the fundamental principles of that technique, a description of the approach to brachiocephalic-artery intervention follows.

Subclavian Artery Intervention

The vast majority of subclavian artery stenoses are caused by atherosclerotic disease. In most series, the incidence of left subclavian artery stenosis far exceeds that of right subclavian artery stenosis. Stenoses typically involve the first portion of the subclavian artery, and occur proximal to the origin of the vertebral artery (Fig. 8-6). Occlusions generally extend from the ostium of the subclavian artery to the origin of the vertebral artery (Fig. 8-4[a]).

Prior to embarking on a subclavian intervention, a high quality arch aortogram, and selective angiography of the brachiocephalic/right subclavian and left subclavian arteries is required, using the technique described above. For the right subclavian artery, the relation of the proximal extent of the lesion to the innominate and right common carotid artery is critical. Similarly, for the left subclavian artery, assessment of the involvement of the true ostium of the vessel off the aortic arch is an important factor. For both vessels, it is necessary to demarcate the relation of the lesion to the origin of its two critical branches (vertebral and IMA). By defining the arch anatomy and the anatomy of the lesion, the interventional strategy may be planned.

Pharmacology

For patients undergoing planned brachiocephalic or subclavian artery intervention, pre-procedural aspirin (325 mg daily) and clopidogrel (300-mg bolus, 75 mg daily for 2 to 3 days) is administered. Currently, all of our procedures are performed using unfractionated heparin to achieve an activated clotting time (ACT) of approximately 250 to 300 seconds. Use of the direct thrombin inhibitor, bivalirudin, is gaining popularity but data to support its use is still preliminary.

Access

The choice of access site for subclavian artery intervention is strongly influenced by the nature of the obstructive lesion. Stenoses are almost always approached using common femoral artery (CFA) access, since crossing the lesion is generally straightforward, and the antegrade approach offers an advantage in visualizing the ostium of the vessel. Additionally, the CFA access site is associated with fewer access site complications. For occlusions, and particularly for flush occlusions, at the origin of the left subclavian artery, most operators prefer an approach from the ipsilateral brachial artery access site. In such circumstances, additional access from the CFA may be useful to help identify the origin of the vessel, and guide successful crossing of the lesion with the wire. For patients with severe aortoiliac disease, the brachial access is the preferred access site for both stenoses and occlusions. In general, avoid radial artery access for subclavian artery intervention, because of its potential for ischemic access site complications.

CFA Access Site Strategy

When using the CFA access site, a 6-Fr sheath (80 cm long) or 7-Fr to 8-Fr guide-based system may be used (Fig. 8-7). The advantage of the guide-based system is that it provides more support and flexibility during the procedure, although support is generally only an issue for occlusive lesions. In patients with significant peripheral vascular disease, the use of the smaller 6-Fr sheath system may offer some advantage. The goal is to deliver the sheath or guide proximal to the lesion without causing atheroembolism. A telescoping technique is employed to achieve this.

Guide-based system

A long (i.e., 125 cm) diagnostic catheter (JR4, Vitek) is advanced through a guide (e.g., JR4, H-1, Multipurpose) (Fig. 8-8) and is engaged in the origin of the subclavian or brachiocephalic artery. A heavy support 0.014″ (Iron Man®, Guidant®, Platinum Plus®, Boston Scientific®), 0.018″ (Flex T®, Mallinckrodt®), or a soft-tipped 0.035″ wire is advanced into the proximal brachial artery. Ideally, the guide is then

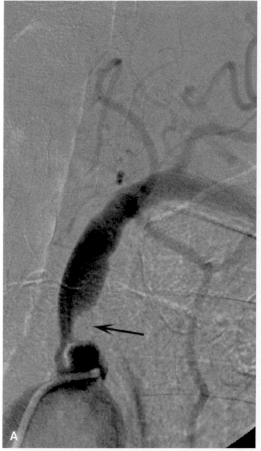

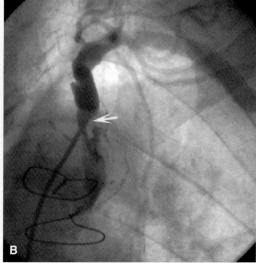

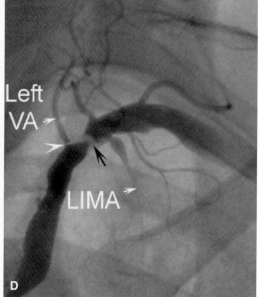

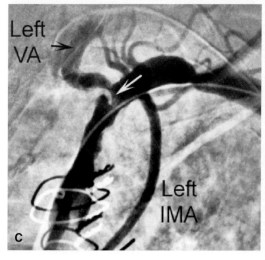

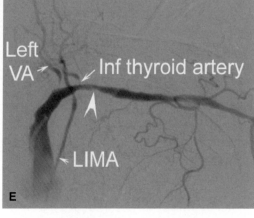

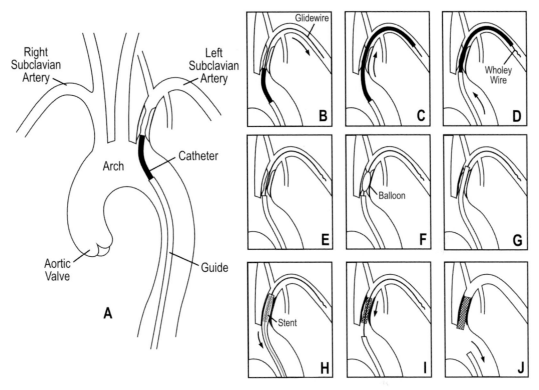

FIGURE 8-7 ● Interventional technique employed for subclavian artery stenosis when using common femoral artery access. See text for details.
Reproduced with permission from Casserly IP, Kapadia SR. Upper extremity intervention. In: Bhatt DL, ed.*The Handbook of Peripheral and Cerebrovascular Intervention*. London; Remedica Publishing: 2004.

advanced over the diagnostic catheter and torqued (e.g., usually counter-clockwise) into the ostium, with subsequent removal of the catheter. Occasionally, the wire will not provide sufficient support for this maneuver, and the diagnostic catheter may have to be advanced across the lesion, prior to advancing the guide. This should not be attempted if the lesion is critical and the risk of atheroembolism with this maneuver is perceived to be high. In this circumstance, the safest option is to engage the guide catheter in the ostium, directly.

Sheath-Based System

When employing a sheath (Fig. 8-8), remove the sheath dilator and telescope the long diag-

nostic catheter through the sheath. The ostium of the brachiocephalic or left subclavian is engaged with the diagnostic catheter, and an 0.035″ wire is passed distally into the proximal brachial artery, as before. The diagnostic catheter is then removed and the sheath dilator combination is advanced proximal to the lesion. It is unlikely that a 0.014″ or 0.018″ wire will provide enough support to allow delivery of the sheath dilator.

Angioplasty

Currently, balloon angioplasty, alone, is rarely performed, as stenting achieves such excellent results. Angioplasty is generally performed prior to stenting to facilitate stent delivery, as most lesions are heavily calcified. It may also provide

FIGURE 8-6 ● **Variation in location of left subclavian artery stenosis. A:** Typical proximal location (*black arrow*); **B:** ulcerated lesion in typical proximal location (*white arrow*); **C:** shelf-like lesion adjacent and proximal to the left vertebral artery (VA); **D:** calcified lesion between the origin of the left vertebral (VA) and left internal mammary (LIMA) arteries; **E:** atypical smooth subclavian stenosis (*white arrowhead*) distal to the left internal mammary branch associated with ostial stenoses in the left vertebral (VA) and inferior thyroid branches in a patient with temporal arteritis.

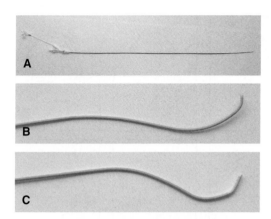

FIGURE 8-8 ● **Sheaths and guides used during subclavian and innominate artery intervention. A:** Shuttle sheath; **B:** JR4 guide; **C:**. H-1 guide

TABLE 8-3

Vessel Size

Vessel	Size (mm)
Innominate	8–11
Subclavian	6–8
Axillary	5–7
Brachial	5–7
Radial	3–4
Ulnar	3–4

some confirmation of the estimated vessel size and length of the lesion. The risk of dissection is minimized by using a conservative approach to balloon sizing, using a balloon diameter approximately 70% of the estimated diameter of the vessel. For most patients this will be approximately 5 mm to 6 mm.

Stenting

Subclavian stenoses proximal to the vertebral artery are usually treated with balloon-expandable stents, owing to the need for accurate stent placement and strong radial force in this location. It should be appreciated that the proximal subclavian artery is an intrathoracic structure and that perforation in this location may result in intrathoracic hemorrhage and significant morbidity or mortality. Therefore, stent sizing should be relatively conservative to minimize this risk. In general, most patients will be treated with 6-mm to 8-mm diameter stents (Table 8-3).

Ostial lesions require attention so that the ostium is fully covered by the stent. This will usually result in 1 mm to 2 mm of free stent in the aortic arch. The ipsilateral oblique view will generally be optimal for this determination. As mentioned above, the use of an antegrade CFA approach is particularly helpful in this setting, as it is very difficult to visualize the ostium when using the brachial approach. Before deployment, it is important to confirm that the origins of the vertebral and IMA branches are not impinged by the stent, which is generally best defined in the

contralateral oblique view. During inflation of the balloon-expandable stent, the patient should be actively questioned as to the presence or absence of pain. Onset of pain is a sign that further expansion may be associated with an increased risk of dissection or perforation and that no further inflation should be performed.

There is some variation in the technique of stent placement. Following angioplasty, some operators will advance the guide or sheath across the lesion and then remove the balloon. The stent is then delivered into the guide and positioned at the site of the lesion, inside the guide or sheath. The guide or sheath is then withdrawn, leaving the stent in position for deployment. This method evolved in an effort to minimize the risk of dislodging the stent from the balloon of the stent-delivery system and subsequent stent embolization. Typically, this occurs when an undeployed stent is withdrawn into the guide or sheath. In our experience, the use of an 0.035″ compatible stent-delivery system, over an 0.014″ wire, increases the risk of stent dislodgement. Therefore, use the appropriately sized wire for the stent-delivery system employed.

For stenoses distal to the vertebral artery, self-expanding stents are generally used. Accurate placement in this location is less critical, and the transition of the subclavian artery into the axillary artery is a flexion point where self-expanding stents are most appropriate.

Brachial Artery Access Site Strategy

The retrograde brachial artery access approach is the preferred strategy for the treatment of the

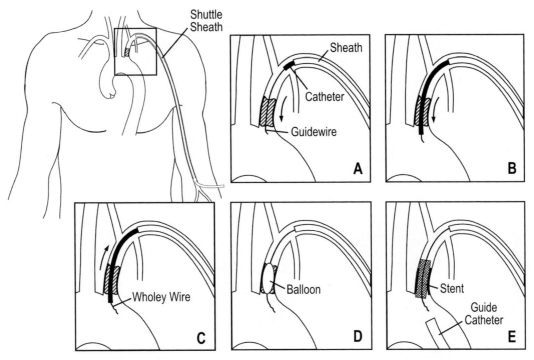

FIGURE 8-9 ● Interventional technique employed for subclavian artery occlusions when using brachial artery access. See text for details.
Reproduced with permission from Casserly IP, Kapadia SR. Upper extremity intervention. In: Bhatt DL, ed. *The Handbook of Peripheral and Cerebrovascular Intervention*. London; Remedica Publishing: 2004.

subclavian artery occlusions, which present a significantly greater technical challenge, as compared to that required for stenoses (Fig. 8-9, Fig. 8-10).

A 6-Fr shuttle sheath (35 mm to 55 mm in length) is advanced with its tip just distal to the occlusion. These occlusions are generally difficult to cross, and will require the use of a 0.035″ stiff-angled glide wire supported by a glide or multipurpose catheter, or an over-the-wire balloon. Occasionally, a stiff 0.014″ wire (e.g., Confianza®, Abbott, Vascular, CROSS-IT® 400XT, Guidant) supported by an over-the-wire balloon may have some utility in crossing these occlusions because these wires have a high degree of directional control. Placement of a diagnostic catheter in the stump of the occlusion may aid in directing the wire toward the true lumen. Finding the true lumen at the ostium of the left subclavian artery is crucial, as dissection at this point will involve the aortic arch and may compromise flow in the other arch branches. Having crossed the lesion, the technique is similar to that outlined above for nonocclusive stenoses.

Accurate positioning of the stent at the ostium of the vessel is again facilitated by injection of contrast agent, via the femoral access site catheter.

Brachiocephalic Artery Intervention

Brachiocephalic artery intervention is more complicated than subclavian artery intervention, owing to the potential for embolization to the anterior cerebral circulation via the right common carotid artery (Fig. 8-11).

The threshold for using embolic protection is, therefore, significantly lowered compared to that of subclavian intervention. Additionally, ensuring patency of both limbs of the brachiocephalic bifurcation, with continued antegrade access, may present a significant technical challenge for true bifurcation lesions.

If the use of an embolic protection device (EPD) is planned, gain right brachial artery access using a 35 cm to 55 cm sheath and CFA access with a short 8-Fr sheath. A 6-Fr IMA guide is advanced through the brachial sheath over an 0.035″ soft-tipped wire, and positioned at the

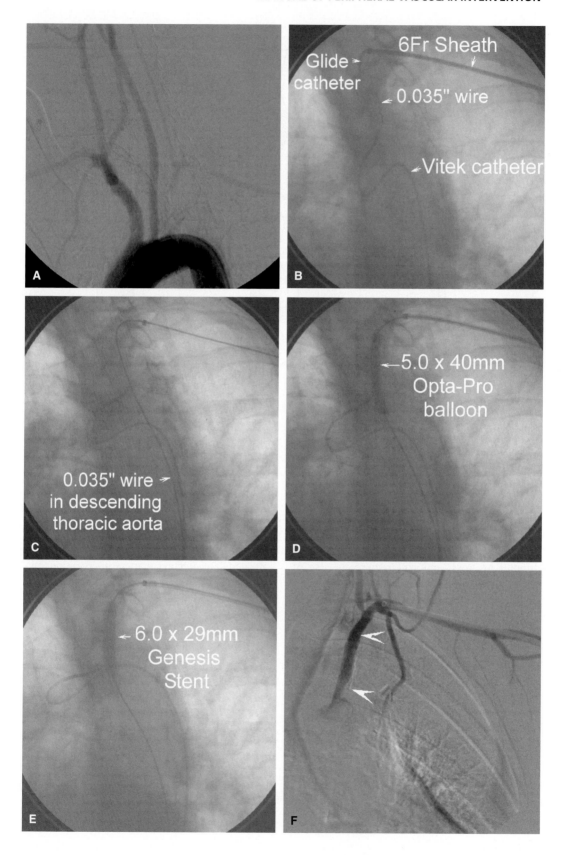

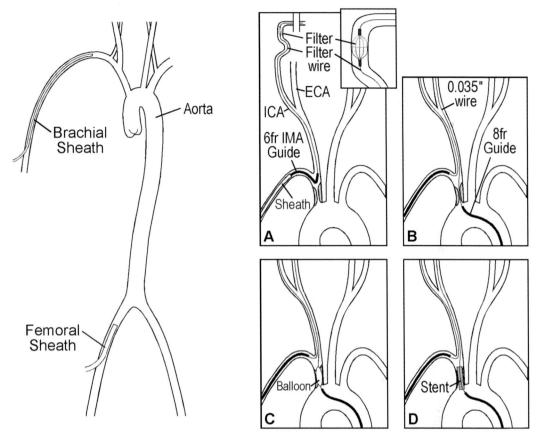

FIGURE 8-11 ● Interventional technique employed for innominate artery stenosis/occlusion when emboli protection is planned. See text for details.

ostium of the right CCA. Through the guide, a filter wire is advanced and the filter positioned in the prepetrous portion of the internal carotid artery (ICA), replicating the position employed during ICA bifurcation interventions. The intervention is then performed from the CFA access site, using a similar technique described above.

For ostial brachiocephalic artery lesions, extra care is required during guide catheter manipulation. Typically, one may employ a multipurpose guide with the intention of staying outside of the ostium of the vessel. Preservation of access to the right CCA will generally

take priority, and the wire from the CFA guide is usually passed toward the right external carotid artery (ECA). Balloon-expandable stents should always be used in this location, and accurate positioning of the stent, with respect to the bifurcation, is usually achieved in the RAO projection. Stent sizes used are typically between 8 mm and 10 mm, in this location (Table 8-3).

OUTCOMES

As with most peripheral vascular interventions, there are no randomized data comparing

FIGURE 8-10 ● **Illustrative case of left subclavian artery occlusion treated using technique outlined in Figure 8-9. A:** arch aortogram showing ostial occlusion of left subclavian artery occlusion; **B:** A Vitek catheter from the right common femoral artery access site is used to engage the ostium of the left subclavian artery to help direct the wire across the lesion toward the true lumen; **C:** wire has successfully crossed lesion and is in descending thoracic aorta; **D:** balloon angioplasty; **E:** stent deployment; **F:** final angiography. Arrows indicate the proximal and distal extent of the stent.

endovascular and surgical revascularization techniques. In addition, there are no randomized data comparing different endovascular strategies. An assessment of the technical success, efficacy, and morbidity and mortality associated with the procedure is derived exclusively from a number of retrospective case series (7–21). These series are now somewhat outdated, in that in some cases angioplasty, alone, was the treatment strategy, or when stents were used, older balloon-expandable (i.e., Palmaz®) and self-expanding (Wallstent®, Strecker®) stents were deployed.

Hadjipetrou et al. reviewed the experience with surgical and endovascular (using stents) revascularization for brachiocephalic and subclavian artery disease (Table 8-4) (10). Despite the limitations of such an observational comparison, the data suggest that endovascular revascularization has equal effectiveness, and is associated with fewer complications, supporting the use of percutaneous revascularization as the therapy of choice for such lesions.

In contemporary series, the technical success for the endovascular treatment of subclavian- and brachiocephalic artery stenosis approaches 100%. Previously, the success rate for total

occlusions in these vessels was significantly less (70 to 80%) (14), but recent series have reported a significant improvement (greater than 90%) attributable to improved technology and the evolution in technique by experienced operators (7,20,21).

The major risk of these procedures is distal embolization. This may occur in the arm (i.e., usually to the digits) or in the posterior cerebral circulation, via the vertebral artery during subclavian or brachiocephalic artery intervention. Embolization to the anterior circulation via the right common carotid artery (CCA) may occur during brachiocephalic intervention. Fortunately, the cumulative rate of significant embolization to these territories has consistently been less than 1% in most series. Previous studies have demonstrated that there is a significant delay (i.e., up to 20 minutes) in the reestablishment of antegrade flow in the vertebral artery following relief of a proximal stenosis (22). This likely explains the low rate of posterior cerebral circulation embolization. It is worth noting that when cerebral events occur, operators have reported a greater relation to manipulation of the aortic arch than to angioplasty or stenting of the subclavian or innominate artery, itself.

Acces site complications are the most common complication reported (0 to 7%). The major risk factor for these events is the use of brachial artery access and highlights the need for particular care when using this access site. Complications include hematoma formation, thrombosis, and pseudoaneurysm formation.

Stent migration is reported in 0 to 6% of case series. This term is often not defined but likely describes both malpositioning of the stent, and the rare occurrence of stent dislodgement from the balloon of the stent-delivery system. Stent malposition may be a problem if critical branch vessels are covered (i.e., vertebral, IMA). Stent dislodgement will require either percutaneous or surgical retrieval. Alternatively, the dislodged stent is occasionally compressed against the vessel wall in a benign location (e.g. common iliac artery).

Prior to the introduction of stents, patients treated with angioplasty, alone, had a reported restenosis rate of 15 to 20% for brachiocephalic- or subclavian artery intervention (16,23). The

TABLE 8-4

Observational Comparison of Endovascular Versus Surgical Revascularization for Innominate and Subclavian Artery Intervention

	Endovascular (n = 108) %	Surgery (n = 2496) %
Technical Success	97 (88–100)	96 (75–100)
Stroke	0	3 (0–14)
Death	0	2 (0–11)
Complications	6 (0–14)*	16 (0–43)†
Recurrence	3 (0–12)	16 (0–50)

Numbers refer to Mean Percent (Range).
* Vascular assess complications and stent dislodgement.
† Stroke/transient ischemic attack, Horner's syndrome, delayed wound healing or infection, graft thrombosis, chylothorax, pneumonia, pleural effusion.
Adapted from Hadjipetrou P, Cox S, Piemonte T, et al. *J Am Coll Cardiol* 1999;33:1238–1245.

advent of stenting has reduced this figure to less than 10% (7,20,21).

A variety of options exist for the management of restenosis, depending largely on the presumed etiology. In cases where restenosis represents a failure to cover the ostium of the vessel adequately, angioplasty of the restenosed area and repeat stenting of the ostium is required. If inadequate stent expansion is suspected, based on the angiographic appearance of the stent or the findings by intravascular ultrasound, more aggressive dilation of the stent may be attempted. If this proves inadequate, re-stenting may be required. In neither of these factors appears operative, repeat angioplasty with gamma-brachytherapy is a reasonable option. Drug-coated stents with a diameter adequate to treat subclavian or brachiocephalic artery stenosis are not available, and are unlikely to be available for the foreseeable future. When endovascular techniques fail, surgical revascularization is an option. Currently, an extrathoracic approach (i.e., carotid-subclavian, axillo-axillary) is the technique employed, owing to the lower morbidity associated with this type of surgical revascularization (Fig. 8-12) (24).

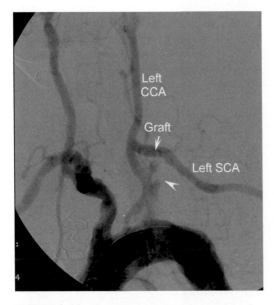

FIGURE 8-12 ● **Arch aortogram demonstrating extrathoracic left common carotid artery (CCA) to left subclavian artery (SCA) graft.** This patient had a prior stent placed in the left subclavian artery that had occlusive restenosis (arrowhead).

POSTPROCEDURAL CARE AND FOLLOW-UP MONITORING

Most patients undergoing subclavian or innominate artery intervention are discharged within 6 to 8 hours of completion of the procedure. High-risk patients are generally admitted overnight for observation. All patients receive prescriptions for life-long aspirin therapy (162 mg to 325 mg daily) and clopidogrel (75 mg daily) for at least 4 weeks. Prior to discharge, blood pressure measurements in both arms should be carefully documented to provide an accurate baseline against which future changes may be compared. During follow-up monitoring, the patients should be assessed for recurrence of symptoms, and any change in upper-extremity blood-pressure measurements. A duplex-ultrasound exam may be performed when these indices suggest recurrence. Early detection of stenosis before progression to occlusion is an important factor in maintaining secondary patency rates above 90 to 95%.

THORACIC-OUTLET SYNDROME

Thoracic-outlet syndrome is a term used to describe the spectrum of clinical presentations caused by compression of the neurovascular structures of the upper extremity (i.e., subclavian artery, subclavian vein, brachial plexus) in the region of the thoracic outlet. In the majority of cases (greater than 90%), symptoms are caused by compression of the brachial plexus and related nerves (25). Arterial and venous compression account for less than 10% of cases, but are responsible for most of the serious morbidity and mortality associated with the condition (26).

Arterial compression in the thoracic outlet usually occurs in the scalene triangle (i.e., bordered by the first rib, scalenus anterior, and scalenus medius muscles) or the subcoracoid space (i.e., bordered by the pectoralis minor muscle, ribs, and coracoid process) and is the least common manifestation of thoracic-outlet syndrome. Extrinsic arterial compression at these sites is typically caused by cervical ribs and congenital fibromuscular bands, and less commonly by anomalies of the first rib, muscular hypertrophy, or excess callus formation following prior clavicular fractures.

Recurrent, chronic, arterial compression leads to intimal and medial vessel injury, producing localized stenosis or occlusion and poststenotic dilation, or occasionally, aneurysmal formation. The formation of collaterals usually minimizes the occurrence of upper-extremity ischemia. Distal thromboembolism is the most typical clinical presentation. Patients are generally young or middle-aged adults.

Angiography is the gold standard for diagnosing extrinsic-arterial compression in the thoracic outlet. Angiography should be performed in the neutral position and repeated in whatever position reproduces the patient's symptoms. Traditionally, these positions will include one or more of the following: depression of the shoulder with the head turned to the symptomatic side (i.e., Adson maneuver), shoulder hyperflexion (i.e., military position), hyperabduction of the arm, and hands above the head (i.e., surrender position). Angiography may reveal normal, smooth, arterial anatomy and compression only with provocative maneuvers (Fig. 8-13).

In addition, angiography may reveal additional features, such as poststenotic dilation, aneurysm formation, thrombosis, or evidence of distal embolization.

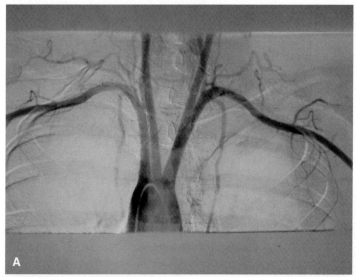

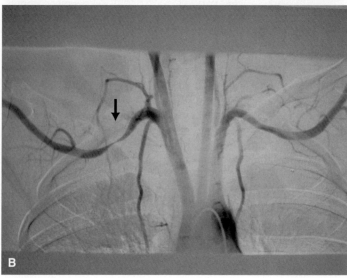

FIGURE 8-13 ● **A:** Arch aortogram with arms in neutral position demonstrating normal angiographic appearance of right subclavian artery; **B:** Arch aortogram from same patients with right arm abducted, externally rotated, and retroverted showing compression of the subclavian artery. (*arrow*)

The treatment of the subclavian arterial compression type of thoracic-outlet syndrome is reserved for patients who are symptomatic or who have evidence of embolization. Surgical decompression of the artery is required and will generally involve resection of the first rib and release of any muscular or ligamentous abnormality. Structural abnormalities of the artery (e.g., aneurysms) are surgically repaired, concomitantly. The presence of unilateral disease should always prompt a search for contralateral involvement and occasionally, prophylactic surgical intervention may be warranted.

REFERENCE

1. Moore KL. The upper limb. In: *Clinically Oriented Anatomy.* 2nd ed. Baltimore, MD: Williams and Wilkins; 1985:626–793.
2. Kadir S. Arteriography of the upper extremities. In: *Diagnostic Angiography.* Philadelphia, PA: Saunders; 1986:172–206.
3. Jaeger HJ, Mathias KD, Kempkes U. Bilateral subclavian steal syndrome: treatment with percutaneous transluminal angioplasty and stent placement. *Cardiovasc Intervent Radiol.* 1994;17:328–332.
4. Chan-Tack KM. Subclavian steal syndrome: a rare but important cause of syncope. *South Med J.* 2001;94:445–447.
5. Elian D, Gerniak A, Guetta V, et al. Subclavian coronary steal syndrome: an obligatory common fate between subclavian artery, internal mammary graft and coronary circulation. *Cardiology.* 2002;97:175–179.
6. Zeitler E, Huttl K, Mathias KD. Subclavian and Brachial Artery Diseases. In: Zeitler E, ed. *Radiology of Peripheral Vascular Diseases.* New York: Springer-Verlag; 2000:591–623.
7. Al-Mubarak N, Liu MW, Dean LS, et al. Immediate and late outcomes of subclavian artery stenting. *Catheter Cardiovasc Interv.* 1999;46:169–172.
8. Angle JF, Matsumoto AH, McGraw JK, et al. Percutaneous angioplasty and stenting of left subclavian artery stenosis in patients with left internal mammary-coronary bypass grafts: clinical experience and long-term follow-up. *Vasc Endovascular Surg.* 2003;37:89–97.
9. Gonzalez A, Gil-Peralta A, Gonzalez-Marcos JR, et al. Angioplasty and stenting for total symptomatic atherosclerotic occlusion of the subclavian or innominate arteries. *Cerebrovasc Dis.* 2002;13:107–113.
10. Hadjipetrou P, Cox S, Piemonte T, et al. Percutaneous revascularization of atherosclerotic obstruction of aortic arch vessels. *J Am Coll Cardiol.* 1999;33:1238–1245.
11. Henry M, Amor M, Henry I, et al. Percutaneous transluminal angioplasty of the subclavian arteries. *J Endovasc Surg.* 1999;6:33–41.
12. Kumar K, Dorros G, Bates MC, et al. Primary stent deployment in occlusive subclavian artery disease. *Cathet Cardiovasc Diagn.* 1995;34:281–285.
13. Martinez R, Rodriguez-Lopez J, Torruella L, et al. Stenting for occlusion of the subclavian arteries. Technical aspects and follow-up results. *Tex Heart Inst J.* 1997;24:23–27.
14. Mathias KD, Luth I, Haarmann P. Percutaneous transluminal angioplasty of proximal subclavian artery occlusions. *Cardiovasc Intervent Radiol.* 1993;16:214–218.
15. McNamara TO, Greaser LE III, Fischer JR, et al. Initial and long-term results of treatment of brachiocephalic arterial stenoses and occlusions with balloon angioplasty, thrombolysis, stents. *J Invasive Cardiol.* 1997;9:372–383.
16. Millaire A, Trinca M, Marache P, et al. Subclavian angioplasty: immediate and late results in 50 patients. *Cathet Cardiovasc Diagn.* 1993;29:8–17.
17. Motarjeme A. Percutaneous transluminal angioplasty of supra-aortic vessels. *J Endovasc Surg.* 1996;3:171–181.
18. Motarjeme A. PTA and stenting of subclavian and innominate arteries. In: White RA, Fogarty TJ, eds. *Peripheral Endovascular Interventions.* 2nd ed. New York: Springer-Verlag; 1999:413–422.
19. Nomura M, Kida S, Yamashima T, et al. Percutaneous transluminal angioplasty and stent placement for subclavian and brachiocephalic artery stenosis in aortitis syndrome. *Cardiovasc Intervent Radiol.* 1999;22:427–432.
20. Rodriguez-Lopez JA, Werner A, Martinez R, et al. Stenting for atherosclerotic occlusive disease of the subclavian artery. *Ann Vasc Surg.* 1999;13:254–260.
21. Sullivan TM, Gray BH, Bacharach JM, et al. Angioplasty and primary stenting of the subclavian, innominate, and common carotid arteries in 83 patients. *J Vasc Surg.* 1998;28:1059–1065.
22. Ringelstein EB, Zeumer H. Delayed reversal of vertebral artery blood flow following percutaneous transluminal angioplasty for subclavian steal syndrome. *Neuroradiology.* 1984;26:189–198.
23. Becker GJ, Katzen BT, Dake MD. Noncoronary angioplasty. *Radiology.* 1989;170:921–940.
24. Paty PS, Mehta M, Darling RC, 3rd, et al. Surgical treatment of coronary subclavian steal syndrome with carotid subclavian bypass. *Ann Vasc Surg.* 2003;17:22–26.
25. Novak CB. Thoracic outlet syndrome. *Clin Plast Surg.* 2003;30:175–188.
26. Hood DB, Kuehne J, Yellin AE, et al. Vascular complications of thoracic outlet syndrome. *Am Surg.* 1997;63:913–917.

The Endovascular Treatment of Acute Ischemic Stroke

Alex Abou-Chebl and Jay S. Yadav

In his essay *Self-Reliance*, Ralph Waldo Emerson wrote, "consistency is the hobgoblin of little minds . . . " In the essay, and this statement in particular, he was expressing his belief that an individual should do what he feels is right, and not what is expected by society. While Mr. Emerson's writings may not apply directly to the treatment and management of patients with cerebrovascular disease, they are not irrelevant.

Cerebrovascular endovascular specialists must, at once, be quite consistent with their meticulous technique and adherence to certain principles related to the nature of the cerebral vasculature, while being willing and able to blaze their own paths with novel approaches to treatments. The wide variety of causes of ischemic stroke (IS), the highly complex clinical manifestations of ischemia, the array of medical conditions that often accompany stroke, and various anatomic and technical factors all conspire to make each patient unique in terms of the endovascular approach to treatment.

Refinements in endovascular techniques and development of novel devices now provide the interventionist with a variety of tools and strategies that may be used to treat the challenging cerebrovascular patient. Creativity and experience are crucial. However, the ability to attempt an invasive treatment must be tempered by the unique qualities of the intracranial cerebral vasculature, which make cerebrovascular interventions very complex and dangerous in ways that are different than other peripheral vascular interventions. What follows is a discussion of these unique qualities, and the endovascular approach to the treatment of acute ischemic stroke.

THE CEREBROVASCULAR CIRCULATION

The major cerebral vessels that are the most amenable to endovascular interventions are also the vessels most commonly involved in the pathogenesis of ischemic stroke. These arteries include the intracranial internal carotid artery (ICA) and its various segments, the middle cerebral artery (MCA), the anterior cerebral artery (ACA), the intracranial vertebral artery (VA), the basilar artery (BA), and the posterior cerebral artery (PCA) (Fig. 9A-1).

These arteries are connected at the base of the brain with three anastomotic channels, the paired posterior communicating arteries, and the single anterior communicating artery, that complete the Circle of Willis, a major source of potential collateral blood supply (Fig. 9A-2).

Cerebral arteries and veins are histologically different from other vessels. The arteries lose their adventitia and external elastic lamina within 1 cm of entering the skull base. As a result, the arteries are more easily damaged with conventional coronary endovascular equipment.

The major cerebral arteries run their courses on the surface of the brain within the subarachnoid space, which is a space constrained by the noncompliant skull, and they supply perforating branches that support the brain tissue.

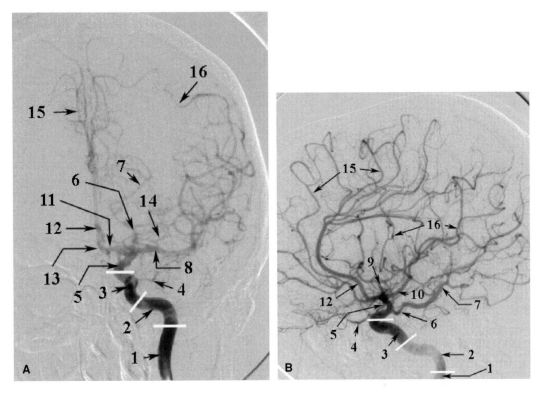

FIGURE 9A-1 ● AP (**A**) and lateral (**B**) cerebral digital subtraction angiograms following selective left internal carotid artery (ICA) injection.

1. Cervical ICA
2. Petrous ICA
3. Cavernous ICA
4. Ophthalmic artery
5. Supraclinoid ICA (ICA terminus)
6. Posterior communicating artery (PCom)
7. Posterior cerebral artery (PCA)
8. Middle cerebral artery, main trunk or M1 segment
9. Superior division of MCA
10. Inferior division of MCA
11. Anterior cerebral artery, pre-communicating/A1 segment
12. Anterior cerebral artery, post-communicating/A2 segment
13. Region of the anterior communicating artery (ACom)
14. Lenticulostriate arteries
15. Distal ACA branches
16. Distal MCA branches   (*continued*)

Perforation of an artery often results in intracranial hemorrhage (ICH), and depending on the location of the perforation, this hemorrhage may occur in the subarachnoid space or cerebral tissue. ICH may lead to a rapid and marked elevation of intracranial pressure (ICP), which in turn may lead to the cessation of cerebral blood flow when the ICP approaches mean arterial pressure (MAP). Intracerebral hemorrhage may lead to tissue disruption and injury, and if large enough, may lead to herniation and brain stem compression. Unlike perforation of a peripheral vessel, which does not lead to immediate tissue injury, subarachnoid and intracerebral hemorrhage may lead to immediate tissue injury and be rapidly fatal. If neurosurgical removal is successfully and safely performed in patients with ICH, the patients' life may be saved but surgery is unlikely to restore normal neurologic function (1,2).

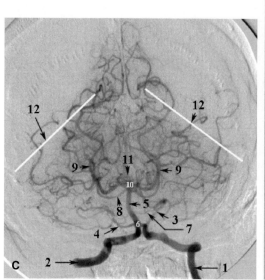
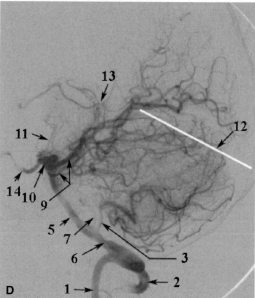

FIGURE 9A-1 ● **C:** and **D:** AP (**C**) and lateral (**D**) cerebral digital subtraction angiograms following selective left vertebral artery (VA) injection.

1. Left VA
2. Right VA
3. Left posterior inferior cerebellar artery (PICA), high but normal origin off left VA
4. Right PICA, anomalous origin from vertebrobasilar junction
5. Basilar artery (BA)
6. Vertebrobasilar junction (VBJ)
7. Left anterior inferior cerebellar artery (AICA)
8. Right superior cerebellar artery (SCA)
9. Bilateral posterior cerebral arteries (PCA),
10. Top-of-the basilar
11. Thalamoperforators
12. Approximate location of the tentorium cerebelli that separates the cerebral hemispheres from the cerebellum (white lines)
13. Posterior choroidal artery
14. Left posterior communicating artery (PCom)

A further, unique characteristic of the cerebral circulation is that the brain is extremely sensitive to embolization. Even minute emboli to a cerebral vessel may cause major clinical syndromes, if a critical area of the brain is affected.

With the above in mind, the following principles should guide all interventional procedures on the cerebral vasculature:

A. Meticulous technique must be used in every aspect of the procedure, in an effort to minimize embolization (i.e., all equipment must be purged of air and kept clean of dried blood and contrast agent, all flushes and contrast should be heparinized unless the patient has a heparin allergy, endovascular tools should not be kept in the cerebrovascular circulation any longer than absolutely necessary, and catheter and wire exchanges should be kept to a minimum).

B. Finesse and gentle technique should be used at all times to prevent vessel perforation. Balloons and stents should be sized accurately to the vessel diameter being treated. One should always err on the side of undersizing rather than oversizing balloons and stents.

ACUTE ISCHEMIC STROKE TREATMENT

The vast majority (85%) of all strokes are ischemic in etiology; the remainder are due to hemorrhage. Ischemic strokes (IS) may be caused by small vessel disease (i.e. lacunar infarcts) or large artery occlusions. It is the patients with large

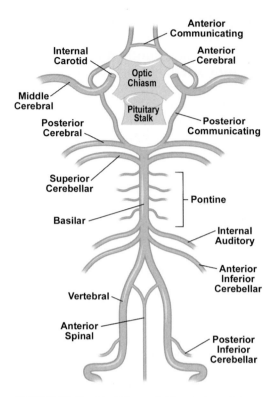

FIGURE 9A-2 ● **Schematic illustration of the anatomy of the Circle of Willis demonstrating the location of the anterior communicating (A Com) and posterior communicating (P Com) arteries.** Note that the A Com branch links the right and left anterior cerebral arteries, and the P Com branch the ipsilateral distal internal carotid artery with the ipsilateral posterior cerebral artery.

artery occlusions who may be treated with endovascular techniques in the setting of an acute event. The goal of endovascular treatment is the rapid recanalization of the occluded vessel, which is the most effective means of preventing neuronal injury and restoring function. This must be accomplished without increasing the risk of ICH.

Unlike the vast numbers of patients enrolled in the various clinical trials of therapies for acute myocardial ischemia, there has been only one randomized study incorporating an endovascular acute stroke treatment (3) and only one successful trial of intravenous thrombolysis (4). Most of the data on various endovascular approaches to acute IS treatment are from small case series and non-randomized safety studies, with marked variation in methodologies and patient populations. The net result is that there are no standardized or widely accepted endovascular techniques for the treatment of acute IS. These

difficulties are attributable not only to the fear of ICH but also to the heterogeneous etiology of stroke.

In contrast to the relatively homogenous mechanism of acute coronary syndromes (ACS) (i.e. atherosclerotic plaque rupture and thrombosis), the mechanism of stroke is highly varied. Within the subset of large artery stroke, large artery occlusion may be caused by embolism from the heart (e.g., left atrial appendage thrombus), aorta (e.g., atheroma), or arterial pathology. In the latter instance, the dominant mechanism of occlusion is atherosclerotic disease that is complicated by localized thrombosis and arterial occlusion, or more distal arterial occlusion resulting from artery-to-artery embolism of thrombus (5). Considering that small artery and cryptogenic (i.e., no definable etiology) strokes account for approximately an additional 25% and 30% of all strokes, respectively, it is clear that no single approach or pharmacologic agent will be effective in all cases. Acute IS treatment must be individualized based on the probable mechanism of ischemia.

The only FDA approved treatment for acute IS is intravenous (IV) recombinant plasminogen activator (rt-PA). Intra-arterial (IA) thrombolysis, although validated to be both safe and effective, is not FDA approved. Non-randomized data suggest that intra-arterial (IA) thrombolysis has superior recanalization efficacy, compared to IV thrombolysis (70% versus 34%) (6), and that this difference is most apparent in larger vessels with greater clot burden. Therefore, IA thrombolysis is generally considered to be the best option for patients with major cerebral vessel occlusions (e.g., occlusions of the internal carotid artery [ICA], middle cerebral artery [MCA], or basilar artery [BA]) (7,8).

As discussed above, there has been only one study that evaluated the safety and efficacy of IA thrombolysis in a placebo-controlled, randomized trial (3). The Prolyse in Acute Cerebral Thromboembolism (PROACT II) trial studied the effects of recombinant prourokinase (r-pro-UK) in 180 patients with MCA occlusions. Compared with IA heparin alone, IA thrombolysis and heparin were associated with improved recanalization rates (defined as TIMI 2 or 3) (66% versus 18%, $P < 0.001$), and a significantly improved neurologic outcome at 90 days (defined as modified Rankin score of less than 2) (40% vs.

25%, $P = 0.04$). These benefits were achieved at the expense of an increased rate of symptomatic hemorrhage in patients treated with IA thrombolysis compared to control patients (10% vs. 2%). For comparison, the ICH rate in the definitive IV rt-PA study that led to FDA approval was 6% (4).

The FDA was unconvinced by these data, and r-pro-UK was not approved for clinical use. In practice however, most clinicians accept the PROACT II results as proof of the safety and efficacy of IA thrombolysis for strokes of less than 6 hours' duration. Many have adopted the "PROACT protocol" using alternative thrombolytic agents in place of r-pro-UK for IA thrombolysis. PROACT II also defined the acceptable rate of symptomatic hemorrhage for IA thrombolysis (i.e., 10%).

The PROACT protocol was remarkable for its stringent inclusion criteria and standardized protocol. All patients received the same doses of peri-procedural heparin, which consisted of a 2,000 U bolus at the start of the procedure, followed by a 500 U per hour infusion for 4 hours only. The total r-pro-UK dose was 9 mg in each of the treatment patients, irrespective of the clot burden, and it was infused over 2 hours. Furthermore, mechanical disruption of the thrombus was not permitted. As a result, although there was approximately a 70% recanalization rate (TIMI 2 and 3) at 2 hours, normal antegrade flow (i.e., TIMI 3 flow) was restored in only 19% of patients (3).

Beyond the currently accepted window for treatment (6 hours for IA thrombolysis and 3 hours for IV thrombolysis), IA thrombolysis may still be useful in circumstances where IV thrombolysis is contraindicated. These include patients with recent nonintracranial hemorrhage, recent surgery or arterial puncture, and patients on systemic anticoagulation; all of these factors increase the risk of ICH and systemic hemorrhage with IV thrombolysis. Although these risks exist with IA thrombolysis as well, the smaller doses of thrombolytics needed for IA thrombolysis minimize the risk (9).

PATIENT SELECTION

The indications and contraindications to IA thrombolysis are listed in Table 9A-1.

TABLE 9A-1

Indications and Contraindications for Intra-arterial Thrombolysis

Indications

Acute, ischemic stroke <6 hours in duration

Stroke is significant, (i.e., disabling or life threatening)

Suspected occlusion of a large artery, (i.e., non-lacunar stroke syndrome)

No hemorrhage on screening computed tomography (CT) scan

Contraindications

Intracerebral hemorrhage is suspected or evident on CT

History of ICH or SAH

History of dementia of Alzheimer's type

Stroke duration is unknown or is > 6 hours, or the patient has had a recent stroke within 3 months

Bleeding diathesis, elevated INR >1.7, or thrombocytopenia <100,000 cells/mm^3

Relative contraindications

Active treatment with heparin or heparinoid, high dose aspirin or clopidogrel, or platelet GP IIb/IIIa receptor antagonist

---

INR, International Normalized Ratio; GP, glycoprotein; ICH, intracranial hemorrhage; SAH, subarachnoid hemorrhage.

In general, the indications for IA thrombolysis are situations in which a patient has a moderate-to-severe deficit but may not receive IV thrombolysis. Patients who present with minor, non-disabling deficits should not be considered for IA thrombolysis, because in those patients, although the prognosis for recovery is relatively better, the probability of finding a large artery occlusion that would potentially be better treated with IA thrombolysis is small. In general, occlusion or severe flow limitation of a major vessel of the Circle of Willis causes at least moderate deficits, whereas occlusion of small, distal, cortical branches or perforating vessels cause more mild deficits.

Although it is beyond the scope of this chapter to delve into the various means for measuring the severity of a stroke, the most accepted and standardized method used is the National Institutes of Health Stroke Scale (NIHSS) (10). This scale, which ranges from 0 (normal) to 42 (no neurologic function), is based on a

12-item, focused, neurologic examination. In general, strokes in the 0 to 3 range are considered minor, those between 4 and 7 are considered mild, those between 8 to 15 are moderate, and strokes with scores of more than 15 are severe.

The NIHSS value may also suggest the size of the vessel involved. For example it is very unusual for lacunar strokes (small vessel) to cause deficits that score more than 8 points. On the other hand, MCA occlusions typically cause strokes with a severity of between 10 to 20 points, and ICA and BA occlusions often cause deficits that score greater than 20 points. In addition the NIHSS value has prognostic value. Deficits with a score of less than 4 are more likely to resolve completely, whereas patients with a score of more than 20 are less likely to derive benefit from any treatment, including IV and IA thrombolysis (3). Patients with a score of 8 to 20 are the most likely to benefit from intervention and are also less likely to have hemorrhagic transformation, so they are the ideal group of patients to select for IA thrombolysis. The assistance of a neurologist, who has particular expertise in cerebrovascular disease, is very helpful in selecting the appropriate patient for intervention.

The time of stroke onset must be known with certainty before an intervention may be performed. This is because of the relationship between time of onset and the risk of ICH (11,12). Six hours appears to be the upper limit for safe intervention. As a rule, the earlier the treatment, the better the prognosis. Treatment should not be delayed needlessly if an intervention is to be performed, it should be considered a medical emergency.

The contraindications to IA thrombolysis are all based on the need to decrease the risk of ICH (Table 9A-1). A history of ICH at any time in the recent, or remote past should be considered an absolute contraindication, in most cases. Similarly, patients with Alzheimer's disease, who are predisposed to ICH, should be considered as very high-risk for IA lysis. The presence of a coagulopathy or bleeding diathesis is an obvious exclusion. It should be stressed that the exclusion of an existing ICH must be performed with certainty (12). A computerized tomographic (CT) scan of the brain is mandatory in all patients presenting with acute IS, owing to its high sensitivity and specificity for ICH.

TECHNIQUE

Diagnostic Angiography

There are three stages in the performance of an acute stroke intervention. The first phase is the screening and preparation stage. The second is the completion of the diagnostic angiogram and its interpretation. The third stage is the actual intervention itself.

Patient screening was described above. During this screening phase, the endovascular team should be made aware that there is a patient for potential intervention. When the decision to proceed with angiography and possible intervention is made, there should be no delay in transferring the patient to the endovascular suite, where all of the equipment should be ready or readily available. The pharmacologic agent of choice (see below) should be ordered from the pharmacy and thawed if needed, in preparation.

Access is obtained via the femoral artery with a 6-Fr short sheath. Ideally, aortic arch angiography should be performed, particularly in older patients, or if selective engagement of the symptomatic vessel is difficult. A 5-Fr diagnostic catheter is used to engage the symptomatic artery rapidly. Ipsilateral common carotid angiography should be performed if the patient has symptoms of anterior circulation ischemia. The carotid bifurcation and ICA origin should be visualized first, followed by intracranial imaging.

The intracranial ICA and MCA are best visualized with both an anteroposterior (AP) image (i.e., with slight cranial angulation) and a lateral image. In both circumstances the entire inner table of the skull should be included in the field of view, so that the venous structures may be visualized as well. Digital subtraction angiography (DSA) is performed with a rapid injection of 4 mL to 5 mL of contrast, and image capture is continued until the end of the venous phase.

The patient should be advised to hold completely still, and not breathe or swallow during the cineangiogram. This is important because the angiographic findings may occasionally be subtle. Occlusion of the ICA or MCA trunk are easily seen but branch occlusions, delayed arterial filling and emptying, and early arteriovenous shunting may be difficult to visualize, and require that close inspection of the angiographic findings be performed (Figs. 9A-3[F] and 9A-3[H]).

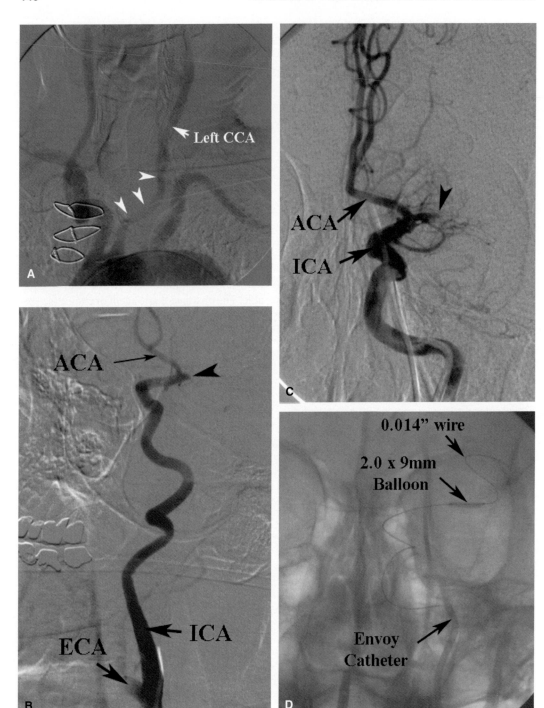

FIGURE 9A-3 ● **An 83-year old man presented within 3 hours of onset of a severe left hemispheric stroke. A:** Aortic arch angiography showed moderate tortuosity of the proximal left common carotid (CCA) (*arrowheads*). **B:** Selective angiography of the left common carotid artery showed marked tortuosity of the left cervical internal carotid artery (ICA), external carotid artery, (ECA). **C:** An AP intracranial angiogram of the left ICA shows an abrupt occlusion in the proximal portion of the M1 segment of the middle cerebral artery (MCA) (*arrowhead*), anterior cerebral artery, (ACA). **D:** Using the technique described in the text, an 8-Fr sheath was placed in the distal CCA and a 6-Fr Envoy guide catheter was placed in the distal, cervical ICA. A Synchro 0.014″ wire was passed through the thrombus and placed distally, permitting passage of a microcatheter into the thrombus, through which 20 mg of rt-PA was infused, with no improvement in flow. A 2 mm diameter × 9 mm length coronary balloon was advanced into the MCA and inflated twice.

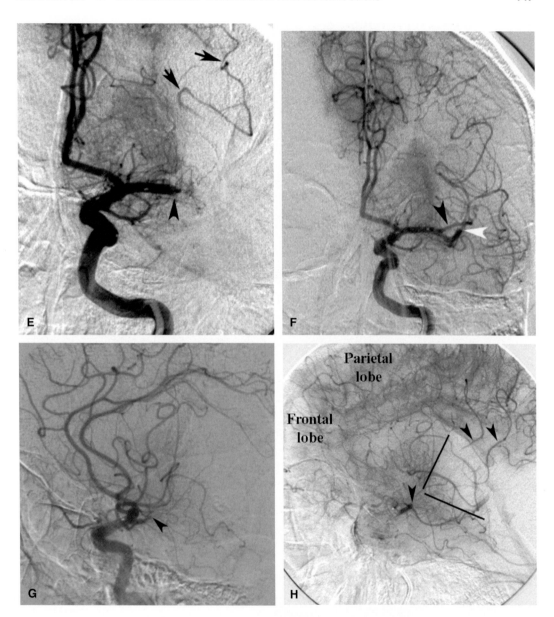

FIGURE 9A-3 ● *(Continued)* **E:** Angiogram following angioplasty demonstrating partial recanalization of the proximal MCA *(arrowhead)*. Note the retrograde flow to the distal MCA territory via pial collaterals from the ACA *(arrows)*. A one-half bolus of abciximab was given directly into the thrombus and angioplasty was repeated twice. **F:** AP intracranial angiogram 10 minutes later demonstrated recanalization of the MCA trunk, with filling of the superior division of the MCA (black arrowhead) and persistent occlusion of the inferior division (white arrowhead). **G:** and **H:** Early **(G)** and late **(H)** image from lateral intracranial angiogram confirming that the inferior division of the MCA is occluded (black arrowheads). Note the absence of a capillary phase in a wedge-shaped distribution in G (delineated by black lines), which is characteristic. Also note the retrograde pial collaterals from the ACA (arrows). An additional 10 mg of rtPA was given with no effect. *(Continued)*

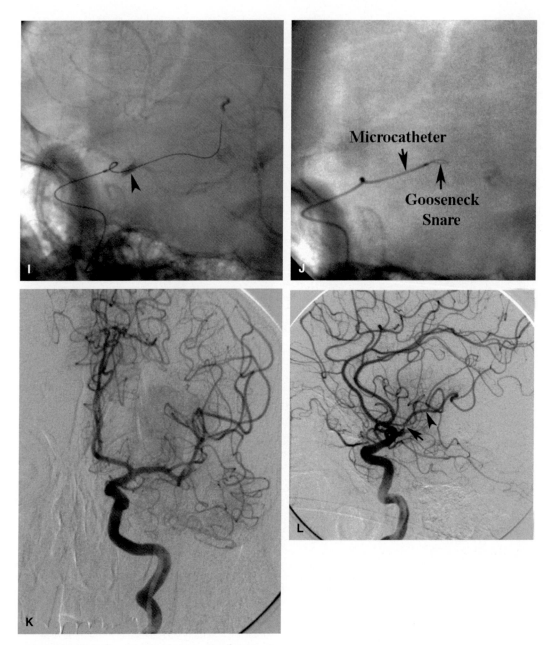

FIGURE 9A-3 ● *(Continued)* **I:** The Synchro wire was passed into the inferior division of the MCA. Note the persistent contrast staining that is characteristic of the presence of thrombus *(arrowhead)*. **J:** A microcatheter was then passed through the thrombus, through which a gooseneck snare was advanced and deployed distal to the thrombus. The snare was withdrawn while suction was applied to the guide catheter with a 60cc syringe. **K:** and **L:** Subsequent AP **(K)** and lateral **(L)** intracranial angiography demonstrated TIMI II flow through the inferior division *(arrowhead in L)*, although there was a persistent filling defect in its proximal portion *(arrow in L)*. The procedure was terminated and intravenous heparin at 500U/hr was continued for 4 hours. The patient began to recover within hours and had only a mild neurologic deficit two days later.

Following angiography of the symptomatic vessel, cannulation of the contralateral carotid artery and at least one vertebral artery (e.g., usually the left or dominant vertebral artery) should be performed, to search for evidence of collateral blood flow from either the anterior communicating artery, the posterior communicating artery, or pial collaterals from the posterior cerebral artery (PCA) to the MCA or ACA, or vice versa. Collaterals are a positive prognostic sign and their absence suggests a high likelihood of infarction of the affected territory, even if rapid recanalization is achieved. The complete absence of collateral blood flow to the affected region should be considered a relative contraindication to thrombolysis, owing to the high likelihood of the existence of complete tissue infarction with subsequent hemorrhagic transformation (13).

In addition, angiography is performed to exclude the presence of large aneurysms or arteriovenous malformations (AVM), or vascular brain tumors, each of which should be considered to be contraindications to thrombolysis, owing to the risk of ICH. If an arterial dissection is found, thrombolysis should be performed with caution. Although most spontaneous dissections are extracranial, some may spread intracranially, or may originate in the intracranial vessels. With intracranial extension, there is a risk of pseudoaneurysm formation and subarachnoid hemorrhage, even without the use of thrombolytics and anticoagulants.

For suspected ischemia in the vertebrobasilar (VB) circulation, angiography of the dominant VA, as defined from the arch aortogram or MR angiography, should be performed. Where there is codominance of the vertebral arteries, angiography of the left VA is preferred because it is technically easier to cannulate. Following engagement of the appropriate subclavian artery, a nonselective angiogram of the VA ostium (i.e., V1 segment) should be performed (i.e., in the contralateral oblique projection), followed by selective engagement of the VA, and selective angiography. One should be aware of the variety of anomalies of the origin of the VA, the most common of which involves the origin of the left VA, directly off the aortic arch from between the origins of the left

common carotid and left subclavian arteries (Fig. 9A-4).

Once the VA is cannulated, digital subtraction angiography should be performed with a gentle rise time and lower injection rates than in the carotid, owing to the smaller size of the VA. An ipsilateral oblique view visualizes the V2 and V3 segments, and lateral and steep PA cranial views visualize the V4 segment, and basilar and posterior cerebral arteries. When using a wire to facilitate delivery of a catheter into the origin of the VA, one needs to be aware that the VA may supply small arterial feeders, which arise medially from its cervical portion, to the anterior spinal artery. Therefore, the wire tip should be pointed laterally, when possible, to avoid precipitation of a spinal cord infarct.

Access

One of the critical factors that determine the chances of procedural success is the ability to achieve stable access to the site of occlusion or stenosis. In elderly patients with tortuosity and sharp angulation of non-compliant cervicocranial vessels, delivery of equipment to the intracranial vessels is very challenging. In general, our practice is to deliver a long, 8-Fr sheath proximal to the area of interest. A 6-Fr Envoy guide is telescoped through the guide to a more distal site, closer to the lesion, to provide additional support. The interventional equipment is then delivered through the guide and the procedure completed, using 0.014″ wires and 0.014″ compatible devices.

Carotid Distribution Intervention

For most carotid distribution stroke interventions, a 55-cm 8-Fr shuttle sheath is delivered from the femoral artery to the distal CCA. The length and diameter of the sheath used is critical. An 8-Fr diameter is required to allow delivery of the 6-Fr envoy, and to provide sufficient support. Sheath length is important to accommodate the limited length of guides (i.e., generally about 100 cm), and balloon and stent delivery systems. Using too long a sheath may limit one's ability to treat distal lesions. In larger individuals with proximal tortuosity in the iliac vessels, aorta, or

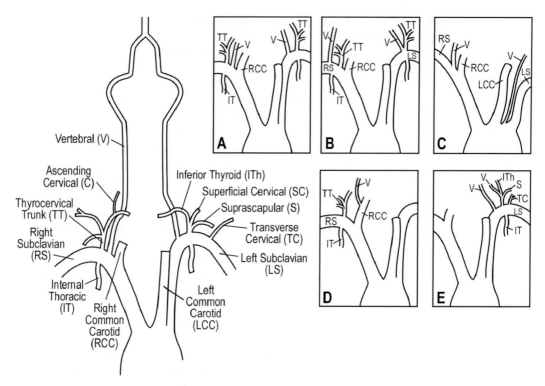

FIGURE 9A-4 ● Normal and variant anatomy of the origin of the vertebral artery. A: Normal origin of the right and left vertebral artery as the first branch from the proximal subclavian artery. **B:** Origin of the vertebral artery lateral to or as common trunk with thyrocervical trunk. **C:** Origin of the left vertebral artery from the aortic arch between the origin of the left common carotid and left subclavian arteries. **D:** Origin of the right vertebral artery from right common carotid artery, typically in patients with anomalous origin of the right subclavian artery. **E:** Dual or accessory origin of the vertebral artery from the aortic arch or thyrocervical trunk.

carotid artery, a 70-cm to 80-cm length sheath may be required, to allow the sheath to reach the distal CCA and provide sufficient support. The method of delivery of the sheath is identical to that for the treatment of carotid artery bifurcation lesions, as described in Chapter 6 (Carotid Intervention).

Having successfully delivered the sheath to the distal CCA, an angiogram should be performed to confirm appropriate placement and the absence of any dissection. A floppy angled GlideWire may be advanced with care, and under roadmap guidance, just beyond the petrous portion of the ICA. Over this wire, the 6-Fr Envoy guide is telescoped through the sheath and advanced to the distal cervical portion of the ICA (i.e. just proximal to the petrous portion of the ICA). This combination of a 6-Fr guide in the distal cervical ICA, supported by an 8-Fr sheath in the distal CCA, provides an ad-

equate platform for most distal ICA and MCA interventions.

Vertebrobasilar Distribution Intervention

For vertebrobasilar (VB) interventions, a variation of the procedure described above is used. The 8-Fr sheath is delivered to the proximal subclavian artery, using the techniques outlined in Chapter 8 (i.e., Subclavian, Brachiocephalic, and Upper Extremity intervention). A floppy GlideWire is then used to wire the vertebral artery, with its tip positioned in the V3 segment. The 6-Fr Envoy guide is then telescoped through the sheath, and advanced over the wire, to the distal portion of the V2 segment. Vertebrobasilar access may be quite difficult if there is severe, proximal tortuosity, as even a rigid sheath may have a tendency to fall out of the subclavian artery, particularly the right subclavian artery. In those cases, there are two options: the first is to place a stiff 0.018″ wire (e.g. IronMan) or 0.035″ nonhydrophilic wire distally, within the axillary or brachial arteries, for added support. Alternatively, the case may be approached using brachial access, with insertion of a 35-cm to 55-cm long, 6-Fr sheath into the subclavian, with its tip positioned just distal to the VA origin.

Anticoagulation

Once the decision has been made to proceed with an endovascular approach to stroke treatment, and access has been obtained, anticoagulation with IV heparin is required. If mechanical interventions are planned (i.e. angioplasty, stenting), a bolus of IV heparin is administered to achieve a target activated clotting time (ACT) of 250 to 300 seconds. If no mechanical manipulations are planned, the PROACT II regimen for heprin dosing (outlined above) is followed.

Recanalization Technique

A necessary prerequisite for recanalization of an occluded or stenotic lesion is the ability to cross the lesion with a 0.014″ wire. Most commonly, either the Synchro wire or occasionally, the Whisper wire is employed. The diseased segment should be crossed very carefully, remembering that the intracranial vessels have no adventitia and are easily perforated. The wire tip should be kept free and mobile at all times. Any buckling or loss of ability to torque the wire tip should raise awareness of the possibility of actual, or impending, subintimal migration. In advancing the wire through the diseased segment, the operator must also be aware of the normal branches arising from that segment, and their usual courses, so that the wire is not directed, inadvertently, into one of the small branches, thereby increasing the risk of perforation.

The essential branches of the ICA that the operator needs to be aware of include the ophthalmic artery arising anteriorly, the posterior communicating artery (PCom) arising posteriorly from the carotid siphon (terminus), and the smaller anterior choroidal artery also arising posteriorly, just distal to the PCom (Figs. 9A-1[A] and 9A-1[B]). The MCA has multiple branches, which arise superiorly (dorsally) along the majority of the main trunk (i.e., M1); therefore, the wire tip should be pointed downwardly in the AP view, when it is being passed through the M1 trunk, to avoid entering these branches. The MCA bifurcation may be variable in its location; the MCA may bifurcate normally, with a long M1 trunk and two main branches arising just as the MCA enters the Sylvian fissure and takes an upward (dorsal) course, or the bifurcation may be early or may even be a tri- or quad-furcation. Often the anterior temporal artery may arise inferiorly (i.e., ventrally) anywhere in the distal third of the M1 trunk.

The VA has several muscular branches in its distal cervical segments and the posterior inferior cerebellar artery (PICA) may often arise extracranially at the C1 level and should not be cannulated inadvertently (Figs. 9A-1[C] and 9A-1[D]). Intracranially, the VA gives off the PICA dorsally, and just before the VB junction, each VA gives off a very small vessel, the anterior spinal artery to the spinal cord, dorsomedially. The BA has multiple, nearly microscopic, perforating branches posteriorly (i.e., dorsally) that supply the pons and midbrain. The large, paired, anterior inferior cerebellar arteries (AICA) arise laterally, at the juncture of the proximal and middle thirds of the BA, and the paired superior-cerebellar arteries (SCA) arise laterally, at the BA terminus, just before the BA bifurcation into the posterior cerebral arteries (PCA).

The wire tip should be carefully maneuvered into the largest possible third-order MCA and PCA branches for adequate support (Fig. 9A-2[D]). Careful shaping of the wire tip is essential; typically, a short primary curve and a longer secondary curve on the wire tip are employed.

Wire placement may be greatly facilitated by loading it first through a microcatheter or over-the-wire balloon angioplasty catheter, which provide support for wire delivery. If there is a low likelihood of underlying atherosclerotic plaque, and thrombolysis is the first planned treatment, then a microcatheter (e.g. RapidTransit or TurboTracker) may be more appropriate, so that thrombolysis may be begun immediately. However if there is a high likelihood of underlying stenosis, then loading the wire through a small, 1.5 mm to 2.5 mm diameter, flexible, over-the-wire balloon catheter (e.g. Maverick, Cross-Sail) will facilitate a more prompt angioplasty. In almost all intracranial interventions, an over-the-wire balloon catheter is preferred to the use of a rapid-exchange system because it permits wire exchanges and is, generally, more deliverable to tortuous segments.

Having successfully crossed the lesion with a wire, there are several approaches to achieve recanalization. Most centers and reported series use thrombolytics alone, essentially replicating the PROACT II protocol but using an alternative thrombolytic agent (14). Some use a combination of pharmacologic agents, while others use a purely mechanical approach (15). The authors prefer a multimodal approach, combining multiple pharmacologic agents and mechanical disruption (Fig. 9A-3) (16). We feel this approach is superior because of the heterogenous nature of IS. Not all thrombi are composed of the same fibrin/platelet ratio and not all emboli are composed of thrombus. For patients with a high likelihood of a cardioembolic cause of the stroke, one may give higher doses of thrombolytics than would be used for patients with an atherothrombotic lesion (i.e., for whom glycoprotein (GP) IIb/IIIa inhibitors may be combined with thrombolytics and angioplasty, or even stenting). In general, the treatment is tailored to the needs of each patient. Again, however, it is emphasized that the technique that has been studied and used the most is the infusion of a thrombolytic agent alone, mostly rt-PA, delivered through a microcatheter. This approach should be considered the first-line treatment for use by operators without much experience in acute IS treatment.

IA thrombolysis

Even among interventionists who perform IA thrombolysis alone, there is some variation in technique. Some operators infuse the thrombolytic agent distal to the occlusion. This approach carries a risk of distal embolization, so another approach is to place the microcatheter within the thrombus and to infuse the pharmacologic agents directly into the thrombus. Even greater sources of variation in IA thrombolysis involve the choices of pharmacologic agent, as well as the bolus doses, and the rates and durations of infusions.

The most widely used thrombolytic agent is rt-PA (17,18). Other commonly used agents

include streptokinase, urokinase, reteplase, and tenecteplase (15,19,20). The only agent whose efficacy and safety were validated in a controlled trial, r-pro-UK, is not commercially available.

One agent in particular, streptokinase, is no longer used and should be avoided because in early studies, it was associated with an excessive risk of ICH (21). Although, rt-PA is the most commonly used agent, there is a suggestion that it may not be ideal because it has some neurotoxic effects, and it may be associated with a higher risk of ICH than other agents (22). The optimal dose of each agent is unknown. The doses that have been used in the various reported series have ranged from 5 mg to 50 mg of rt-PA, 250,000 units to 1,000,000 units of urokinase, and 1 unit to 8 units of reteplase. In general, lower doses of thrombolytics are used for stroke thrombolysis than are used for coronary thrombolysis, and the IA doses of rt-PA average between 20 to 50% of those used for IV coronary thrombolysis. The adage "it is easier to add than it is to remove" should be kept in mind when dosing these agents, owing to the risk of ICH. The dosing of each agent is adjusted to the needs of each patient rather than adhering to a fixed-dose schema. The dose is based on the presence, or absence, of several patient characteristics that are associated with higher risks of ICH or poor prognosis, namely: increasing patient age (i.e., older than 80 years), hypertension, duration of ischemia (i.e., more than 4 hours), the absence of collateral blood flow, underlying brain infarct greater than one-third to one-half of MCA territory, and associated coagulopathy or thrombocytopenia. The presence of several of these factors would lead the authors to avoid thrombolytics completely, and to use a purely mechanical approach, whereas the absence of all of the factors would favor an aggressive approach, particularly if the clinical deficit is severe. The dose is further modified based on the estimated clot-burden size, and the intended use of other agents or aggressive mechanical manipulation during the intervention (23).

A rapid infusion of thrombolytics is given in two to three boluses, over a 30-minute period, directly into the thrombus. Slow infusions, as practiced in the PROACT II trial, take an inordinately long time to achieve thrombolysis.

In addition, between boluses of thrombolytics, it is possible to perform mechanical disruption to facilitate thrombolytic diffusion and thrombolysis. This is yet another aspect of IA thrombolysis that has not been studied systematically, and no approach has been proved superior to another.

Glycoprotein IIb/IIIa Inhibitors

Platelet GP IIb/IIIa receptor antagonists are a mainstay in the treatment of acute coronary syndromes. In addition, there are new data on their efficacy and safety, in the setting of acute IS (24). GP IIb/IIIa receptor antagonists have been used in combination with IA thrombolytics quite successfully, without significantly increasing the risk of ICH (15,16). These agents may facilitate thrombolysis when combined with a thrombolytic agent because thrombi are often composed of a combination of aggregated platelets bound with fibrin strands (25). The two most commonly used agents are abciximab and eptifibatide. We typically administer a GP IIb/IIIa receptor antagonist early, particularly if planning to perform balloon angioplasty. The typical bolus doses employed are similar to those used to treat acute coronary syndromes, although the preference is to start slowly and give more as needed (e.g., divide conventional abciximab bolus into four boluses, administered 5 to 10 minutes apart). The GP IIb/IIIa inhibitor doses are alternated with boluses of thrombolytic agent. These agents are typically infused intravenously, but IA administration directly into the thrombus, through the microcatheter, has occasionally facilitated thrombolysis (16). The authors have used abciximab more frequently than eptifibatide, but there are no data showing that one is superior to the other in this setting. A continuous infusion is rarely administered following successful thrombolysis, but if a stent is placed, or there is an underlying atherosclerotic plaque and small doses of thrombolytics were used, one may continue a peripheral IV GP IIb/IIIa antagonist infusion for 12 hours. The risk of ICH appears to be low with this approach, but this has not been studied in a randomized fashion; therefore extreme caution must be exercised and the interventionist should have prior experience using these agents before using them for the first time to treat an acute IS.

Mechanical Clot Disruption—Wires, Angioplasty, Stenting, Embolectomy

One may combine a mechanical approach with pharmacologic thrombolysis for the treatment of acute stroke. In the PROACT II trial, mechanical disruption was prohibited and that may account for the generally low rate of TIMI-3 flow at 2 hours (19%). Mechanical manipulation may consist of something as simple as repeated passes of the guidewire or microcatheter through the thrombus or a more elaborate approach, with embolectomy, angioplasty, and stenting. Mechanical manipulation adds complexity to the procedure and may increase the risk of vessel perforation and embolization, so great care should be taken to avoid traumatizing the underlying vasculature.

Wire manipulation of the thrombus works best for smaller amounts of fresh thrombus, whereas larger clot burdens, or occlusions caused by atherothrombosis, are unlikely to be disrupted sufficiently with wire manipulation. Adjunctive balloon angioplasty for acute stroke has been reported, both in combination with other techniques, or as the sole treatment (16,26–28). Gentle balloon angioplasty with undersized coronary balloons, may be performed in most patients who do not respond quickly to thrombolysis (Figs. 9A-2[D] and 9A-2[E]). In particular, individuals in whom a thrombotic occlusion has formed over an underlying stenosis may benefit greatly from angioplasty. Patients of African or Asian descent and those with diabetes mellitus are particularly prone to intracranial atherosclerosis and this mechanism should be considered in the treatment decision process (29). Since many of these thrombi often have a gelatinous consistency, the inflations should be somewhat prolonged, typically of 1 to 2 minutes' duration, and multiple inflations may be required. As mentioned previously, angioplasty is generally performed between boluses of pharmacologic agents, as this represents the most efficient use of the time delay between drug boluses. The use of adjuvant GP IIb/IIIa antagonists should be given strong consideration in patients treated with angioplasty, owing to the likelihood of iatrogenic endothelial injury.

In some circumstances, stenting of the occluded vessel may be required. The authors have treated several patients with stents in the acute phase of a stroke; some were treated with stenting alone (i.e. without thrombolysis [unpublished data]). All of these patients and the few reported in the literature have had severe, underlying stenoses, either of the intracranial or extracranial vessels (30). These lesions are thought to have a high propensity for both early, and delayed, reocclusion. Stenting may result in optimal recanalization in the acute phase, and may reduce the risk of subsequent reocclusion. Adequate platelet inhibition is absolutely essential in these cases, and patients should receive GP IIb/IIIa antagonists intraprocedurally, in addition to clopidogrel and aspirin, as soon as possible after the intervention if they have not already received it. This approach is quite novel and should not be considered as standard of care. However, in the authors' experience, it may be safely performed in carefully selected patients.

Mechanical embolectomy (i.e., clot removal) is an alternative to thrombolysis. An alternative is needed because the major limitation of thrombolysis is the speed of recanalization. Furthermore, thrombolysis is performed under the assumption that all thrombi and emboli may be pharmacologically lysed. In some circumstances, pharmacologic thrombolysis may be contraindicated or ineffective. By physically removing the clot in one piece, thrombolysis may not be required, or the doses may be greatly reduced. Unfortunately, although there are several devices under investigation, none are approved for the treatment of acute stroke (31,32). There are commercially available snares, which are designed for the removal of foreign bodies, that have been used by some to remove thrombi successfully (33,34). One such snare is the GooseNeck snare. Snaring is reserved for patients who have probable cardioemboli, because such emboli are often resistant to thrombolysis, and are less likely to be attached to an underlying plaque. The technique of snaring is straightforward. A 0.014″ guidewire and microcatheter are passed just distal to the occlusion and the wire is then exchanged for the snare, which is slightly oversized for the occluded artery. The snare is pushed through the microcatheter, which opens the loop on the snare (Fig. 9A-2[I]). At this point, the snare and microcatheter are withdrawn together into the thrombus and the snare is "tightened" slightly. The microcatheter/snare unit is then withdrawn into the guide catheter. Negative pressure proximal to the occlusion facilitates thrombus removal and decreases the likelihood of distal embolization. This may be achieved by using a balloon-guide catheter, which consists of a balloon just proximal to the guide catheter tip. Inflation of the balloon results in interruption of antegrade flow. Application of negative pressure, using a 20-mL to 60-mL syringe to the side arm of the guide, may then create a suction effect. When it works, this approach may lead to very rapid recanalization. The major disadvantage of this technique is the loss of wire position, if the snaring is unsuccessful, and the potential for vascular injury caused by the oversized snare.

PERIPROCEDURAL MEDICAL MANAGEMENT

Basic measures to maintain a patient's airway, breathing, and circulation must not be neglected in the rush to obtain access and recanalize the occluded vessel. Patients with a depressed level of consciousness are unable to protect their airways and are at risk for aspiration and hypoventilation. These patients should be intubated and mechanically ventilated, prior to beginning the intervention. When patients are breathing spontaneously and are alert, it is the authors' practice *not* to intubate the patient for the procedure. No sedation is administered, so we may monitor for complications and a response to treatment. Headache is an important sign of vascular irritation and intracerebral bleeding, and its occurrence during an intervention always necessitates a re-evaluation of the patient, and a reassessment of the operative technique and equipment positioning, particularly with regard to the wire.

Brain tissue oxygenation is greatly increased with supplemental oxygen, and although there is some concern that high oxygen levels may worsen reperfusion injury, preserving the ischemic penumbra is essential. The most important medical management issue, periprocedurally, is blood pressure control. Under ischemic conditions, the cerebral vessels maximally vasodilate to maintain cerebral blood flow (CBF) in the optimal range (a process termed *cerebral autoregulation*); as a result, CBF becomes linearly proportional to the mean arterial pressure (MAP). Therefore, iatrogenic or spontaneous declines of MAP may potentiate cerebral ischemia in the ischemic penumbra by decreasing CBF below the critical levels for tissue survival (35). Similarly, excessive elevations of MAP may lead to marked elevations of CBF and increase the risk of reperfusion injury and hemorrhage.

The optimal range for the MAP is different in each patient, but in general, blood pressures should be maintained below a MAP of 135 mmHg (i.e., 185/110 mmHg) threshold for patients receiving thrombolytics but above 110 mmHg (i.e., 150/90 mmHg) (36). Beta-blockers are the preferred method for controlling BP, but nitroprusside should be used for persistently elevated blood pressures. Although nitroglycerin is effective, it may cause headache, which may mimic or mask the headache of ICH.

Following the procedure, all patients should be sent to a neurologic intensive care unit (NICU) for monitoring. Frequent neurologic checks should be performed (i.e., every 15 minutes), and particular attention should be paid to the occurrence of headache, with or without nausea and vomiting, the worsening of deficits, or the development of a decreased level of consciousness, all of which could be the signs of ICH. An urgent CT scan of the brain should be obtained if any of the above symptoms and signs develops.

The management of ICH following thrombolysis is quite difficult and the prognosis is poor. If ICH is present, any remaining doses or effects of anticoagulants, thrombolytics, or antiplatelets should be reversed, if possible. Neurosurgical consultation should be obtained immediately. It is unclear if there is, in fact, a role for neurosurgical decompression in this setting (1,2). A full discussion of the critical care management of post-stroke and ICH patients is beyond the scope of this text; however the assistance of an experienced neurointensivist and stroke neurologist is invaluable with these patients. Ideally, a neurologic specialist should be involved in the care of the stroke patient from the outset. Interested readers may reference more detailed text on these matters (36,37).

REFERENCES

1. Juvela S, Heiskanen O, Poranen A, et al. The treatment of spontaneous intracerebral hemorrhage. A prospective randomized trial of surgical and conservative treatment. *J Neurosurg*. 1989;70(5):755–758.
2. Batjer HH, Reisch JS, Allen BC, et al. Failure of surgery to improve outcome in hypertensive putaminal hemorrhage. A prospective randomized trial. *Arch Neurol*. 1990;47(10):1103–1106.
3. Furlan A, Higashida R, Wechsler L, et al. Intra-arterial prourokinase for acute ischemic stroke. The PROACT II study: a randomized controlled trial. Prolyse in Acute Cerebral Thromboembolism. *JAMA*. 1999;282(21):2003–2011.
4. Tissue plasminogen activator for acute ischemic stroke. The National Institute of Neurological Disorders and Stroke rt-PA Stroke Study Group. *N Engl J Med*. 1995;333(24):1581–1587.
5. Foulkes MA, Wolf PA, Price TR, et al. The Stroke Data Bank: design, methods, and baseline characteristics. *Stroke*. 1988;19(5):547–554.
6. Moskowitz M, Caplan LR, eds. *Thrombolytic Treatment in Acute Stroke: Review and Update of Selective Topics. Cerebrovascular Diseases. Nineteenth Princeton Stroke Conference*. Boston, Mass: Butterworth-Heinemann; 1995.
7. del Zoppo GJ, Ferbert A, Otis S, et al. Local intra-arterial fibrinolytic therapy in acute carotid territory stroke. A pilot study. *Stroke*. 1988;19(3):307–313.
8. del Zoppo GJ, Poeck K, Pessin MS, et al. Recombinant tissue plasminogen activator in acute thrombotic and embolic stroke. *Ann Neurol*. 1992;32(1):78–86.
9. Katzan IL, Masaryk TJ, Furlan AJ, et al. Intra-arterial thrombolysis for perioperative stroke after open heart surgery. *Neurology*. 1999;52(5):1081–1084.
10. Brott T, Adams HP, Jr., Olinger CP, et al. Measurements of acute cerebral infarction: a clinical examination scale. *Stroke*. 1989;20(7):864–870.
11. Adams HP, Jr., Brott TG, Furlan AJ, et al. Guidelines for thrombolytic therapy for acute stroke: a supplement to the guidelines for the management of patients with acute ischemic stroke. A statement for healthcare professionals from a Special Writing Group of the Stroke Council, American Heart Association. *Circulation*. 1996;94(5):1167–1174.
12. Hacke W, Ringleb P, Stingele R. How did the results of ECASS II influence clinical practice of treatment of acute stroke. *Rev Neurol*. 1999;29(7):638–641.
13. Barr J. Cerebral angiography in the assessment of acute cerebral ischemia: guidelines and recommendations. *J Vasc Intervent Radiol*. 2004;15[1]:S57–S66.
14. Furlan AJ. Acute stroke therapy: beyond I.V. tPA. *Cleve Clin J Med*. 2002;69(9):730–734.
15. Lee DH, Jo KD, Kim HG, et al. Local intraarterial urokinase thrombolysis of acute ischemic stroke with or without intravenous abciximab: a pilot study. *J Vasc Intervent Radiol*. 2002;13(8):769–774.
16. Abou-Chebl A, Krieger D, Bajzer C, et al. Multimodal therapy for the treatment of severe ischemic stroke combining GP IIb/IIIa antagonists and angioplasty after failure of thrombolysis. *Stroke*. 2003;34[1]:312.
17. Hacke W, Kaste M, Fieschi C, et al. Intravenous thrombolysis with recombinant tissue plasminogen activator for acute hemispheric stroke. The European Cooperative Acute Stroke Study (ECASS). *JAMA*. 1995;274(13):1017–1025.
18. del Zoppo GJ, Sasahara AA. Interventional use of plasminogen activators in central nervous system diseases. *Med Clin North Am*. 1998;82(3):545–568.
19. Qureshi AI, Ali Z, Suri MF, et al. Intra-arterial third-generation recombinant tissue plasminogen activator (reteplase) for acute ischemic stroke. *Neurosurgery*. 2001;49(1):41–48.
20. Arnold M, Schroth G, Nedeltchev K, et al. Intra-arterial thrombolysis in 100 patients with acute stroke due to

middle cerebral artery occlusion. *Stroke.* 2002;33(7): 1828–1833.

21. Thrombolytic therapy with streptokinase in acute ischemic stroke. The Multicenter Acute Stroke Trial—Europe Study Group. *N Engl J Med.* 1996;335(3):145–150.

22. Figueroa BE, Keep RF, Betz AL, et al. Plasminogen activators potentiate thrombin-induced brain injury. *Stroke.* 1998;29(6):1202–1207.

23. Yokogami K, Nakano S, Ohta H, et al. Prediction of hemorrhagic complications after thrombolytic therapy for middle cerebral artery occlusion: value of pre- and post-therapeutic computed tomographic findings and angiographic occlusive site. *Neurosurgery.* 1996;39(6):1102–1107.

24. Abciximab in acute ischemic stroke: a randomized, double-blind, placebo-controlled, dose-escalation study. The Abciximab in Ischemic Stroke Investigators. *Stroke.* 2000;31(3):601–609.

25. Collet J, Montalescot G, Lesty C, et al. Disaggregation of in vitro preformed platelet-rich clots by abciximab increases fibrin exposure and promotes fibrinolysis. *Arterioscler Thromb Vasc Biol.* 2001;21:142–148.

26. Ringer AJ, Qureshi AI, Fessler RD, et al. Angioplasty of intracranial occlusion resistant to thrombolysis in acute ischemic stroke. *Neurosurgery.* 2001;48(6):1282–1288.

27. Nakano S, Iseda T, Yoneyama T, et al. Direct percutaneous transluminal angioplasty for acute middle cerebral artery trunk occlusion: an alternative option to intra-arterial thrombolysis. *Stroke.* 2002;33(12): 2872–2876.

28. Qureshi AI, Siddiqui AM, Suri MF, et al. Aggressive mechanical clot disruption and low-dose intra-arterial third-generation thrombolytic agent for ischemic stroke: a prospective study. *Neurosurgery.* 2002;51(5):1319–1327.

29. Sacco RL, Kargman DE, Gu Q, et al. Race-ethnicity and determinants of intracranial atherosclerotic cerebral infarction. The Northern Manhattan Stroke Study. *Stroke.* 1995;26(1):14–20.

30. Li SM, Miao ZR, Zhu FS, et al. [Combined intraarterial thrombolysis and intra-cerebral stent for acute ischemic stroke institute of brain vascular diseases]. *Zhonghua Yi Xue Za Zhi.* 2003;83(1):9–12.

31. Bellon RJ, Putman CM, Budzik RF, et al. Rheolytic thrombectomy of the occluded internal carotid artery in the setting of acute ischemic stroke. *AJNR Am J Neuroradiol.* 2001;22(3):526–530.

32. Gomez CR, Misra VK, Terry JB, et al. Emergency endovascular treatment of cerebral sinus thrombosis with a rheolytic catheter device. *J Neuroimag.* 2000;10(3):177–180.

33. Wikholm G. Mechanical intracranial embolectomy: A report of two cases. *Intervent Neuroradiol.* 1998;4:159–164.

34. Chopko BW, Kerber C, Wong W, et al. Transcatheter snare removal of acute middle cerebral artery thromboembolism: Technical case report. *Neurosurgery.* 2000;46(6):1529–1531.

35. Ahmed N, Nasman P, Wahlgren N. Effect of intravenous nimodipine on blood pressure and outcome after acute stroke. *Stroke.* 2000;31:1250–1255.

36. Adams HP Jr, Brott TG, Crowell RM, et al. Guidelines for the management of patients with acute ischemic stroke. A statement for healthcare professionals from a special writing group of the Stroke Council, American Heart Association. *Circulation.* 1994;90(3):1588–1601.

37. Management of nontraumatic brain hemorrhage. In: Ropper A, Gress D, Diringer M, et al, eds. *Neurological and Neurosurgical Intensive Care.* Philadelphia, Pa: Lippincott Williams & Wilkins; 2004: 217–230.

Intracranial Angioplasty and Stenting

Alex Abou-Chebl and Jay S. Yadav

Intracranial atherosclerosis is a difficult clinical entity to diagnose and to treat. The difficulty arises from the relative lack of knowledge of the natural history of atherosclerotic disease involving the cerebral vessels. The vessels involved include the distal internal carotid arteries (ICA), vertebral arteries (VA), and the vessels of the Circle of Willis, namely, the middle cerebral artery (MCA), basilar artery (BA), anterior cerebral artery (ACA) and posterior cerebral artery (PCA). The small size of the vessels, their location within the calvarium, their proximity to delicate brain tissue and cranial nerves, and the presence of small perforators further complicate and limit the therapeutic options.

Surgical bypass has been used in selected patients, but in a randomized trial, patients who were treated surgically fared worse than the control group (1). Recent advances in endovascular techniques and equipment now make it possible to recanalize the intracranial vessels, using percutaneous transluminal angioplasty (PTA) and stenting. What follows is a discussion of the natural history of this disease and the interventional techniques used to treat it.

EPIDEMIOLOGY AND NATURAL HISTORY

Intracranial atherosclerosis causes 8 to 10% of all ischemic strokes (2). Patients at particular risk include those who have diabetes mellitus or hypercholesterolemia, and those of African-American, Hispanic, Asian, or Middle-Eastern descent (2). The pathophysiology of most intracranial stenoses is thought to be atherosclerosis. Uncertainty as to the pathophysiology exists because of the small number of available postmortem studies and the lack of tissue from surgical specimens (2–5). In the evaluation of such patients, consideration should be given to other causes of intracranial arterial narrowing, such as vasculitis, dissection, embolism, Moyamoya arteriopathy (a rare, progressive cerebrovascular disorder, typically seen in young females, characterized by the narrowing or occlusion of major blood vessels leading into the brain, and the formation of abnormal blood vessels called moyamoya vessels), postradiation arteriopathy, and infection.

The most common locations for intracranial atherosclerosis are the petrous ICA, the cavernous ICA, the clinoid or terminal ICA, the MCA trunk, the distal VA (i.e., V4 segment), the vertebrobasilar junction, and the mid-BA (3). Of these locations, the BA is the most commonly affected (3).

Until recently, the data on the risks of stroke or transient ischemic attack (TIA) in patients with intracranial atherosclerosis have been obtained from small retrospective series (4–8). Annual rates of stroke or TIA recurrence range from 3% to 22.3%, with most series reporting an annual risk of recurrence of between 6% and 10%.

The investigators of the Warfarin-Aspirin Symptomatic Intracranial Disease (WASID) study recently presented their results (9). WASID is the only large study to date that prospectively followed patients with angiographically proven intracranial stenoses of greater than 50%. The risk of recurrent stroke was approximately 12 per 100 patient years, which is approximately the equivalent of a 12% annual risk. The highest risk was in the first year following the initial event, and there was no difference in stroke recurrence rates between the aspirin- and warfarin-treated groups.

In our own series of patients with vertebrobasilar stenoses, the presence of multifocal stenoses involving both the BA and VA or both VAs was associated with nearly a 50% risk of stroke over 4.8 years of follow-up monitoring (8). Such strokes were also twice as likely to be fatal or disabling. Thijs and Albers found that patients who fail any medical regimen are at a particularly high risk of recurrent ischemia, when compared to patients who are not taking an antithrombotic medicine at the time of initial presentation (8,10). These data suggest there may be differences in stroke risk, based on the affected vascular territory and patterns of atherosclerosis.

Arteries such as the MCA and BA which are channels may be associated with higher risks of stroke (11). The ICA and VA, on the other hand, terminate proximal to major potential sources of collateral blood supply, namely, the anterior communicating artery and the contralateral VA, respectively. The origins of small perforating arteries from the mainstem MCA and BA, the ostia of which may be occluded by atherosclerosis, may further increase the risk of ischemia. In addition, the risks of lesion progression may vary depending on location.

Akins et al. have reported that in 21 patients followed with serial angiograms over a mean of 26.7 months, 20% of intracranial ICA stenoses progressed by more than 10% (12). Of patients with MCA or VB stenoses, approximately 60% progressed to a degree seen angiographically. Approximately 20% of lesions regressed and the remainder were stable. The risk of TIA or stroke in asymptomatic patients who have intracranial stenoses, found incidentally, is unknown.

STROKE MECHANISMS AND THE GOALS OF ENDOVASCULAR THERAPY

The intracranial vasculature is most similar to the coronary vasculature in size, but unlike acute myocardial infarction, platelet aggregation and thrombus formation upon an area of acute plaque rupture is not the predominant mechanism of stroke (13). Hypoperfusion and embolism are the most common mechanisms of ischemia associated with intracranial stenosis (14,15).

Hypoperfusion may occur in the territory of the parent artery, resulting in ischemia of the cortical borderzones. In the case of the MCA and BA, atherosclerotic occlusion of the ostia of the perforating vessels that arise from the main trunks of both arteries may cause deep borderzone or large lacunar strokes (16). It is likely that in many patients, a combination of these mechanisms is responsible for ischemia.

Caplan and Hennerici have put forth the concept that impaired clearance of emboli stemming from decreased flow through a region of stenosis or thrombosis is prominent in the genesis of cerebral ischemia (13). An understanding of these concepts is crucial to determining what the goals of revascularization therapy should be. Improving flow through the stenosis should be the primary aim of any endovascular procedure. Not only will the improvement in flow decrease the risk of hypoperfusion, or so-called "watershed" strokes, but also increase the clearance of emboli from the downstream vessels. An additional benefit is that the creation of a larger channel will decrease turbulent flow and shear effects, and therefore decrease the risk of platelet aggregation and thrombus formation. The increase in lumen diameter need not be large, since flow is proportional to the fourth power of the radius. Even small changes in diameter will have a great effect on flow through the stenotic segment (18,19). This is an important point because an angiographic endpoint of a smooth lumen of normal caliber, while desirable, is not essential to help the patient, and the pursuit of such a goal may lead to a poor outcome. With time, the site of angioplasty or stenting will undergo remodeling and reduce the thrombogenic potential of the plaque surface (19).

For proper patient selection, it is also important to understand the pathophysiology of ischemia in each patient. For example, it has been the experience of the authors that patients who develop recurrent, transient ischemia in the distribution of a single, perforating vessel or branch that originates from a stenotic segment of the parent artery, are at a very high risk of completely occluding that branch vessel and completing the infarct, if the parent artery segment is treated. This is because they have branch atheromatous disease i.e., the atherosclerotic plaque in the parent vessel is encroaching on the ostium of the branch vessel and compromising flow into it (16). Angioplasty and stenting of the parent vessel is very likely to cause plaque shift, further occluding the ostium of the branch. Unless these patients also have ischemia in the territory of the parent vessel distal to the stenosis, they are unlikely to derive benefit from revascularization. This emphasizes the need for a careful, clinical history and examination in every patient, as well as the need for a consultant neurologist who has experience with cerebrovascular disease to be involved in the decision process.

The indications for endovascular repair of intracranial stenosis are controversial (20,21). Most neurologists and interventionists would probably disagree with the opinion that the presence of a symptomatic, intracranial stenosis is, by itself, an indication for endovascular repair. Neurologists generally recommend angioplasty or stenting only for those patients who have failed maximal medical therapy. What is maximal medical therapy? There is no universally accepted definition, but the most common criterion for failure is recurrent symptoms despite a combination of warfarin and low-dose aspirin therapy. As discussed previously, failure of any medical regimen appears to place the patient at a very high risk for recurrent stroke (10). This would suggest that recurrent symptoms on any regimen of anticoagulant or antiplatelet agent should be considered a medical failure. Clearly more research into the area of medical therapy of intracranial stenoses is needed, and a direct comparison of medical treatment

with endovascular treatment will help answer the issue.

INTRACRANIAL ANGIOPLASTY AND STENTING OUTCOMES

The technical and clinical outcomes of intracranial angioplasty and stenting are generally favorable (18,19,22–37). As of yet, however, there have been no controlled, clinical trials comparing these invasive therapies with medical therapy. Angioplasty, alone, has a technical success rate of approximately 80%. The stroke and death rates with angioplasty are 13% and 1.6%, respectively. In the largest series to date (combined n = 259), dissection and arterial rupture occurred in 8.7% of patients. Data on restenosis has not been consistently obtained in all series and there is significant variation in the duration of follow-up monitoring, between series. From the series that do report these data, the restenosis rate is approximately 12%.

Although it is not possible to make general statements based on the small number of patients treated with stenting, some have suggested that the technical success rate appears to be greater with stenting, compared with angioplasty alone and that complications may be lower (38). The authors agree that stenting, particularly that performed with the latest generation of highly flexible coronary stents, is superior to angioplasty alone and is likely associated with more durable results. However, there are a distinct lack of data to support this opinion. In published series of intracranial stenting, the periprocedural stroke and death rates range from 0 to 45.5% and 0 to 18%, respectively (18,19,23–26,28–37). Restenosis data for intracranial stenting are even more scarce, and no worthwhile conclusion may be made at this time.

Many factors may affect the technical and clinical success of intracranial interventions. Patient and lesion selection, lesion characteristics, operator experience, availability of equipment, periprocedural antithrombotic and antiplatelet medical regimens, and method and duration of follow-up monitoring will all affect actual, and measured, outcomes.

Intracranial angioplasty and stenting are certainly feasible and are appropriate therapeutic options in selected patients. They should be reserved for symptomatic patients who have failed medical therapy, and not used as the primary mode of therapy for intracranial atherosclerosis (20,21). Intracranial interventions are very complicated procedures that require great technical skill, and knowledge of the unique physiology and anatomy of the brain and its vessels. The morbidity and mortality risks associated with these techniques are significant. In particular, intracranial hemorrhage is the most feared complication, as it is almost universally fatal. Follow-up monitoring and appropriate medical management are also critical to successful outcome. There is a pressing need for prospective clinical trials of intracranial angioplasty and stenting.

ANGIOPLASTY AND STENTING: TECHNIQUE

Patient Selection

In 1980, Sundt et al. performed angioplasty on two patients with BA stenosis, through a surgical cut down to the VA (40). Their success encouraged others and to date, there have been many published case reports and series of endovascular interventions of the major intracranial vessels (18,19,22–37). Most of these reports have shown favorable outcomes but all have been retrospective, and are for the most part, anecdotal. Furthermore, these reports differ significantly in criteria for patient selection, location of stenoses, endovascular technique, use of adjuvant medical therapy, and methods of follow-up monitoring. Direct comparisons between them are problematic and definitive conclusions about the efficacy, safety, and superiority of particular techniques or equipment may not be made. This early experience is nonetheless crucial. Several concepts and techniques have been learned from this experience, and form the basis for the safe and successful performance of intracranial intervention.

Appropriate patient selection is the first and most crucial step in ensuring success. The interventionalist must assess the feasibility of obtaining access and achieving a technically successful outcome at the lesion site. An unfriendly aortic arch (i.e., Type III arch), tortuous cervical vessels, proximal stenoses, or the need for a brachial approach will each make access to the intracranial stenosis difficult, if not impossible in some cases. An arch aortogram and selective angiography of the culprit vessel are crucial to decision making in this regard.

Multiple orthogonal views to define the stenosis (i.e., length of lesion, vessel diameter at lesion site) and its relationship to critical adjacent branches, are also imperative (Fig. 9A-1).

An accurate assessment of vessel diameter will guard against overly aggressive balloon or stent sizing, and may reduce the risk of vessel perforation. The close association of adjacent side branches to the culprit lesion is important if plaque shift from angioplasty is anticipated. All of these angiographic data provide the interventionist with the information required to plan arterial access and the interventional strategy.

Mori et al. have described a classification scheme, based on the angiographic characteristics of the stenosis, that may help predict the chances of technical success as well as the risks of complications (23). In this schema, lesions of less than 5 mm in length that are concentric, and less than totally occlusive, are classified as type A. These lesions had a success rate with angioplasty of 92%, and a stroke risk or need for extracranial or intracranial bypass rate of 8%. Type-B lesions are those that are tubular, 5 mm to 10 mm in length, and eccentric or totally occluded for less than 3 months. In this intermediate group technical success occurred in 86% of the patients, but the rate of stroke, death or need for bypass was 26%. Type-C lesions are either diffuse, more than 10 mm in length and extremely angulated (i.e., greater than 90°), with excessive tortuosity of the proximal segment, or they are totally occluded for more than 3 months. This last group of patients was successfully recanalized in one-third of cases, but the rate of periprocedural stroke, death, or need for bypass was 87%. These data provide an assessment of the risk-versus-benefit ratio for various lesion types, based on the angiographic findings. Only the most experienced operators should attempt an intervention on type-B or type-C lesions.

Recent symptoms, especially those associated with an infarct, may increase the risk of postintervention complications, particularly of

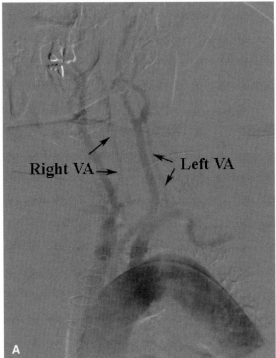
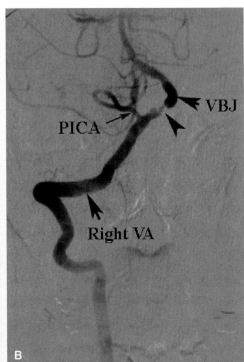
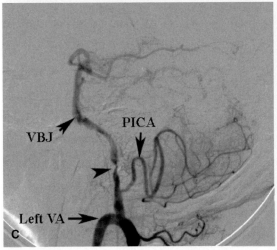
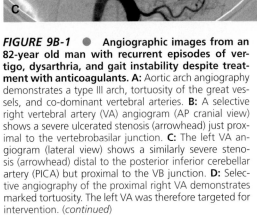
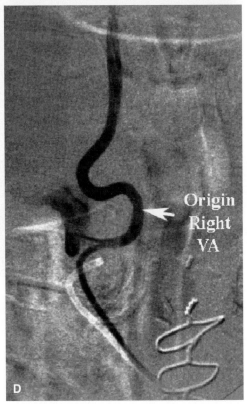

FIGURE 9B-1 ● **Angiographic images from an 82-year old man with recurrent episodes of vertigo, dysarthria, and gait instability despite treatment with anticoagulants. A:** Aortic arch angiography demonstrates a type III arch, tortuosity of the great vessels, and co-dominant vertebral arteries. **B:** A selective right vertebral artery (VA) angiogram (AP cranial view) shows a severe ulcerated stenosis (arrowhead) just proximal to the vertebrobasilar junction. **C:** The left VA angiogram (lateral view) shows a similarly severe stenosis (arrowhead) distal to the posterior inferior cerebellar artery (PICA) but proximal to the VB junction. **D:** Selective angiography of the proximal right VA demonstrates marked tortuosity. The left VA was therefore targeted for intervention. (*continued*)

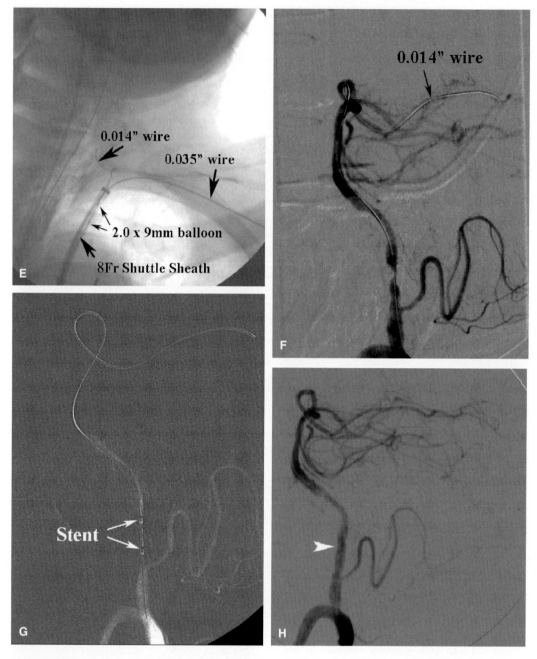

FIGURE 9B-1 ● **E:** An 8-Fr shuttle sheath was positioned in the proximal left subclavian artery. Stability of the sheath position required that a 0.035″ wire be placed through the sheath into the distal axillary artery. With stable access, the VA was engaged with the 0.014″ soft, hydrophilic wire, which was loaded through a 2-mm diameter X 9-mm length coronary balloon. A 6-Fr Envoy® guide catheter was then advanced over the wire and ballon into the distal cervical VA. **F:** The wire was placed distally in the posterior cerebral artery for added support and predilation was performed, but repeat angiography demonstrated marked recoil. **G:** Using the road-map function, a 3.0 × 12 mm Multilink Vision® stent was positioned across the lesion in the distal VA, taking care not to jail the PICA branch. **H:** Final angiography following stenting demonstrates a widely patent stent at the lesion site in the distal VA and a widely patent PICA branch.

hemorrhagic transformation. Some clinicians have excluded or delayed treatment for 6 weeks, or more, in patients with a large stroke (19,26). The basis for this approach is anecdotal and, in part, reflects the common practice of delayed carotid endarterectomy following stroke. Theoretically, hemorrhagic transformation occurs upon reperfusion of a previously ischemic vascular bed that has had recent injury to the endothelium and breakdown of the blood-brain barrier (BBB). The vessels in ischemic areas of brain do not have intact autoregulation and, therefore, flow through them is entirely dependent on blood pressure. Recanalization of a proximal stenosis increases the pressure head through those injured regions and, therefore, may lead to hemorrhagic conversion. The use of multiple antithrombotic medicines, during endovascular treatment, may further increase the risk. A delay in recanalization may allow for healing and restoration of the BBB, permit restoration of some degree of autoregulation, and decrease the risk of hemorrhagic conversion. This is a reasonable approach and the authors advocate delaying therapy if there is a large, completed stroke; as discussed in the section on acute stroke treatment, stenting may be carried out acutely but at a much higher risk of intracranial hemorrhage (ICH) than is acceptable for an elective procedure. If hemorrhagic conversion is already present, then endovascular repair should definitely be delayed. Preprocedural computed tomographic (CT) scans should be considered in all patients, especially in those with recent symptoms. These factors must all be taken into account when evaluating a patient for potential intervention.

Preprocedural Management – Pharmacotherapy and Sedation

Preprocedural management centers on two critical issues: antithrombotic therapy (Table 9A-1) and sedation and anesthesia.

Platelet inhibition has been shown to be critical in preventing acute thrombus formation at the site of plaque injury from angioplasty and stenting. Platelet deposition on the damaged endothelium occurs within minutes of plaque disruption (44). The presence of a foreign body, such as a stent, is associated with a further elevation in the risk of vessel thrombosis.

TABLE 9B-1

Summary of Pharmacological Agents Used Prior to and During Intracranial Intervention

Drug	Dose
Preprocedural	
Aspirin	325 mg qd po
Clopidogrel	300–600 mg load, 75 mg qd po
Ticlopidine	500 mg load, 250 mg bid po
Intraprocedural	
Heparin	Weight-adjusted bolus (~50 units/kg) to achieve target ACT of 250–300 seconds
Argatroban	Weight-adjusted (2μcg/Kg/min infusion) to achieve lengthen aPTT to 2–3 times control
Miscellaneous	
Abciximab	0.125–0.25 mg/kg IV bolus, 0.125μcg/Kg/min infusion × 12 hours
Eptifibatide	180μcg/Kg bolus, 2μcg/Kg/min infusion × 18 hours
Dextran 40/70	Variable dosing

qd - once daily, po - by mouth, bid - twice daily, IV - intravenous, ACT - activated clotting time, aPTT - activated partial thromboplastin time.

The use of preprocedural aspirin and a thienopyridine (e.g., clopidogrel or ticlopidine) is established in coronary intervention involving stents, and has been empirically applied to intracranial stenting procedures. The authors prefer clopidogrel because of its superior safety profile. If angioplasty, alone, is planned, pretreatment with aspirin only is sufficient. These therapies should be administered for at least 3 to 4 days prior to the procedure to ensure therapeutic levels of platelet inhibition at the time of the procedure.

The role of platelet glycoprotein IIb/IIIa receptor (GP IIa/IIIa) antagonists in the setting of intracranial endovascular stenting procedures is unclear (28). The lack of evidence supporting a beneficial effect, and the potential risk of ICH weigh heavily against the routine use of such agents for intracranial procedures. On the other hand, abciximab, in combination with aspirin and low-dose heparin, did not increase the risk of ICH following percutaneous coronary intervention (47). There are also reports of the safe use of these drugs in patients undergoing cervical carotid artery PTA and stenting (48), and the risk of ICH has been very low in several reports of the treatment of acute stroke patients with abciximab (49–51).

Based on this indirect evidence, some operators have used abciximab during intracranial intervention. In combination with aspirin, clopidogrel, and heparin, Levy and colleagues used abciximab therapy in the performance of stenting of the vertebrobasilar system in 11 patients (33). Four (36.3%) of these patients died; two of vessel rupture and one of sudden brain death. What the authors defined as vessel rupture is not clear, but likely they were describing subarachnoid hemorrhage. These rates of rupture and death are very high, compared with other published series. In a separate series of 50 patients undergoing intracranial angioplasty, who were treated with adjunctive abciximab therapy, there were no cases of ICH (19). Based on these conflicting results, it seems reasonable not to use GP IIb/IIIa agents, routinely, during intracranial intervention. Instead, their use should be reserved for specifically selected patients, such as patients who are not adequately pretreated with oral antiplatelet agents, or in the setting of acute ischemic stroke.

Heparin is the anticoagulant of choice for intracranial intervention. This is given either as a bolus followed by an infusion, or as a bolus followed by intermittent boluses, to achieve a target activated clotting time (ACT) of between 250 and 300 seconds. Mori and his group in Japan have reported using a dextran infusion, at a rate of 1 L to 2 L per day, in addition to heparin (23–25). Some groups continue a heparin infusion for 12 to 24 hours following the procedure. There is no consensus on the optimal regimen. The authors favor weight-adjusted heparin boluses to keep the ACT at 250 to 300 seconds. The use of a fixed-dose bolus of heparin is not appropriate and should not be used if the interventionist has the means to measure the ACT. In addition to anticoagulants, some clinicians pretreat patients with antivasospasm regimens, including sublingual nifedipine (18), or intraarterial nitroglycerin (52). In earlier series, vasospasm was frequent

and associated with poor outcomes (53). Routine pretreatment for vasospasm is not required, but intraarterial nitroglycerin must be available, if needed.

The second issue in preprocedural management is sedation and anesthesia. Some groups commonly perform intracranial procedures under general anesthesia (19,33,54). The benefits are touted to be a secure airway, reliable control of physiologic parameters, and no interference by patient movements. If our practice is to perform procedures under local anesthesia, with low-dose, intravenous, conscious sedation available if needed. While it is certainly true that patient movement may be distracting, patient feedback during angioplasty is quite helpful in assessing clinical status and in gauging whether or not the angioplasty is too aggressive (28). The cerebral vessels are richly innervated with pain fibers, even though the brain itself is not. If patients complain of headache or neck pain during balloon inflation, the inflation pressure should be decreased. Once again, there are no objective data to favor either approach. As experience with intracranial intervention grows, local anesthesia will likely replace general anesthesia, since it may be safer and is less invasive and costly.

Technique

Access is perhaps the most important technical factor ensuring a successful procedure. The cerebral vessels are quite tortuous and without adequate and stable access to the stenotic segment, an otherwise straightforward case may be impossible to complete. A femoral approach is ideal but a brachial or radial approach is feasible, although technically challenging, especially for MCA and ICA procedures (28). One may use the same technique described in the chapter on acute ischemic stroke treatment (Chapter 9B) to obtain access. For carotid distribution interventions, the sheath is placed in the distal CCA, and the Envoy guide in the distal cervical ICA, at about the C1-C3 level, just below the skull base (26,28,38). For vertebrobasilar intervention, the sheath is placed in the subclavian artery, and the Envoy guide placed in the distal portion of the V2 segment of the VA. This usually provides a sufficient platform for most intracranial interventions.

After stable access is obtained, the lesion should be crossed with a 0.014″ hydrophilic, soft wire with an atraumatic tip, such as a Synchro®, Transcend®, or Whisper® wire (65,71). If excessive tortuosity is not present and delivery of the balloon or stent appears to be feasible, the intervention may proceed over the soft wire, ensuring that the wire is placed sufficiently distal to the lesion to provide sufficient support.

If stent delivery seems unlikely without more support, then a hydrophilic microcatheter such as the Rapid Transit®, or an over-the-wire angioplasty balloon catheter such as the Maverick® should be advanced over the wire across the lesion. The wire is then exchanged for a nonhydrophilic wire that will give more support, such as a Balance Trek®, BMW®, or Dasher-14® wire.

Hydrophilic wires are generally easier to pass through the stenotic segment and are better at negotiating tortuous segments, but are more likely to cause perforation or dissection, compared to nonhydrophilic wires. Great care should be taken to avoid placing the wire in small branches or perforators originating from the distal ICA, M1 segment of the MCA, or the BA. For carotid distribution intervention, the wire should be passed into the sylvian branches, (i.e., after the genu) in the second-order branches (i.e., from the M2 segment) or proximal third-order branches (from M3 segment). In the posterior circulation, the PCAs serve as good conduits for the wire, and placing the wire in a second- or third-generation branch is usually straightforward (Fig. 9A-1[G]). Imaging in orthogonal planes is very helpful with making correct wire positioning.

Having successfully crossed the lesion with the wire, angioplasty is performed. In general, most centers undersize the diameter of the angioplasty balloon by 10% to 20% of the vessel diameter, which should be assessed using digital measurement techniques (18,52,55). In addition to the need for undersizing, balloon-inflation rates and pressures have an effect on the risk of dissection and rupture. Many authors advocate slow inflations, at low-to-moderate pressures (4 to 8 atm) for 45 to 60 seconds (24,26,55), while others advocate a very slow, low-pressure inflation (2 to 4 atm) over 2 to 5 minutes (19). Very rapid inflation is thought to increase the risk of vessel rupture, particularly in calcified, noncompliant vessels. Connors et al. have published reports on the largest series of intracranial angioplasty (n = 70), to date (19), and found that their slow-inflation technique resulted in fewer dissections and fatalities but with more technical failures.

The current generation of coronary balloon catheters are optimal for use during intracranial angioplasty. These balloons have a low profile, may be maneuvered through the tortuous cervico-cranial vessels, and are compliant. The balloon lengths used should be as short as possible to facilitate delivery, and to limit the risk of vessel perforation (19). Balloons that have been used with success include the Open-Sail®, Predator XL® or Ninja®, Ranger®, Stealth®, and Stratus®. In the practice of the authors, the Maverick® balloon is the balloon of choice. Over-the-wire balloons are preferred to monorail balloons because of their improved tracking capability, particularly in the presence of vessel tortuosity.

An angiogram should be performed immediately after angioplasty, to examine for recoil (Fig. 9A-1[G]), dissection, vasospasm, or embolization. Some authors advocate repeat angiography over a 1-hour period following angioplasty, to monitor for delayed vasospasm or thrombotic occlusion (19). Repeat angioplasty should be considered where stent deployment is contraindicated or not feasible and angioplasty produces no significant increase in lumen diameter or is associated with significant recoil. The immediate postangioplasty angiographic appearance may not reflect the delayed angiographic appearance, owing to acute vasospasm or delayed healing of the intima and subintimal layers. This delayed healing may sometimes lead to scar retraction and an increase in luminal diameter (57), and explains why some operators advocate delaying repeat angioplasty until weeks later, when intimal and endothelial healing has occurred.

Whether to deploy a stent, or not, is controversial and the experience, to date, with stenting is limited. A few case reports and small series constitute the current published data on intracranial stenting (18,19,23–26,28–37). It is important to understand the three different stenting strategies: (1) direct stenting, which is the placement of the stent without an initial angioplasty of the lesion; (2) primary stenting, which is the a priori decision to stent after angioplasty, even if the angioplasty results are excellent; and (3) provisional stenting which is the a priori decision to stent only if the angioplasty results are suboptimal.

The potential risks of direct stenting are: (1) the inability to deliver the stent because the lesion is too severe, (2) the inability to fully dilate the stent in a rigid lesion, and (3) distal embolization if the stent is forced through the lesion. Offsetting these risks is the potential advantage that with direct stenting, the lesion is only crossed once, possibly decreasing the risk of embolization and dissection associated with predilation. Some authors advocate provisional stent deployment, if there is a flow-limiting dissection or elastic recoil (19,26,28). The authors agree with other groups that stents should be deployed whenever possible (i.e., primary stenting) (20,25). Extrapolating from the experience with stenting in the coronary circulation, it is felt that stents improve the short- and long-term patency rates, compared to angioplasty alone, by nullifying the effect of vasospasm at the treatment site, tacking up dissections, and preventing elastic recoil and negative vessel remodeling.

The potential drawbacks of stenting include: (1) added technical complexity, (2) greater difficulty in delivery as compared to balloons only, and (3) the potential for stent-strut occlusion of the ostia of small and microscopic perforators leading off the MCA and BA. Furthermore, there may be a higher risk of vessel perforation, caused by the higher pressures needed for full stent deployment and opposition with the vessel wall. Stents that are not fully deployed and well opposed to the arterial wall have a higher risk of subacute thrombosis.

At present, there are no commercially available stents specifically designed for the intracranial circulation. Coronary stents that have been used intracranially include the Bx Velocity®, GFX2®, Multilink Duet®, Pixel®, Tetra®, Penta®, Express2®, and Multilink Vision®. The authors have had the most success, in terms of deliverability, with the Express2®, and the Multilink Vision®.

Stent delivery remains the most challenging single aspect of intracranial stenting. Although the newer generation stents have been a major advance and have made stent delivery easier, it may still be very difficult, and sometimes impossible.

Severe tortuosity and atherosclerosis, proximal to the site of the stenosis, are challenging obstacles to surmount. As emphasized previously, adequate and stable access to the culprit vessel is essential, and during the intervention, the operator frequently must assess that the guide and sheath have not slid back, particularly if significant forward pressure is required to advance the stent. By applying constant forward pressure on the guide and sheath, one may gain extra support in delivering the stent.

Occasionally, if there is sufficient wire length distal to the stenosis, pulling back on the wire as the stent is advanced may improve the deliverability of the stent. If the stent still does not track, then changing the wire to a more supportive wire, as was discussed, may facilitate stent delivery. More supportive wires occasionally hinder the deliverability of a stent by creating pseudostenoses and increasing the friction between the stent and the vessel wall.

Like balloon sizing and positioning, stents should never be oversized, and care must be taken to avoid occluding any critical branches or perforating vessels. If patients develop pain during stent inflation, then further inflation should be avoided, until the vessel and patient are reassessed. In most circumstances, the stenting result is adequate, even if the nominal inflation pressures are not achieved. Although further inflation might improve the angiographic result, this should be reconsidered if the patient develops severe headache with the initial inflation. Meticulous attention to stent placement decreases the risk of "jailing" or shifting plaque into adjacent branches. In some cases, there is no choice but to stent across the branch (e.g., with the MCA and BA perforators, and the anterior inferior cerebellar artery, which often arises from the middle of a BA stenosis). In these cases, the patient must be made aware of that possibility and the potential for stroke. If there is a high likelihood of this occurring, the interventionist must also be certain that an intervention is the optimal therapy.

Following successful stenting, a diagnostic angiogram should be performed in multiple planes, to assess for subtle signs of dissection, plaque shifting, dye extravasation, vasospasm, or distal embolization. The wire should be removed cautiously, and only if there is no obvious dissection. Before removing the supporting sheath and guide, the patient should be assessed neurologically.

Periprocedural Management

Patients should be transferred immediately to a neurological intensive care unit or similar nursing unit with nursing staff experienced in neurologic assessment and vascular access site care. Strict bedrest should be maintained for 6 to 8 hours and vital signs, in particular blood pressures, should be recorded continuously.

There is no consensus on optimal blood pressure management postprocedurally. In patients who had critical stenoses with poor cerebrovascular reserve, as documented by a functional study (i.e., acetazolamide single positron emission computed tomography (SPECT) or transcranial Doppler [TCD]), or those who had poor angiographic collaterals, there is a potential risk of hyperperfusion syndrome and intracranial hemorrhage (59–61). In such patients, especially if they have received GP IIb/IIIa receptor antagonists, blood pressure should be maintained in the low-to-normal range. Certainly hypertension should be avoided, as in most other patients. In some circumstances, such as when multiple stenoses are present, or if there is concern about the occlusion of a branch vessel or perforator secondary to stent placement, blood-pressure management becomes very complex and the risk of ICH must be balanced against the risk of ischemia if blood pressure is lowered. Care must be individualized in each case.

Frequent neurologic assessments are carried out immediately following the intervention, to monitor for the two most serious and likely complications with intracranial interventions, those of intracranial hemorrhage and ischemia. The former is the most devastating and has been the most common cause of death in published reports. Sudden severe headache, nausea and vomiting with a rapid decline in consciousness associated with extreme hypertension and possibly bradycardia, are common clinical findings with ICH. The bleeding is usually into the subarachnoid space, since all of the intracranial cerebral vessels that are amenable to intervention, except

for the petrous and cavernous ICAs, run through that space. ICH occurs in this setting from either rupture or dissection of the treated vessel or tearing of branches or perforators. If ICH is suspected, it is urgent that a CT of the brain be obtained when the patient is stabilized.

Frequently, endotracheal intubation becomes necessary, and medical measures should be instituted to control elevated intracranial pressure and to decrease bleeding. Anticoagulants and antiplatelets should be reversed, immediately, with protamine, fresh-frozen plasma, and platelet transfusions, as needed. Unfortunately, such measures are often futile because the effects of clopidogrel and aspirin are difficult to reverse, and if abciximab was used, platelet transfusion is only partially effective. Urgent neurosurgical intervention may be lifesaving but is unlikely to restore function (62,63). A lateral ventricular drain should be considered as a means to rapidly decrease intracranial pressure, particularly if there is hydrocephalus from intraventricular or subarachnoid hemorrhage. Neurosurgical intervention in this setting is fraught with significant risk of surgical-bed bleeding, owing to the antiplatelet effects of aspirin and clopidogrel. As a result, despite all of these interventions, few patients will survive a significant subarachnoid or intraparenchymal hemorrhage, in this setting.

Cerebral ischemia may develop during the intervention, or shortly thereafter. Intraprocedural ischemia may be related to vasospasm, which is common in the cerebral vasculature. Thrombosis and embolism may occur if adequate levels of anticoagulation and platelet inhibition were not maintained during the procedure, especially following stent deployment. Other mechanisms of ischemia include plaque shifting and occlusion of microscopic perforators, especially those of the BA and MCA.

Postprocedural ischemia is occasionally caused by acute thrombosis of the treated vessel, as a result of unrecognized dissection or inadequate platelet inhibition. Delayed vasospasm is unusual. If encountered, ischemia should be treated with measures to improve perfusion, such as blood pressure elevation, hydration and hemodilution, and continuation of antithrombotic agents. If symptoms develop after the procedure, reassessment of the treated vessel must be considered, to assess for acute thrombosis or vasospasm. The latter may be treated with nitroglycerin given intra-arterially. Acute thrombosis may be treated with repeat angioplasty or with GP IIb/IIIa inhibitors alone. These agents may be particularly useful, especially if they were not used during the intervention, itself. Intraarterial thrombolytics may be used in this setting, but at a significantly increased risk of ICH. Unfortunately, in either ICH or acute ischemia, treatments are not ideal and these complications are easier to avoid than they are to treat.

If patients are asymptomatic and their blood pressures were not difficult to control, they may be discharged 24 to 48 hours following the procedure. Aspirin and clopidogrel or ticlopidine are continued for 30 days, after which aspirin is continued indefinitely. In those at risk for hyperperfusion, blood pressures should be monitored daily for at least 14 days following the procedure. Pressures should be kept in the low-normal range. Patients should be instructed to seek medical attention if they develop hypertension, headache, nausea, vomiting or focal neurologic signs, as these may all indicate the occurrence of the hyperperfusion syndrome.

Follow-up assessment is performed at 30 days and 6 months. Vessel patency should be assessed at 6- to 12-month intervals. Angiographic follow-up evaluation may be performed at 1 year following the intervention, but does carry some risk.

Unless the patient is symptomatic, noninvasive methods of vascular assessment should be used, such as magnetic resonance angiography (MRA), computed tomography angiography (CTA), or transcranial Doppler (TCD) ultrasound. Unfortunately both MRA and CTA are unable to adequately image the intracranial vessels if a stent is present. CTA may be adequate if the stented vessel is larger than 3.5 mm. TCD is a noninvasive, rapid, economical, and relatively sensitive method of following most ICA siphon, MCA, VA, and BA stenoses. TCD may be obtained the day following the procedure. Acutely, blood-flow velocities, as measured by TCD, may be elevated and unless the patient is symptomatic, should rarely be acted upon. If the noninvasive studies suggest the presence of restenosis, then angiography is justified.

REFERENCES

1. Failure of extracranial-intracranial arterial bypass to reduce the risk of ischemic stroke. Results of an international randomized trial. The EC/IC Bypass Study Group. *N Engl J Med.* 1985;313(19):1191–1200.
2. Sacco RL, Kargman DE, Gu Q, et al. Race-ethnicity and determinants of intracranial atherosclerotic cerebral infarction. The Northern Manhattan Stroke Study. *Stroke.* 1995;26(1):14–20.
3. Hass WK, Fields WS, North RR, et al. Joint study of extracranial arterial occlusion. II. Arteriography, techniques, sites, and complications. *JAMA.* 1968;203(11):961–968.
4. Moufarrij NA, Little JR, Furlan AJ, et al. Vertebral artery stenosis: long-term follow-up. *Stroke.* 1984;15[2]:260–263.
5. Craig DR, Meguro K, Watridge C, et al. Intracranial internal carotid artery stenosis. *Stroke.* 1982;13[6]:825–828.
6. Caplan LR, Babikian V, Helgason C, et al. Occlusive disease of the middle cerebral artery. *Neurology.* 1985;35:975–982.
7. Chimowitz MI, Kokkinos J, Strong J, et al. The Warfarin-Aspirin Symptomatic Intracranial Disease study. *Neurology.* 1995;45(8):1488–1493.
8. Abou-Chebl A, Rensel M, Krieger D, et al. Long-term outcome in symptomatic intracranial vertebrobasilar occlusive disease. *Stroke.* 2000;31(1):294. Abstract.
9. Chimowitz M, Lynn M, Howlett Smith H, et al. Warfarin-Aspirin Symptomatic Intracranial Disease (WASID) trial: final results. *Stroke.* 2004;35(1):235.
10. Thijs VN, Albers GW. Symptomatic intracranial atherosclerosis: outcome of patients who fail antithrombotic therapy. *Neurology.* 2000;55(4):490–497.
11. Caplan LR. Large-vessel occlusive disease of the anterior circulation. In: ed(s). *Stroke: A Clinical Approach.* Boston: Butterworth-Heinemann; 1993:195–236.
12. Akins PT, Pilgram TK, Cross DT III, et al. Natural history of stenosis from intracranial atherosclerosis by serial angiography. *Stroke.* 1998;29(2):433–438.
13. Caplan LR, Hennerici M. Impaired clearance of emboli (washout) is an important link between hypoperfusion, embolism, and ischemic stroke. *Arch Neurol.* 1998;55(11):1475–1482.
14. Hinton RC, Mohr JP, Ackerman RH, et al. Symptomatic middle cerebral artery stenosis. *Ann Neurol.* 1979;5(2):152–157.
15. Adams HP, Gross CE. Embolism distal to stenosis of the middle cerebral artery. *Stroke.* 1981;12:228.
16. Caplan LR. Intracranial branch atheromatous disease: a neglected, understudied, and underused concept. *Neurology.* 1989;39:1246–1250.
17. Topol EJ, Yadav JS. Recognition of the importance of embolization in atherosclerotic vascular disease. *Circulation.* 2000;101(5):570–580.
18. Callahan AS, III, Berger BL. Balloon angioplasty of intracranial arteries for stroke prevention. *J Neuroimaging.* 1997;7(4):232–235.
19. Connors JJ III, Wojak JC. Percutaneous transluminal angioplasty for intracranial atherosclerotic lesions: evolution of technique and short-term results. *J Neurosurg.* 1999;91(3):415–423.
20. Gomez CR, Orr SC. Angioplasty and stenting for primary treatment of intracranial arterial stenoses. *Arch Neurol.* 2001;58(10):1687–1690.

21. Chimowitz MI. Angioplasty or stenting is not appropriate as first-line treatment of intracranial stenosis. *Arch Neurol.* 2001;58(10):1690–1692.

22. Clark WM, Barnwell SL, Nesbit G, et al. Safety and efficacy of percutaneous transluminal angioplasty for intracranial atherosclerotic stenosis. *Stroke.* 1995;26(7):1200–1204.

23. Mori T, Fukuoka M, Kazita K, et al. Follow-up study after intracranial percutaneous transluminal cerebral balloon angioplasty. *AJNR Am J Neuroradiol.* 1998;19(8):1525–1533.

24. Mori T, Fukuoka M, Kazita K, et al. Follow-up study after percutaneous transluminal cerebral angioplasty. *Eur Radiol.* 1998;8(3):403–408.

25. Mori T, Kazita K, Chokyu K, et al. Short-term arteriographic and clinical outcome after cerebral angioplasty and stenting for intracranial vertebrobasilar and carotid atherosclerotic occlusive disease. *AJNR Am J Neuroradiol.* 2000;21(2):249–254.

26. Marks MP, Marcellus M, Norbash AM, et al. Outcome of angioplasty for atherosclerotic intracranial stenosis. *Stroke.* 1999;30(5):1065–1069.

27. Alazzaz A, Thornton J, Aletich VA, et al. Intracranial percutaneous transluminal angioplasty for arteriosclerotic stenosis. *Arch Neurol.* 2000;57(11):1625–1630.

28. Ramee SR, Dawson R, McKinley KL, et al. Provisional stenting for symptomatic intracranial stenosis using a multidisciplinary approach: acute results, unexpected benefit, and one-year outcome. *Catheter Cardiovasc Interv.* 2001;52(4):457–467.

29. Abou-Chebl A, Krieger D, Bajzer C, et al. Intracranial angioplasty and stenting in the awake patient. *Stroke.* 2003;34(1):312. Abstract.

30. Gondim FA, Cruz-Flores S, Moore J, et al. Angioplasty and stenting for symptomatic basilar artery stenosis. *J Neuroimaging.* 2002;12(1):55–58.

31. Miao Z, Ling F, Li S, et al. Stent-assisted angioplasty in treatment of symptomatic intracranial artery stenosis. [Chinese]. Chung-Hua i Hsueh Tsa Chih *Chinese Medical Journal.* 2002;82(10):657–660.

32. Lylyk P, Cohen JE, Ceratto R, et al. Angioplasty and stent placement in intracranial atherosclerotic stenoses and dissections. *AJNR Am J Neuroradiol.* 2002;23(3):430–436.

33. Levy EI, Horowitz MB, Koebbe CJ, et al. Transluminal stent-assisted angioplasty of the intracranial vertebrobasilar system for medically refractory, posterior circulation ischemia: early results. *Neurosurgery.* 2001; 48(6):1215–1221.

34. Morris PP, Martin EM, Regan J, et al. Intracranial deployment of coronary stents for symptomatic atherosclerotic disease. *AJNR Am J Neuroradiol.* 1999;20(9):1688–1694.

35. Al Mubarak N, Gomez CR, Vitek JJ, et al. Stenting of symptomatic stenosis of the intracranial internal carotid artery. *AJNR Am J Neuroradiol.* 1998; 19(10):1949–1951.

36. Rasmussen PA. Transluminal stent-assisted angioplasty of the intracranial vertebrobasilar system for medically refractory, posterior circulation ischemia: early results. *Neurosurgery.* 2001;49(6):1489–1490.

37. Gupta R, Schumacher HC, Mangla S, et al. Urgent endovascular revascularization for symptomatic intracranial atherosclerotic stenosis. *Neurology.* 2003;61(12): 1729–1735.

38. Gomez CR, Misra VK, Campbell MS, et al. Elective stenting of symptomatic middle cerebral artery stenosis. *AJNR Am J Neuroradiol.* 2000;21(5):971–973.

39. Dotter CT, Judkins MP. Transluminal treatment of arteriosclerotic obstruction. Description of a new technic and a preliminary report of its application. 1964. *Radiology.* 1989;172(3)(Pt 2):904–920.

40. Sundt TM Jr, Smith HC, Campbell JK, et al. Transluminal angioplasty for basilar artery stenosis. *Mayo Clin Proc.* 1980;55(11):673–680.

41. Samuels OB, Joseph GJ, Lynn MJ, et al. A standardized method for measuring intracranial arterial stenosis. *AJNR Am J Neuroradiol.* 2000;21(4):643–646.

42. North American Symptomatic Carotid Endarterectomy Trial Collaborators. Beneficial effect of carotid endarterectomy in symptomatic patients with high-grade carotid stenosis. *N Engl J Med.* 1991;325:445–453.

43. Bhatt DL, Kapadia SR, Yadav JS, et al. Update on clinical trials of antiplatelet therapy for cerebrovascular diseases. *Cerebrovasc Dis.* 2000;10(suppl 5):34–40.

44. Wilentz JR, Sanborn TA, Haudenschild CC, et al. Platelet accumulation in experimental angioplasty: time course and relation to vascular injury. *Circulation.* 1987;75(3):636–642.

45. Bhatt DL, Kapadia SR, Bajzer CT, et al. Dual antiplatelet therapy with clopidogrel and aspirin after carotid artery stenting. *J Invasive Cardiol.* 2001;13(12):767–771.

46. Mori T, Mori K, Fukuoka M, et al. Percutaneous transluminal cerebral angioplasty: serial angiographic follow-up after successful dilatation. *Neuroradiology.* 1997; 39(2):111–116.

47. Akkerhuis KM, Deckers JW, Lincoff AM, et al. Risk of stroke associated with abciximab among patients undergoing percutaneous coronary intervention. *JAMA.* 2001;286(1):78–82.

48. Kapadia SR, Bajzer CT, Ziada KM, et al. Initial experience of platelet glycoprotein IIb/IIIa inhibition with abciximab during carotid stenting: a safe and effective adjunctive therapy. *Stroke.* 2001;32(10):2328–2332.

49. Abciximab in acute ischemic stroke: a randomized, double-blind, placebo-controlled, dose-escalation study. The Abciximab in Ischemic Stroke Investigators. *Stroke.* 2000;31(3):601–609.

50. Lee DH, Jo KD, Kim HG, et al. Local intraarterial urokinase thrombolysis of acute ischemic stroke with or without intravenous abciximab: a pilot study. *J Vasc Interv Radiol.* 2002;13(8):769–774.

51. Abou-Chebl A, Krieger D, Bajzer C, et al. Multimodal therapy for the treatment of severe ischemic stroke combining GPIIb/IIIa antagonists and angioplasty after failure of thrombolysis. *Stroke.* 2003;34(1):312. Abstract.

52. Suh DC, Sung KB, Cho YS, et al. Transluminal angioplasty for middle cerebral artery stenosis in patients with acute ischemic stroke. *AJNR Am J Neuroradiol.* 1999;20(4):553–558.

53. Takis C, Kwan ES, Pessin MS, et al. Intracranial angioplasty: experience and complications. *AJNR Am J Neuroradiol.* 1997;18(9):1661–1668.

54. Phatouros CC, Higashida RT, Malek AM, et al. Carotid artery stent placement for atherosclerotic disease: rationale, technique, and current status. *Radiology.* 2000; 217(1):26–41.

55. Higashida RT, Halbach VV, Tsai FY, et al. Interventional neurovascular techniques for cerebral revascularization in the treatment of stroke. *AJR Am J Roentgenol.* 1994;163(4):793–800.

56. Ohman EM, Marquis JF, Ricci DR, et al. A randomized comparison of the effects of gradual prolonged

versus standard primary balloon inflation on early and late outcome. Results of a multicenter clinical trial. Perfusion Balloon Catheter Study Group. *Circulation*. 1994;89(3):1118–1125.

57. Higashida RT, Hieshima GB, Tsai FY, et al. Transluminal angioplasty of the vertebral and basilar artery. *AJNR Am J Neuroradiol*. 1987;8(5):745–749.

58. Altmann DB, Racz M, Battleman DS, et al. Reduction in angioplasty complications after the introduction of coronary stents: results from a consecutive series of 2242 patients. *Am Heart J*. 1996;132(3):503–507.

59. Bando K, Satoh K, Matsubara S, et al. Hyperperfusion phenomenon after percutaneous transluminal angioplasty for atherosclerotic stenosis of the intracranial vertebral artery. Case report. *J Neurosurg*. 2001;94(5):826–830.

60. Meyers PM, Higashida RT, Phatouros CC, et al. Cerebral hyperperfusion syndrome after percutaneous transluminal stenting of the craniocervical arteries. *Neurosurgery*. 2000;47(2):335–343.

61. Abou-Chebl A, Yadav J, Reginelli J, et al. Intracranial hemorrhage and hyperperfusion syndrome following carotid artery stenting: risk factors, prevention, and treatment. *J Am Coll Cardiol*. 2004;43(9):1596–1601.

62. Juvela S, Heiskanen O, Poranen A, et al. The treatment of spontaneous intracerebral hemorrhage. A prospective randomized trial of surgical and conservative treatment. *J Neurosurg*. 1989;70(5):755–758.

63. Batjer HH, Reisch JS, Allen BC, et al. Failure of surgery to improve outcome in hypertensive putaminal hemorrhage. A prospective randomized trial. *Arch Neurol*. 1990;47(10):1103–1106.

CHAPTER 10

Renal Artery Intervention

Joel P. Reginelli, MD and Christopher J. Cooper, MD

INDICATIONS AND PIVOTAL TRIALS

Natural History of Renal Artery Stenosis

The prevalence of renal artery stenosis (RAS) in patients with hypertension has been estimated at 1 to 5%; however, angiographic studies suggest this may be an underestimate (1). Among patients with documented atherosclerotic disease in other peripheral vascular beds, the prevalence of RAS may be as high as 30 to 40% (2). Fibromuscular dysplasia (FMD) and atherosclerosis are the two primary pathologic etiologies of renal artery stenosis. Fibromuscular dysplasia accounts for about 10% of all RAS cases, typically occurs in younger (i.e., younger than 50 years) women, and has the classic "beads on a string" appearance at angiography (Fig. 10-1).

A young woman with new-onset hypertension that is accelerating or refractory to antihypertensive therapies suggests FMD. Atherosclerosis is responsible for approximately 90% of all RAS cases, and generally occurs in an older population (i.e., older than 50 years) with vascular risk factors. There is no gender preference observed in atherosclerotic RAS, and these patients may present in a myriad of ways: refractory or accelerating hypertension, worsening renal function, ACE inhibitor-induced renal failure, congestive heart failure, or as an incidental finding during other testing. The natural history of RAS depends largely upon the underlying etiology. FMD may involve the intimal, medial, or adventitial layer of the vessel, but medial FMD accounts for the

overwhelming majority of cases (i.e., about 90%) (3). Progressive narrowing occurs in one-third of patients with medial FMD; however, progression to complete occlusion is an extremely rare event. In contrast, atherosclerotic RAS is a progressive disease that may culminate in occlusion of the vessel. In one series, patients with RAS of less than 60% severity had a rate of progression to significant disease (i.e., greater than 60% severity) of approximately 20% per year. Among patients with vessels that had an initial stenosis of greater than 60% severity, there was progression to complete occlusion in 5% of patients at one year, and 11% at two years; however, some investigators have been unable to demonstrate a relationship between stenosis severity and renal function (4–6). While one might conclude from this that stenoses do not cause renal dysfunction, such a conclusion would be unfounded. Fundamentally, the kidney requires blood flow to function. Thus, it is absolutely clear that severe stenoses and occlusions yield a nonfunctioning kidney.

Why then is there difficulty relating stenosis severity to function? Clearly, there are factors beyond the degree of stenosis that influence function. Some are intrinsic to RAS, including the duration of the insult, atheroemboli, hypertensive nephrosclerosis of the contralateral kidney, activation of the renin-angiotensin system, and finally the characteristics and effects of the stenosis (including lesion length, minimal lumen diameter, etc) on renal blood flow and intrarenal pressure. This is the reasoning behind the hemodynamic requirement in the inclusion criteria. Additionally, other factors, such as

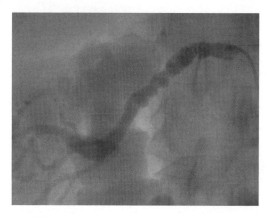

FIGURE 10-1 ● Right renal artery angiogram in a 40 year old female demonstrating 'beaded' appearance of vessel lumen, consistent with a diagnosis of fibromuscular dysplasia.

essential hypertension, diabetes, concomitant medications, generalized atherosclerosis progression, and aging, play roles in determining overall renal function.

Renal Artery Revascularization Procedures

An early, nonrandomized comparison suggested a benefit of surgical revascularization of severely narrowed renal arteries; however, surgery has been associated with significant perioperative complications and mortality (7). Most patients with RAS have lesions in other vascular beds, making them high-risk operative candidates; therefore, percutaneous transluminal renal angioplasty (PTRA) became an attractive alternative. Notably, the results of PTRA and surgery appear equivalent, when compared directly (8). PTRA was associated with improved blood-pressure (BP) control and a decrease in need for antihypertensive medications in retrospective studies; however, PTRA is associated with a high restenosis rate for ostial lesions, and 80 to 85% of all atherosclerotic RAS lesions involve the ostium. With the advent of stents, the problems associated with angioplasty may be circumvented.

Rees et al. reported 96% technical success rate with Palmaz® stents in ostial lesions (9), and perhaps more importantly, stents appear to be superior to PTRA, when compared directly (10). For these reasons, stents have become the favored mode of revascularization for ostial-atherosclerotic lesions of the renal artery.

Indications for Treatment of Renal Artery Stenosis

The goals of treatment in RAS are to improve the management of refractory hypertension (HTN) or congestive heart failure, and to preserve or improve renal function (Table 10-1).

While there is general agreement that PTRA/stent procedures offer benefits for patients with the aforementioned conditions, who are found to have bilateral renal artery stenoses, the indications for PTRA/stent procedures in similar patients with unilateral disease is more contentious.

In three randomized trials that compared balloon angioplasty to medical therapy, in the treatment of HTN in patients with RAS, there was no difference in BP control or serum creatinine among the two treatment groups; however, the need for fewer antihypertensive medications

TABLE 10-1

Indications for Percutaneous Revascularization for Renal Artery Stenosis

---

Indication

Medically refractory hypertension
  Requiring ≥3 antihypertensive medications at maximal doses
Significant hypertension in the setting of fibromuscular dysplasia
Acute renal failure after the initiation of angiotensin converting enzyme (ACE) inhibitors
Recurrent flash pulmonary edema in setting of uncontrolled hypertension
Severe renal artery stenosis in a solitary kidney
Severe bilateral renal artery stenoses
Severe unilateral renal artery stenosis with
  Evidence of decreased filtration in the affected kidney
  Hyperfiltration in the contralateral kidney (ie, lateralization)
Subacute renal failure (< 6 months),
  Particularly if creatinine < 3.0 and kidney size ≥ 9 cm in length

---

in patients treated with angioplasty was a consistent finding in each of the studies (11–13). These trials were limited by the high rate of crossover in treatment arms—from medical to angioplasty treatment—the small number of patients enrolled, the treatment of patients with stenoses that may not have been physiologically significant, and the use of angioplasty without stenting. A well designed, prospective, randomized trial comparing state-of-the-art interventional therapy to maximal medical therapy in this patient population is needed.

The ASTRAL trial will evaluate the effect of renal angioplasty or stenting on blood pressure control, while the CORAL trial will evaluate the effect of renal artery stenting on cardiovascular and renal events. In normotensive or mildly hypertensive patients with unilateral RAS, percutaneous revascularization is generally not recommended; however, in patients with preocclusive disease (i.e., greater than 90% stenosis), it may be considered. This subset of patients has a high rate of progression to complete occlusion, and stenting in this patient group may serve as a preventative measure to preserve renal function (4,14).

PATIENT SELECTION

Screening for RAS is often based on the clinical presentation. If a young woman presents with medically refractory hypertension, this should raise suspicion for RAS caused by FMD. Likewise, in patients with vascular risk factors, the presence of any of the following should prompt screening: refractory hypertension, ACE inhibitor-induced renal failure, recurrent flash pulmonary edema in the setting of hypertension, unexplained hypokalemia, subacute (i.e., 6 months) onset of renal insufficiency, or an incidental finding of decreased kidney size on imaging studies obtained for other reasons (15). The most common modes of screening for RAS are measurement of serum creatinine and the performance of a renal duplex ultrasound, although tomographic imaging with magnetic resonance or computed tomography are accepted alternatives in many centers. Unfortunately, serum creatinine is a highly unreliable marker of renal function. In the case of unilateral RAS, as disease progresses in one kidney, there is often lateraliza-

tion or hyperfiltration of the unaffected kidney, which maintains the serum creatinine within a relatively normal range despite significant renal impairment.

The renal duplex scan (i.e., 2D imaging and Doppler) is the most widely available, and most frequently employed, noninvasive test for assessing renal artery stenosis. While it provides important information regarding stenosis severity and kidney size, it does not provide a measure of overall renal function. Many facilities advocate magnetic resonance angiography (MRA) or computed tomography (CT) angiography; however, both are more expensive and less readily available than renal duplex scanning. In addition, CT angiography requires the administration of a contrast agent load, and MRA is limited in patients following stent placement, owing to image artifact. To assess overall glomerular filtration rate (GFR) and the differential GFR of each kidney, nuclear scanning with technetium-labeled diethylene-triaminepertaacetic acid (DTPA) may be performed. The combination of renal duplex scanning, followed by a DTPA scan in patients with RAS, provides both anatomic and functional data to assist in therapeutic decision making. A typical screening and treatment algorithm is outlined in Fig. 10-2.

ANATOMY (FIG. 10-3)

The bilateral renal arteries arise from the lateral aspect of the descending aorta at the level of the 1st and 2nd lumbar vertebrate, just inferior to the anterior origin of the superior mesenteric artery. The origin of the right renal artery is often slightly higher than that of the left renal artery. The takeoff point of the renal arteries is slightly posterior, and the main renal artery remains intact for a variable length, prior to subdividing into segmental arteries. These segmental arteries further subdivide into interlobar arteries that subsequently divide into the arcuate and interlobular arteries. The arcuate and interlobular arteries provide the smaller arterioles that penetrate the renal cortex and medulla. There are a number of variations in renal artery anatomy that warrant mention. The most common variant is the presence of an accessory renal artery. This is a second, generally smaller caliber, renal artery that typically arises inferior to the main renal artery (Fig. 10-4).

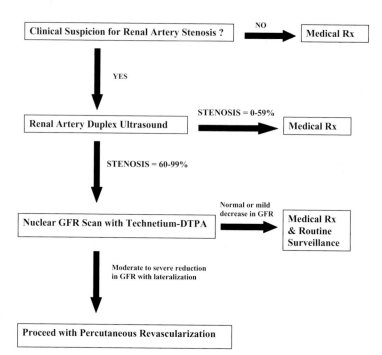

FIGURE 10-2 ● Algorithm for diagnosis and management of patients with suspected renal artery stenosis.

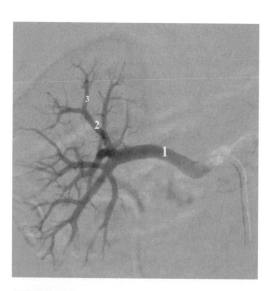

FIGURE 10-3 ● Digital subtraction angiogram of right renal artery demonstrating: **1.** main renal trunk, **2.** segmental artery, and **3.** interlobar artery.

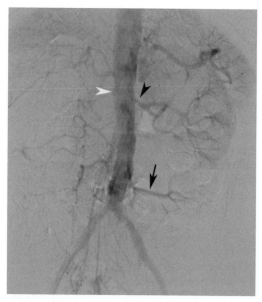

FIGURE 10-4 ● **Abdominal aortogram demonstrating accessory left inferior renal artery (black arrow).** This patient has a proximal lesion in the left upper renal artery (black arrowhead) and an occlusion of the right renal artery (white arrowhead), most likely caused by atherosclerosis.

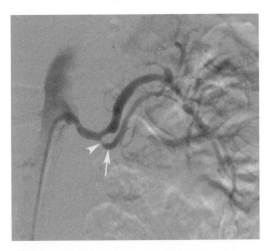

FIGURE 10-5 ● Left renal artery digital subtraction angiogram demonstrating early origin of a segmental branch of the renal artery (white arrow). There is a severe stenosis at the origin of this branch (white arrow head).

In some instances, the accessory renal artery may be of similar caliber to the main renal artery, thus supplying a large portion of the renal blood supply. In these circumstances, revascularization of stenosed accessory renal arteries has been performed.

A second anatomic variant is early subdivision of the main renal artery (Fig. 10-5). Normally, a main renal artery remains intact for several millimeters prior to dividing into a variable number of segmental branches. In some cases, a main renal artery may immediately subdivide into segmental branches just beyond its origin, thus making optimal percutaneous revascularization more challenging.

ACCESS

In most cases, arterial access for renal angiography is retrograde, via either common femoral artery, using a modified Seldinger technique to place a 4-Fr to 6-Fr arterial sheath. If there is moderately severe atherosclerotic disease in the iliofemoral vascular tree, a long sheath (i.e., about 35 cm) may be placed to avoid additional trauma to these vessels during catheter exchanges. In cases where there is severe bilateral aortoiliac disease, severely downgoing orientation of the proximal segment of the renal arteries, or when an abdominal aortic aneurysm is present, an antegrade approach via the brachial artery may be the preferred approach.

DIAGNOSTIC ANGIOGRAPHY

As a general rule, it is a good idea to obtain an abdominal aortogram prior to performing selective renal artery angiography (Fig. 10-6). The abdominal aortogram will provide important information regarding: the location of the renal artery ostia, the presence of high-grade ostial stenosis, the presence of accessory renal arteries or other anomalies, the degree of aortic calcification and atherosclerotic disease adjacent to the renal artery ostia, and the presence and degree of aneurysmal dilation of the abdominal aorta. Frequently, an optimal image of the renal arteries may be obtained in a shallow (10° to 15°) left-anterior oblique or AP projection.

To engage the renal arteries selectively, the authors recommend the use of 4-Fr to 6-Fr diagnostic catheters. Commonly employed diagnostic catheters include the internal mammary (IMA), renal double curve, Judkins Right® (JR4), SOS®, and Cobra® catheters. As a result of the posterior take-off point of the renal arteries, angiography sometimes may be done in an ipsilateral oblique projection (15° to 30°) to optimize visualization of the ostium and proximal segment of the vessel. Cineangiography should be performed long enough to allow visualization of contrast in the renal cortex (i.e., a nephrogram), in order to gain additional information on overall kidney size and regional function. The choice of contrast medium is at the discretion of the operator; however, low-osmolar and nonionic contrast media are recommended. For patients with severe renal insufficiency (i.e., creatinine clearance of less than 20 mL per minute), consideration should be given to using gadolinium or carbon dioxide imaging, in place of standard contrast imaging.

GENERAL STRATEGY

The goal of renal artery intervention is to achieve a durable result with minimal manipulation of catheters within the aorta and the ostium of the renal artery. Balloon angioplasty, without stenting, is sufficient in most patients with fibromuscular dysplasia; however, atherosclerotic narrowing of the arteries, particularly that involving the ostium

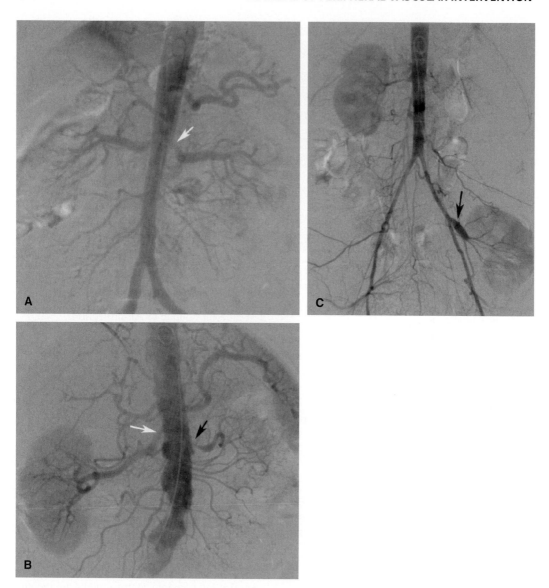

FIGURE 10-6 ● **Selection of abdominal aortograms highlighting the utility of this study prior to renal artery angiography. A:** Abdominal aortogram demonstrating a relatively smooth aortic lumen, a mild stenosis of the proximal right renal artery, and a severe stenosis at the origin of the left renal artery *(white arrow)*. **B:** Abdominal aortogram demonstrating an ostial left renal artery stenosis *(black arrow)* with a delayed left nephrogram, a mild-to-moderate proximal right renal artery stenosis *(white arrow)* with a normal right nephrogram, and diffuse irregularity of the lumen of the aorta consistent with significant atherosclerosis. **C:** Abdominal aortogram in a patient with known fibromuscular dysplasia. Prior left renal artery stenting resulted in occlusion of the vessel, necessitating surgical transposition of the kidney and its renal artery to the pelvis, where the renal artery was attached to the left common iliac artery *(black arrow)*. There is evidence of stenosis at the origin of the right renal artery.

of the renal artery, requires stent placement for an optimal result.

INTERVENTION

In general, patients should receive full-dose aspirin (i.e., 325 mg) and intravenous hydration prior to arriving in the catheterization lab. Once

arterial access has been obtained, heparin should be administered to achieve a goal activated clotting time (ACT) of 250 to 300 seconds. The routine use of platelet glycoprotein IIb/IIIa inhibitors is not recommended; however, these agents may be useful in cases complicated by the development of acute thrombus or distal embolization. Following the intervention, patients should receive dual antiplatelet therapy with aspirin and clopidogrel, for at least 30 days; however, presumably arising from the high flow in the renal arteries, treatment with aspirin, only, also has been associated with good outcomes (16).

Guide Catheter

The choice of guide catheter depends upon several factors: the location of the stenosis, the angle at which the renal artery comes off the aorta, and operator preference. A 6-Fr guide is used in most interventions, and commonly employed guide catheters include the IMA, JR4, renal standard curve (RSC), renal double curve (RDC), and hockey stick. Some operators prefer not to directly engage the ostium of the renal artery with a guide catheter, and they may opt to use a shuttle sheath, or multipurpose guide, placed just outside the ostium of the renal artery. There are two basic techniques for guide-catheter engagement: direct engagement and telescoping engagement.

Direct Engagement

The guide catheter is gently manipulated until it is seated in the ostium of the renal artery. This is a safe approach for most lesions; however, with high-grade ostial lesions or severe adjacent aortic disease, there is an increased risk of guide catheter-induced dissection, embolization, or abrupt closure, using this technique. A variation that may be safer is to use the "no touch" technique, wherein a guide wire is positioned extending up the abdominal aorta, while the guiding catheter is manipulated toward the ostium of the renal artery. When the renal artery is approximated, the wire is retracted, allowing the guiding catheter to engage the artery.

Telescoping Engagement

A long 4-Fr or 5-Fr diagnostic catheter is telescoped through a shorter 6-Fr guide catheter. The two catheters are advanced into the abdominal aorta over a 0.035″ guide wire, and the diagnostic catheter is used to engage the ostia of the renal artery. Once a wire has been placed across the stenosis, the diagnostic catheter is used as a monorail to bring the guide into the ostium, after which the diagnostic catheter is removed. This minimizes guide-catheter manipulations within the aorta and the renal artery ostium.

Wire

The choice of wire is based, primarily, on operator preference. Renal interventions may be performed over 0.035″, 0.018″, or 0.014″ wires. Irrespective of diameter, the wire chosen to cross the stenosis should be one with torque capabilities, with a soft tip to minimize distal embolization and to avoid unroofing the lesion. Recent trends suggest a movement toward 0.014″ wires (e.g., BMW®, Balance Trek®, Spartacore®, Guidant Corporation, Santa Clara, CA) for renal interventions. Emboli protection devices (EPDs) are being used more frequently in renal intervention, as will be discussed later, and these devices are generally mounted onto a 0.014″ wire.

Balloons and Stents

The choice of angioplasty balloon depends upon the size of the renal artery. The average diameter of a renal artery ranges from 5 mm to 7 mm; however, there may be a significant degree of variation from this average range. It is recommended that measurements be performed on a nonstenotic segment of vessel, free of poststenotic dilation, adjacent to the area of interest using the diagnostic- or guide catheter as a reference diameter. Many operators suggest an initial balloon diameter that is approximately 1 mm less than the measured diameter of the vessel. As mentioned previously, optimal results are often obtainable with angioplasty, alone, for RAS caused by FMD; however, stent placement is often required for patients with atherosclerotic RAS, particularly if the stenosis involves the ostium.

Ostial lesions are best managed with balloon-expandable stents, whereas consideration may be given to the use of self-expanding stents for stenoses that are in the midportion of the vessel. After deployment of a stent for ostial RAS, the authors recommend 'flaring' the ostium by retracting the balloon approximately one-half the balloon's length, and inflating it to a higher pressure. It is important to be sensitive to any pain (i.e., usually back pain) reported by the patient during either stent deployment or postdilation of the stent, as this reflects stretch of the renal artery, and further dilation may increase the risk of renal artery or aortic perforation.

Two stents are approved for use with failed renal-artery angioplasty: the Palmaz® stent

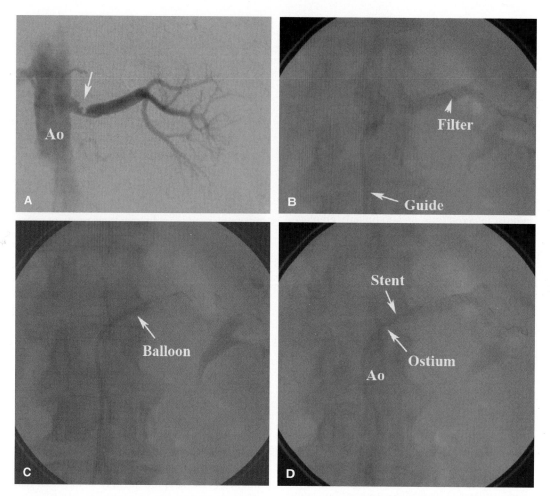

FIGURE 10-7 ● **Fluoroscopic images from left renal artery intervention. A:** Baseline angiogram demonstrating irregular ulcerated lesion in the proximal portion of the left renal artery *(white arrow)*. **B:** FilterWire placed in the distal portion of the main renal artery with good apposition of the loop of the filter with the vessel wall. **C:** Predilation of the lesion with 4.0 × 15 mm Maverick balloon. **D:** Stent placement to cover the ostium of the left renal artery. *(continued)*

(Cordis Corp.) and the Double Strut® stent (Medtronic Corp.); however, these older stents are relatively inflexible and many operators use other balloon-expandable stents, often those approved for biliary indications, for the purpose of renal artery revascularization (Fig. 10-7).

Emboli Protection

Balloon angioplasty or stent placement within an atherosclerotic lesion may result in embolization of particulate debris into the distal vasculature. During complex coronary cases (i.e., thrombus-laden lesions or saphenous vein-graft interven-

tions), the risk of embolization is high, and myocardial necrosis or no-reflow effects are common. Likewise, embolization during peripheral interventions may be associated with end-organ ischemia or infarction.

Several emboli protection devices (EPD) have recently been developed to reduce the embolic burden during endovascular procedures. These EPDs fall into one of two categories: balloon occlusive devices (e.g., Percusurge Guardwire®, Medtronic Inc.) or filter devices (e.g., FilterWire® EX, Boston Scientific). To date, these devices have only been approved for saphenous vein-graft interventions; however,

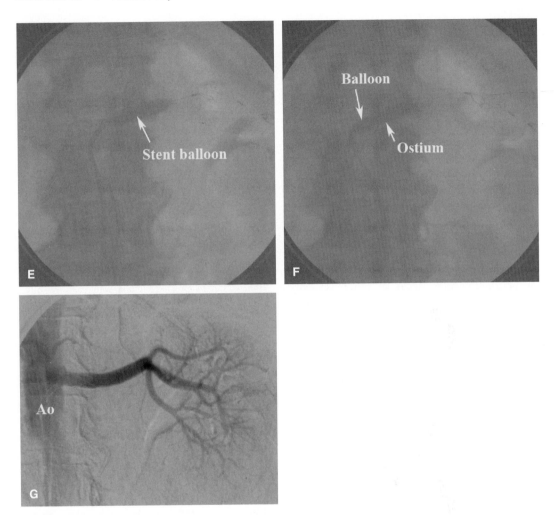

FIGURE 10-7 ● **E:** Deployment of balloon-expandable stent (6.5 × 18 mm Genesis). **F:** Flaring of the ostium with the stent balloon. **G:** Final digital subtraction angiogram of left renal artery.

many investigators have employed these devices in an 'off-label' use for peripheral interventions. At the time of this writing, a third EPD (Angioguard® XP, Cordis) is in the final stages of the approval process, for an indication of carotid interventions, and it is anticipated that the choices of, and indications for, EPDs will increase over the next few years. Distal embolization during renal intervention may result in ischemic nephropathy, and thus result in a deterioration of renal function, rather than achieving the intended goals of improvement or stabilization of renal function.

The role for these devices in renal artery interventions has not been studied in a prospective manner; however, case reports suggest a high rate of technical success with significant particulate debris retrieved (15). The use of EPDs during renal artery intervention may be limited by the underlying anatomy. If the main renal artery has a proximal branch point, often one must choose the largest segmental artery in which to place the EPD, recognizing that full protection is not possible in that setting. Additionally, the diameter of the mid- or distal segment of the main renal artery exceeds the maximal diameter of current iterations of approved EPDs (i.e., 5.5 mm). Once carotid EPDs become approved, the available EPD sizes will more appropriately match the renal artery diameter.

Complications

There are a number of complications that may arise during renal-artery intervention (Table 10-2).

Damage to the renal artery in the form of dissection or abrupt closure may occur as a complication of guide catheter engagement, wiring, or balloon or stent deployment. In abrupt occlusions, attempts should be made to cross the occlusion with a wire. Dissections involving the renal artery ostium generally require stent placement, whereas focal dissections that occur more distally may respond favorably to balloon inflation (Fig. 10-8).

Aneurysmal renal arteries are felt to be at higher risk for perforation, though rare cases of perforation may occur in otherwise normal vessels from an oversized stent, aggressive stent postdilation, or spearing of calcium plaque through the vessel wall. Oftentimes these may be managed with prolonged balloon inflation with, or without, reversal of anticoagulation. In nearly all circumstances, a low-pressure inflation should be performed, often with an oversized balloon, simply to stop bleeding. In cases that do not respond to balloon inflation tamponade, consider-

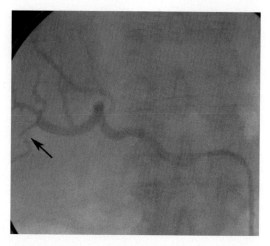

FIGURE 10-8 ● Focal dissection compromising the vessel lumen in an interlobar branch of the renal artery caused by the interventional wire.

ation may be given to placing a stent graft; however, if percutaneous sealing cannot be achieved with these measures, emergency surgery may be necessary.

Wire perforations in the parenchyma of the kidney may respond to particle or coil embolization and reversal of anticoagulation. Distal embolization in renal artery interventions may result in renal infarction or worsening ischemic nephropathy. Recognizing the salutary effects of glycoprotein IIb/IIIa inhibitors on embolization during coronary interventions, some operators advocate the administration of these agents when there is evidence of renal artery embolization; however, supportive data are lacking for the use of these agents in renal artery intervention. In heavily atheromatous aortas, cholesterol embolization to the lower extremities and splanchnic vessels may occur, as a result of catheter manipulation. As with any interventional procedure, bleeding or access site difficulties are the complications most commonly encountered.

Long-Term Outcomes

Restenosis following angioplasty, in patients with FMD, is generally caused by elastic recoil and occurs in approximately 10% of the cases. These restenotic lesions often respond favorably to repeat balloon angioplasty. In-stent restenosis (ISR) caused by neointimal hyperplasia

---

TABLE 10-2

Complications of Renal Artery Intervention

Complication

Renal infarction
Deterioration in renal function
Distal embolization to renal artery
Renal artery dissection
Cholesterol embolism
　To lower extremity circulation
　To mesenteric circulation
Renal artery/aortic perforation
Perinephric hematoma
Occlusion or thrombosis of renal artery
Bleeding complications
Stent embolization
Infection

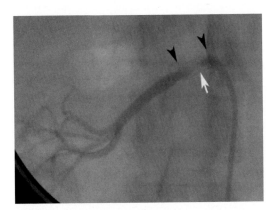

FIGURE 10-9 ● Right renal artery angiogram demonstrating severe in-stent restenosis (white arrow) in a previously placed stent (margins shown by black arrow heads) in the proximal segment of the vessel.

occurs in approximately 10 to 20% of renal interventions (Fig. 10-9). The mainstay treatment for renal artery ISR has been balloon angioplasty. Some centers employed gamma brachytherapy, in an off-label use, as an adjunct to balloon angioplasty; however, this treatment modality is no longer readily available. The application of drug-eluting technology to peripheral vascular stents holds great promise for reducing the rate of restenosis, although a drug-eluting peripheral-vascular stent is not currently available.

LONG-TERM FOLLOW-UP MONITORING

After renal artery intervention, patients should be followed, long-term, by a physician knowledgeable in renal artery stenosis and the syndromes of renovascular hypertension and ischemic nephropathy. Patients may develop delayed renal dysfunction stemming from embolization, restenosis, or progression of other causes of nephropathy; therefore, long-term follow-up assessment of renal function is advisable. Similarly, those patients who present with hypertension are certainly at risk for continued hypertension, or recurrence of hypertension if restenosis is encountered; therefore, regular blood pressure (BP) monitoring is recommended.

Anatomic follow-up evaluation to detect restenosis is somewhat controversial. Some operators follow only blood pressure and renal func-

tion, reserving anatomic evaluation for those patients with worsening of one or both parameters. Other clinicians perform a surveillance anatomic assessment at between 6 months and 1 year after treatment, to detect restenosis. Currently, duplex ultrasonography with careful interrogation of velocities along the renal artery, from the aortic origin to the kidney proper, is the preferred strategy. It does not require contrast medium, involves no ionizing radiation, and may provide diagnostic data regarding the stented segment; however, not all centers are adept at this technology and some patients have body shapes that preclude adequate ultrasound evaluation. Under these circumstances, CT angiography is a reasonable alternative. MRA is of limited value in this instance, as metallic artifact compromises visualization of the stented segment.

KEY PRINCIPLES (PEARLS, DO'S AND DON'TS)

Do

1. Document clinical indications and results of noninvasive anatomic and functional testing, prior to proceeding with revascularization.
2. Administer periprocedural hydration and N-acetylcysteine in patients with documented renal insufficiency.
3. Confirm stent placement in two views (i.e., anteroposterior and ipsilateral oblique) before deployment, to avoid missing the ostium.

Don't

1. Do not intervene routinely on stenoses discovered during incidental renal angiography obtained at the time of cardiac catheterization. Anatomic and functional testing is indicated prior to intervention.
2. Do not perform bilateral renal artery stenting during one procedure. There will be exceptions to this rule; however, in the vast majority of cases where bilateral renal stenting is indicated, the procedures should be performed in a staged manner.
3. Do not routinely stent lesions caused by FMD. Balloon angioplasty is equally efficacious and stenting should be reserved for use if dissection occurs.

REFERENCES

1. Harding MB, Smith LR, Himmelstein SI, et al. Renal artery stenosis: prevalence and associated risk factors in patients undergoing routine cardiac catheterization. *J Am Soc Nephrol.* 1992;2:1608–1616.
2. Olin JW, Melia M, Young JR, et al. Prevalence of atherosclerotic renal artery stenosis in patients with atherosclerosis elsewhere. *Am J Med.* 1990;88:46N–51N.
3. Safian RD, Textor SC. Renal-artery stenosis. *N Engl J Med.* 2001;344(6):431–434.
4. Zierler RE, Bergelin RO, Isaacson JA, Strandness DE. Natural history of atherosclerotic renal artery stenosis: A prospective study with duplex ultrasonography. *J Vasc Surg.* 1994;19:250–258.
5. Wright JR, Shurrab AE, Cheung C, et al. A prospective study of the determinants of renal functional outcome and mortality in atherosclerotic renovascular disease. *Am J Kidney Dis.* 2002;39(6):1153–1161.
6. Suresh M, Laboi P, Mamtora H, et al. Relationship of renal dysfunction to proximal arterial disease severity in atherosclerotic renovascular disease. *Nephrol Dial Transplant.* 2000;15(5):631–636.
7. Hunt JC, Sheps SG, Harrison EG Jr, et al. Renal and renovascular hypertension. A reasoned approach to diagnosis and management. *Arch Intern Med.* 1974;133(6): 988–999.
8. Weibull H, Bergqvist D, Bergentz SE, et al. Percutaneous transluminal renal angioplasty versus surgical reconstruction of atherosclerotic renal artery stenosis: a prospective randomized study. *J Vasc Surg.* 1993; 18:841–852.
9. Rees CR, Palmaz JC, Becker GJ, et al. Palmaz stent in atherosclerotic stenoses involving the ostia of the renal arteries: preliminary report of a multicenter study. *Radiology.* 1991;181(2):507–514.
10. van de Ven PJ, Kaatee R, Beutler JJ, et al. Arterial stenting and balloon angioplasty in ostial atherosclerotic renovascular disease: a randomised trial. *Lancet.* 1999:353:282–286.
11. van Jaarsveld BC, Krijnen P, Pieterman H, et al. The effect of balloon angioplasty on hypertension in atherosclerotic renal artery stenosis. Dutch Renal Artery Stenosis Intervention Cooperative Study Group. *N Engl J Med.* 2000;342:1007–1014.
12. Webster J, Marshall F, Abdalla M, et al. Randomised comparison of percutaneous angioplasty vs continued medical therapy for hypertensive patients with atheromatous renal artery stenosis. Scottish and Newcastle Renal Artery Stenosis Collaborative Group. *J Hum Hypertens.* 1998;12:329–335.
13. Plouin PF, Chatellier G, Darne B, et al. Blood pressure outcome of angioplasty in atherosclerotic renal artery stenosis: a randomized trial. Essai Multicentrique Medicaments vs Angioplastie (EMMA) Study Group. *Hypertension.* 1998;31:823–829.
14. Jaff MR, Olin JW. Atherosclerotic stenosis of the renal arteries: indications for intervention. *Texas Heart Inst J.* 1998;25:34–39.
15. Tan WA, Yadav JS, Wholey MH, et al. Endovascular Options for Peripheral Arterial Occlusive and Aneurysmal Disease. In:Topol EJ, ed. *Textbook of Interventional Cardiology.* 4th ed. Philadelphia: Saunders; 2003: 481–522.
16. Burket MW, Cooper CJ, Kennedy DJ, et al. Renal artery angioplasty and stent placement: predictors of a favorable outcome. *Am Heart J.* 2000;139(1)(Pt 1):64–71.

CHAPTER 11

Endovascular Treatment of Abdominal and Thoracic Aortic Aneurysms

Takao Ohki and Mahmoud B. Malas

T he first successful surgical repair of an abdominal aortic aneurysm (AAA) was performed by Dubost in 1952 (1). Since then, significant improvements related to the surgical repair of AAAs have been made. Modern series have reported an impressive 1 to 5% surgical mortality rate following open repair. However, it is important to note that there are other risks besides mortality in performing a major laparotomy. These include high rates of major complications (i.e., 20 to 40%), prolonged hospitalization (i.e., 5 to 10 days), prolonged recuperation (i.e., 2 to 5 months), and sexual dysfunction (i.e., 60 to 80%). Moreover, there are patients that are not surgical candidates, owing to comorbid conditions. As a result, there was a significant unmet need for a better way to treat patients with AAAs. This led to the development of endovascular repair of aneurysms (EVAR), with the first such procedure being performed and reported by Juan Parodi in the early 1990s (2). Since that time, significant improvements in both technique as well as devices have been made. Currently, three endografts are approved by the Food and Drug Administration (FDA) for AAA repair, and EVAR has become one of the standard treatment options. Similarly, endografts for thoracic pathologies including aneurysms, dissections and penetrating ulcers are being developed with promising early results.

This chapter includes a description of the general indications for AAA therapy, the specific indications for EVAR, the various types of endovascular grafts that are currently available for AAA and thoracic aortic aneurysms (TAAs), as well as the techniques employed for EVAR.

GENERAL INDICATION FOR AAA THERAPY

At the present time, the same size criteria for open repair should be used for EVAR as there are no data to justify performing EVAR for smaller aneurysms. In 1966, the first paper discussing the size of AAA as an indication for open operative repair was published. Measurement on physical exam of more than 6.0 cm was used as a cut-off to proceed with the repair. Since then extensive studies have been done to define the standards for management. The first two prospective randomized multi-centre studies were the United Kingdom Small Aneurysm Trial (3) and the Aneurysm Detection and Management trial (the ADAM trial) (4). Each study prospectively randomized patients (i.e., n = 1090, and 1136, respectively) with asymptomatic AAAs 4.0 cm to 5.5 cm in diameter to undergo early elective open surgery, or surveillance with ultrasonography or computed tomography, every 3 to 6 months. Patients were followed up for a mean of 4.6 years in the UK trial and a mean of 4.9 years in ADAM trial. If the diameter of an aneurysm exceeded 5.5 cm, or the aneurysm expanded by more then 1.0 cm in 1 year, or the patient became symptomatic (i.e., in the surveillance groups), surgical repair was recommended. The primary end-point was death, and analysis was done by intention-to-treat. Both groups had similar cardiovascular risk factors at baseline.

At the end of the trial, surgical repair was performed in 90% of the patients in the immediate-repair groups, and in 60% of the surveillance groups (i.e., similar for both studies). The 30-day operative mortality rate in the early surgery group for the UK trial was 5.8%, which led to a survival disadvantage for these patients early in the trial. Mortality rates did not differ significantly between the two groups at 2 years, 4 years, or 6 years. Age, sex, or initial aneurysm size did not modify the overall hazard ratio. Although the immediate post-operative mortality rate in the ADAM trial (i.e., 2.7%) is significantly less then the UK trial (i.e., 5.8%), there was no reduction in the rate of death related to AAA in the immediate-repair group (i.e., 3.0%), as compared with the surveillance group (i.e., 2.6%). The conclusion for both studies was that radiographic surveillance with delayed surgery, for small, abdominal aortic aneurysms (i.e., 4.0 cm to 5.5 cm) is safe,

and immediate surgery does not provide a long-term survival advantage.

As a result of these recent findings, the Society for Vascular Surgery Guidelines for the treatment of AAA have recently been modified. The previous guidelines recommended surgical treatment for an AAA greater than 4.0 in diameter, in an average patient. This size threshold has been modified to 5.5 cm (5).

For aneurysms larger than 5.5 cm, there are no prospective studies published yet. The decision to operate should be made when the risk of rupture exceeds the operative risks. The patient, and his or her family, should participate actively in making the decision, after knowing all the facts. There is a significant variation among vascular surgeons regarding the concept of rupture risk based on size (i.e., when AAA is larger than 5.5 cm). However, the general consensus is that size is the most important predictor of rupture. Also most vascular experts agree that there is a significant increase in rupture rate when AAA diameter increases from 5 cm to 6 cm. Table 11-1 summarizes rupture risks, based on size.

This significant variation in experts' opinions, as well as the available data for rupture risk, suggest that although size is a very important factor, there are other factors that play important roles.

TABLE 11-1

Estimated Rupture Risk Per Year According to Abdominal Aortic Aneurysm Diameter Alone

AAA Diameter (cm)	Nevitt[1]	Reed[2]	UK[3]	Scott[4]	Jones[5]	ADAM[6]	Experts Consensus[7]
<4.0	0%	0% (0 to 5%)	0.3%	0.7%	—		0%
4–4.9	0%	1% (0 to 5%)	1.5%	1.7%	—		0.5 to 5%
5–5.9	5%	11% (1 to 21%)	6.5%	10%	12%	9.4%	3 to 15%
6–6.9	—	26% (7 to 46%)	—	—	14%	10.2%	10 to 20%
7–8.0	—	—	—	—	—	32%	20 to 40%
>8.0	—	—	—	—	—	—	30 to 50%

[1]Nevitt MP et al. N Engl J Med 1989;321:1009–14.
[2]Reed WW et al. Arch Intern Med 1997;157:2064–8.
[3]Brown LC et al. J Vasc Surg 1998;28:124–8.
[4]Scott RA et al. J Vasc Surg 1998;28:124–8.
[5]Jones A et al. Br J Surg 1998;85:1382–4.
[6]Lederle FA et al. JAMA 2002;287:2968–72.
[7]Brewster DC et al. Guidelines for the treatment of abdominal aortic aneurysms report of a subcommittee of the Joint Council of the American Association for Vascular Surgery and Society for Vascular.

Each of the following has been found to be an independent risk factor for AAA rupture: (4,6)

1. Chronic obstructive pulmonary disease (COPD)
2. Hypertension (HTN)
3. Female gender
4. Smoking
5. Symptoms—abdominal or back pain

Other non-independent risk factors include:

1. First degree relative with AAA (i.e., 15 to 35% increase based upon the number of first-degree relatives).
2. The ratio of the AAA diameter to the diameter of the native aorta.
3. The shape of the aneurysm. Saccular aneurysms have a higher risk than more cylindrical (i.e., fusiform) aneurysms. This is probably related to the significant increase in wall stress with eccentric aneurysms leading to rapid expansion and rupture.
4. The degree of expansion continues to be regarded as a significant risk factor for rupture. Aneurysms that grow more then 0.6 cm in diameter in 1 year are at higher risk for rupture, and thus require earlier repair. Smoking, HTN, and thrombus within the aneurysm are each associated with rapid expansion.

EVAR VS. OPEN REPAIR

The first prospective randomized study, the European EVAR trial, comparing endovascular versus open repair of AAA, completed enrollment in December 2003. The aim of this study is to assess the efficacy and durability of endovascular repair in terms of morbidity, mortality, and cost effectiveness. Inclusion criteria were age 60 years and older, with an established diagnosis of an AAA with a diameter of 5.5 cm, or larger. All patients underwent computed tomography (CT) prior to randomization to evaluate anatomic suitability for EVAR. Patients that were anatomically suitable for endovascular repair were assigned to either the EVAR I or EVAR II trial, based on their physiologic ability to withstand an open repair or not, respectively. The EVAR I trial prospectively randomized patients to either conventional open repair or endovascular repair. EVAR II prospectively randomized patients to either endovascular repair with best medical management, or best medical management alone.

Enrollment has been completed for both studies (i.e., over 1100 patients for EVAR I, over 300 patients for EVAR II). Patients will be followed up for at least 1 year.

Recently, the early outcome results were published (7). The 30-day mortality rate was 4.7% for those randomized to open surgery and 1.7% for those receiving EVAR (p < 0.05). The final report is expected in mid-2005. The Open Versus Endovascular Repair trial (OVER), conducted by the Veterans Affairs Medical System in the United States, follows in the footsteps of the European EVAR trial. The enrollment started in October 2003, with a target of 1200 patients. The conclusions of this trial are expected to be announced in 2009. The Dutch Randomized Endovascular Aneurysm Management trial (DREAM) prospectively randomized patients to undergo either endovascular or open repair. The goal of this trial is to evaluate the cost effectiveness of the endovascular repair compared to conventional open surgery.

The recently published early results were identical to the EVAR trial with lower 30-day mortality in the endovascular arm (open repair 4.6%, EVAR 1.2%) (8). A recent registry study also strongly suggests that EVAR is safer in the short term (9).

In December, 2003, the FDA Public Health Notification (PHN) committee announced the update on the AneuRx device, which has the longest follow-up data, among all other devices (i.e., 942 patients treated between March 1996 and October 2002). The report mentions that EVAR results in reduced peri-operative death, compared to open surgery (10). The mortality rate following EVAR is 1.5%, which compares favorably to 3 to 5% in most of the reliable, published data for open repair (i.e., UK trial, (3) and US Medicare data (11)). In their report, however, the FDA estimates that the aneurysm-related death rate is higher for EVAR (i.e., 0.4% per year), compared to open surgery (i.e., 0.1% per year), as a result of late endograft failures. Therefore, the survival curve may cross in the long-term, if the patient lives long enough. The operative mortality rate for open repair is significantly higher if one of the following factors is present (Canadian aneurysm study, (12) UK trial (3)):

1. Electrocardiographic changes indicating ischemia

2. Congestive heart failure
3. COPD with a forced expiratory volume in 1 minute (FEV1) of less than 1.
4. Elevated serum creatinine greater than 1.8.
5. Age older than 75 years

The 30-day operative mortality rates may range between 2 to 50%, based on the number of the above factors that are present. The presence or absence of these risk factors might be helpful in selecting the optimal treatment modality.

Morbidity rates are significantly lower with EVAR. The relative reduction in complication rate approaches 30 to 70% (5). This may be attributed to the significant reduction in anesthesia time, blood loss, and fewer cardiac complications. Minimal invasiveness (i.e., avoiding the abdominal or the retroperitoneal cavity) and a smaller incision result in significantly fewer gastrointestinal complications and less post-operative pain, allowing early mobilization and feeding. Reducing anesthesia time and incisional pain, and early mobilization, ultimately reduce post-procedural pulmonary complications. The end result is a shorter length of stay (13). The most striking difference between EVAR and open repair is the remarkable recovery time. Up to 30% of patients with open repair did not recover at 34 months postoperatively, and 18% indicated that they would not have the open repair again, knowing the recovery process. Sexual dysfunction following open repair approaches 60 to 80%, in some studies (14). This is obviously significantly less with EVAR because there is no dissection of the pelvic nerves. Even in the case of intentional coverage of the internal iliac artery, the incidence of post-operative sexual dysfunction is less then 1% with EVAR.

Early conversion of EVAR to open surgery has significantly decreased from 10% to 2%, as patient selection improved, devices became more flexible, and surgeons became more experienced. Reported late conversion rates of 1 to 2% per year, secondary to aneurysm enlargement, device migration, graft structural failure, or late AAA rupture, are typical (15,16). However, secondary conversion is associated with higher morbidity and mortality rates. All of these factors make open repair ideal for younger patients who have a minimal number of high-risk characteristics. Adequate patient understanding of the follow-up requirements, and the incidence of secondary

intervention and open conversion, are crucial issues in a properly informed consent. Until data from prospective randomized trials are available, patient choice remains the most important factor in selecting the treatment modality (5).

INDICATION FOR EVAR FOR TREATMENT OF AAAs (17,18)

Since its first introduction in 1991, EVAR has gained significant popularity. However, not all patients are anatomically suitable for EVAR. Inclusion criteria include (Fig. 11-1):

1. A patent SMA or celiac trunk.
2. An infrarenal neck diameter of less than 28 mm, as the graft chosen is over-sized by 10 to 20%, and the largest graft available has a 32-mm diameter neck (e.g., Cook, Zenith, see Table 11-2).

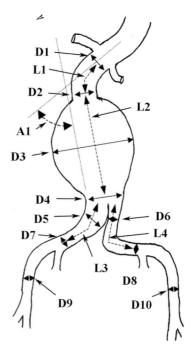

FIGURE 11-1 ● **Diameter and length measurements for abdominal aortic aneurysms.** In order to evaluate the patient's eligibility for EVAR and also to select the appropriate endograft and sizes, all the measurements listed should be obtained. This is best done with 3-D reconstructed CT scan images. Diameters: D1 and D2 – proximal neck of aneurysm, D3 – aneurysm, D4- distal neck of aneurysm, D5 and D7 – right common iliac, D6 and D8 – left common iliac, D9 – right external iliac, D10 – left external iliac. Lengths: L1 – length of proximal neck, L2 – length of aneurysm, L3 – length of right iliac limb, L4 –length of left iliac limb.

TABLE 11-2

Endograft Main Body Specifics

Company	Device	Main Body Length (cm)	Main Body Diameter (mm)	Iliac Leg Length (cm)	Iliac Leg Diameter (mm)	Delivery System Profile OD	Delivery System Profile ID	Fixed Location	Stent Expansion	Stent Material	Graft Material	Markets Available
Cook	Zenith	7.4, 8.8, 10.3, 11.7, 13.2	22, 24, 26, 28, 30, 32	3.7, 5.4, 7.1, 8.8, 10.5, 12.2	8, 10, 12, 14, 16, 18, 20, 22, 24	20, 22 F	18, 20 F	Suprarenal	Self-Expanding	Stainless Steel	Woven Polyester	US, Europe, Asia, Australia, Latin America
Cordis	Fortron†	8	26, 30, 34	10, 12, 14	16, 22	Info not provided		Suprarenal crown stent	Self-expanding & infrarenal barbs	Nitinol	Woven Polyester	Europe
Edwards	Lifepath†	8.7, 8.9, 9.2	21, 23, 25, 27, 29, 31	7.5, 7.7, 8.0	15		21F	Infrarenal	Balloon-Expanding	Elgiloy	Woven Polyester	Europe, Australia
Edologix	Powerlink	8, 10	25, 28, 34†	4, 55	16	21F		Infrarenal or Suprarenal	Self-Expanding	Stainless steel alloy	e-PTFE	Europe, Filed in Japan and US
Gore	Excluder	14, 16, 18	23, 26, 28.5, 31†	10, 12, 14	12, 14.5, 16, 18, 20	20F	18F	Infrarenal	Self-Expanding	Nitinol	e-PTFE	US, Europe, Asia, Filed in Japan, Australia, Latin America
Medtronic	AneuRx	13.5, 16.5	20, 22, 24, 26, 28	85, 115	12, 13, 14, 15, 16	21F		Infrarenal	Self-Expanding	Nitinol	Woven Polyester	US, Europe, Australia, Latin America
Medtronic	Talent*,†	15.5, 17	24, 26, 28, 30, 32, 34	7.5, 9, 105	12, 14, 16, 18, 20	22.24F		Suprarenal	Self-Expanding	Nitinol	Woven Polyester	Europe, Asia, Australia, Latin America
NanoEndo-luminal	Apolo†	135–180	25, 28, 31, 34	75–115	12, 14, 16, 18	19, 23 F	16, 20 F	Suprarenal	Self-Expanding	Nitinol	e-PTFE	Latin America, EU pending

*Additional sizes available through custom order; † Not available in the US.
OD-outer diameter, ID-internal diameter.

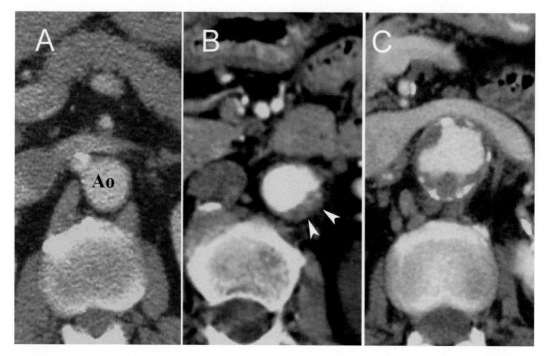

FIGURE 11-2 ● **Quality of the proximal neck. A:** Ideal proximal neck with absence of plaque or mural thrombus. **B:** Acceptable neck for EVAR with thrombus (*arrowheads*) occupying 90° of the circumference. **C:** Extensive mural thrombus is a contraindication for EVAR.

3. The length of the proximal neck has to be at least 10 mm to 15 mm, to allow for a proper seal of the stent graft against the aortic wall.

4. Ideally, the neck angulation should be less than 45° to 60°, as this is associated with a lower incidence of endoleak.

5. Calcification and mural thrombus encompassing more than 90° of the circumference of the proximal neck is unfavorable. (Fig. 11-2.)

6. A contour change of the proximal neck of more than 10% (i.e., flared neck) is associated with a higher incidence endoleak.

7. The minimal diameter of the external iliac artery should be 6 mm to 7 mm, to allow the passage of the device delivery system. The smallest delivery system in the US market, currently, is 20 Fr (Excluder).

8. Distal fixation requires a 10-mm to 15-mm length in the iliac vessels, similar to that required for proximal fixation.

PRE-OPERATIVE IMAGING AND WORK UP

Computed Tomography

A spiral contrast-enhanced computed tomography (SPECT) scan is the standard pre-operative imaging modality for EVAR and endovascular thoracic aneurysm repair (ETAR). A high-quality scan may be reconstructed in three dimensions.

Advantages of 3D CT scan:

1. Ability to evaluate vessel wall calcification and mural thrombus

2. Non-invasive study

3. Enables accurate measurement of all the dimensions needed to perform EVAR including the diameter, length, and angle of the proximal neck as well the iliac vessels. If one uses the MMS® (i.e., Medical Media System) reconstruction, these measurements are more precise. A 3-D reconstruction allows one to rotate the images on sagittal, coronal, or axial axes,

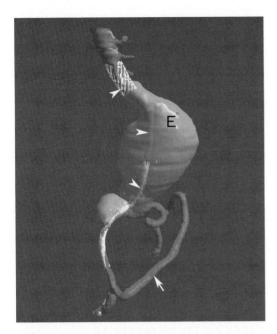

FIGURE 11-3 ● **Example of 3-D reconstruction of an abdominal aortic aneurysm.** 3-D reconstruction of a spiral CT scan along with axial images provides all the information needed to plan for EVAR. In this example, an aorto-uni-iliac endograft (*arrowheads*) was placed along with a femoral-iliac bypass (*arrow*) and an occluder in the left common iliac artery. Note the presence of a type 2 endoleak arising from the inferior mesenteric artery (**E**).

and to obtain all measurements required for the proper graft selection (Fig. 11-3). An additional advantage is that it provides aneurysmal volume measurements. This is particularly beneficial for future follow-up studies.

Disadvantages of CT scan:

1. 1 to 2% of patients might experience contrast-induced allergic reactions.
2. Risk of Contrast nephropathy.
3. A major pitfall of axial imaging is not taking aortic neck deviation into consideration. As the vessels enlarge, they also elongate, resulting in tortuosity and deviation. This may result in an over-estimation of neck diameter (i.e., when the aortic lumen is oval rather than round) and an under-estimation of neck length. This may be overcome by image processing with curved linear reformatting, perpendicular to an imaginary line inserted in the center of the vessel lumen. If reformatting is not available, one may estimate the angula-

tion and factor in the extra length. The minor diameter of the neck should always be used, to avoid overestimation.

Angiography

In the vast majority of cases, high-resolution CT-scan imaging should be sufficient for thorough evaluation of the anatomy of the AAA, and for accurate graft selection. On rare occasions, a pre-operative angiogram may be beneficial. However, this may always be done at the time of EVAR. A pre-operative angiogram may be beneficial for beginner interventionists.

The advantages of the aortogram include better evaluation of aorto-iliac occlusive disease and major branch stenoses, including main and accessory renal and mesenteric arteries. However, angiography is not as good as CT for evaluating vessel calcification, and may not be able to measure the neck diameter accurately, owing to the inability to detect thrombus within the neck.

Protocol for angiogram for AAA:

1. After insertion of a short femoral sheath, a 0.035″ guidewire is advanced under fluoroscopy into the aorta, taking care to avoid branches.
2. A 5 Fr pigtail catheter is advanced over the wire to a point 3 cm above the level of the renal arteries (L1-L2).
3. Using a power injector (i.e., 30 mL, 600 psi, 15 mL per second), a AP angiogram of the abdominal aorta is obtained, encompassing the renal arteries down to the iliac bifurcation, bilaterally. Appropriate oblique views are necessary for patients with an angulated proximal aneurysmal neck.
4. A pelvic angiogram is then obtained with the pigtail catheter placed in the distal abdominal aorta, just above the aortic bifurcation.

Magnetic Resonance Angiography

Magnetic resonance angiography (MRA) is an alternative diagnostic modality to CT angiography, with the following advantages:

1. It eliminates the use of nephrotoxic contrast agents.
2. It eliminates the use of radiation.

3. It is non-invasive.
4. It also generates 3-D reconstructions of the abdominal aorta and run-off vessels.

The disadvantages of MRA are:

1. MRA is inferior to SPECT scan in terms of spatial resolution. It may miss collateral vessels.
2. In 10 to 15% of patients, MRA may not be performed, owing to metal implants that produce artifacts, or patient intolerance stemming from claustrophobia.
3. MRA is more expensive than CT scanning.
4. MRA does not demonstrate vessel wall calcification.
5. MRA is technician dependent and a standard AAA protocol has yet to be developed.

Ultrasound Imaging

Ultrasound is useful mainly for screening purposes, as it is readily available, and relatively inexpensive. However it may not provide accurate information on vessel diameter and length. It is also operator dependent.

Medical Evaluation

Although EVAR may be performed safely under local or regional anesthesia, one may not be sure that EVAR will be successful. If difficulties are encountered during the course of EVAR, one needs to decide whether to proceed with EVAR or to stop and convert to an open repair. Without knowing the risk of open repair in the individual patient, a sound decision regarding conversion may not be made and therefore, it is important to obtain thorough pre-operative cardiac and pulmonary evaluation.

Physical Examination

It is important to document the presence or absence of pulsatility in the aneurysm, pre-operatively. Once EVAR is performed, an abdominal examination should be performed and compared with the pre-operative exam. This will provide insight into the effectiveness of the aneurysm exclusion. For the same reason, one should make a full examination of the lower extremity, including pulses.

TYPES OF ENDOVASCULAR GRAFTS

Initially, the authors and others used a physician-made device constructed from Gianturco or Palmaz stents. Although there were several different types and configurations, each of these hand-made devices consisted of a single unit, and most of them were made either in a tube or an aorto-uni-iliac configuration. More recently, a number of industry-made endovascular grafts (EVGs) have been approved by the FDA, and have become available in the United States, including the AneuRx, Excluder, and Zenith (Fig. 11-4[A, B]).

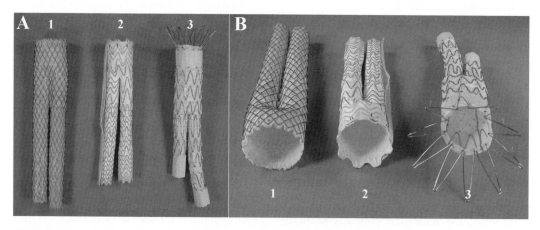

FIGURE 11-4 ● **Longitudinal (A) and oblique view (B) of FDA approved endografts**. 1. Medtronic AneuRx, 2. WL Gore Excluder, 3. Cook Zenith.

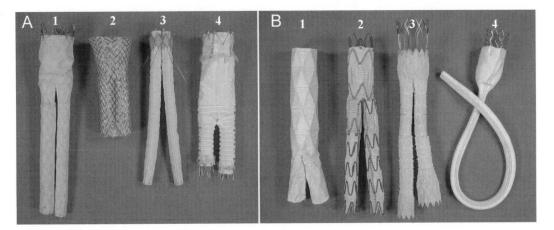

FIGURE 11-5 ● **A:** Endografts that were pulled from the market or whose clinical trials were prematurely terminated: 1. Boston Scientific Corp. Vanguard, 2. Covita endograft, 3. Cordis Quantum, 4. Guidant Ancure. **B:** Endografts that are expected to obtain FDA approval in the near future. 1. Endologix PowerLink, 2. Medtronic Talent, the Cordis Fortron, 3. Nano Endoluminal Apollo, 4. Vascular Innovation Parodi endograft.

For a number of reasons, some devices have been taken off of the market, or the clinical trials were prematurely aborted. These include the Ancure, Corvita, Quantum, and the Vanguard (Fig. 11-5[A]).

Others are awaiting FDA approval, or are undergoing clinical trials, including the TALENT®, LifePath, PowerLink, Fortron, Anaconda, Enovus, and the Parodi VI endograft (Fig. 11-5[B]). The currently available, industry-made devices are all bifurcated endovascular grafts, and most are modular grafts that consist of two or more components (Tables 11-2 and 11-3).

Self-Expanding versus Balloon-Expandable Stents

Basically, EVGs are a combination of vascular stents and prosthetic grafts, with the stents serving as fixation devices. Depending on the type of stent that is used, EVGs may be classified into two distinct types, self-expanding or balloon-expandable. Most EVGs use a self-expanding stent. The advantages of self-expanding devices include ease of deployment and the ability to accommodate some degree of aortic neck enlargement. The disadvantages include the risk of neck enlargement, as well as stent migration. A balloon-expandable stent has been used for the Lifepath graft and the Parodi endograft. The latter uses an extra-large Palmaz® stent. Although balloon-expandable stents may be more demand-

ing, technically, to deploy accurately at the desired location, in general they have stronger radial strength, as compared to self-expanding stents. This is especially advantageous in treating aneurysms with a short, and angulated, proximal neck.

Most EVGs, with the exception of Ancure, Enovus, and Parodi endografts, are fully supported (i.e., have a stent that supports the entire length of the graft). This feature is advantageous when endovascular grafts are deployed in tortuous arteries, as it helps to prevent compression or kinking of the graft, a phenomenon that has been encountered more frequently in grafts that lack this support.

Single Component versus Multiple Components (Modular)

As the anatomy, length, and diameter of aneurysms vary significantly from patient to patient, it is advantageous for an endovascular graft to have a certain dimensional adaptability, to accommodate this variability. Variability in length, between the proximal and the distal ends or termination points, may be managed by changing the amount of overlap between each of the two components. In the bifurcated grafts, the additional limb of a modular bifurcated graft and extenders will serve to achieve this form of lengthwise dimensional adaptability. The distal landing

TABLE 11-3

Ancillary Products

Company	Product	Main Body Extension		Iliac Extension		Aorto-Uni-Iliac Convertor		Occluder Diameter
		Length (cm)	Diameter (mm)	Length	Diameter	Length	Proximal Diameter	
Cook	Zenith	3.6	22, 24, 26, 28, 30, 32	5.5	8, 10, 12, 14, 16, 18, 20, 22, 24	8	24, 28, 32	14, 16, 20, 24
Endologix	Powerlink	5.5, 7.5	25, 28, 34†	5.5, 8.8	16, 20	20, 22	25, 28	25
Gore	Excluder	3.3, 4.5†	23, 26, 28.5, 32†	7, 10, 12, 14, 15, 16	10, 12, 14.5, 16, 18, 20	N/A	N/A	N/A
Medtronic	AnueRx	3.75	20, 22, 24, 26, 28	5.5	12, 13, 14, 15, 16	N/A	N/A	N/A
Medtronic	Talent	2.6	22, 24, 26, 28, 30, 32, 34, 36	7.4, 8.1	8, 10, 12, 14, 16, 18, 20, 22, 24	1 piece AUI: 15.7, 17 2 piece AUI: Proximal 124–126 Distal 7.5, 8, 14	22, 24, 26, 28, 30, 32, 34, 36	8, 10, 12, 14, 16, 18, 20, 22, 24
NanoEndoluminal	Apollo	4	25, 28, 31, 34	6, 0–11, 5	12, 14, 16, 18	115 (AUI device)	25, 28, 31, 34	12, 14, 16, 18

* Additional sizes available through custom order; †Not available in the US.

zone of the limb may be adjusted by changing the amount of overlap between the main body and the limb. In addition, the length of the ipsilateral limb may be extended with an extender stent graft. All EVGs, with the exception of the Ancure, Enovus, and the Parodi endografts, are modular in design.

DESCRIPTION OF INDIVIDUAL DEVICES APPROVED BY THE FDA FOR EVAR

For a list of these devices, see Tables 11-2 and 11-3. A detailed description follows below.

Ancure

Unlike other devices, the Ancure EVG secures the graft to the proximal and distal aneurysm necks with stents that have hooks. A balloon is used to ensure seating of the stent hooks into the aortic wall. The Ancure graft is made from a single component (Fig. 11-5[A]). This means that the graft lacks the ability for intraprocedural customization; therefore, precise pre-operative length measurement is of paramount importance when using this device. In addition, as the size of the introducer sheath is 24 Fr in outer diameter, difficulties in inserting the device through the femoral and iliac arteries, and injures to these vessels, have been encountered. Ancure is the only industry-made device that lacks a stent in the mid-portion of the graft. This has led to compression or kinking of the graft limb, which has resulted in graft occlusion. Placement of an additional stent has been effective in preventing such complications. Production of this device, however, was terminated as of October 2003.

AneuRx

The AneuRx EVG employs a nitinol stent as a fixation device and also as the structural support of the body of the graft. It is a modular device composed of a main graft and a separate contralateral limb component (Fig. 11-4). The stent is located on the outside of the graft, which is believed to increase the fixation capabilities to the native artery. The chief advantage of this device includes its versatility. The company provides a full line of proximal and distal extension cuffs (i.e., 12-mm to 28-mm diameter) that may be used to accommodate a wide range of distal landing-zone diameters. Following deployment of the main graft, a contralateral limb is inserted, via the contralateral femoral artery, and deployed. Recently, an enhanced version of the AneuRx has been introduced. Improvements include the Xpedient delivery system for accurate and easy deployment, the use of high-density Dacron that eliminates type-4 endoleaks, and larger sizes for the proximal and distal stents.

Excluder

The Excluder also employs a nitinol stent, as a fixation device and as the structural support of the body of the graft. It is a modular device, composed of a main graft and a separate, contralateral limb component (Fig. 11-4). The chief advantages of this device include the smaller crossing profile (i.e., 20 Fr) and its flexibility. This aspect has been extremely helpful in treating patients who have diseased, and small, iliac vessels. In addition, as the stent is attached to the graft material with thin layers of polytetrafluoroethylene (PTFE), this endograft does not have sutures, a feature in some devices that has been responsible for some endograft failures. The main graft is constrained by an outer wrap, and is deployed by pulling a rip cord that releases the outer wrapping. Recent 3-year follow-up data show that over 20% of patients had sac enlargements, but without a demonstrable endoleak (i.e., endotension). Although this has not resulted in any clinical sequelae so far, it has been of concern for physicians and patients.

Zenith

The Zenith is another modular EVG, but unlike the others, it uses a stainless steel stent (Fig. 11-4). Also, it has a large supra-renal stent that is designed to be deployed across the renal orifices. The supra-renal stent has 16 barbs that are believed to decrease the risk of stent migration. Such features may be beneficial in treating patients whose aneurysms have shorter necks. In addition, the Zenith has a wide range of iliac diameters, allowing treatment of AAAs with large iliac arteries. The US clinical trial has shown an impressive 0% migration (i.e., migration greater than 10 mm) and a 98% sac shrinkage/stabilization rate, at 2 years. Fenestrated and branched endografts that may treat peri-renal aneurysms are in the research pipeline.

REQUIRED EQUIPMENT FOR EVAR

The vast majority of endograft procedures are currently performed in an operating room, using a portable C-arm and digital fluoroscope with subtraction capabilities. The rationale for performing the procedure in the operating room include:

1. The need to be able to convert rapidly to an open major surgical procedure when necessary, without any delay
2. A sterile environment is mandatory, as all the devices currently require surgical exposure of the femoral artery, and the risk of graft infection must be minimized
3. The ability to perform a simultaneous open procedure, such as creation of a conduit for iliac access, or a femoral-femoral bypass in conjunction with an endovascular graft insertion.

However, with improved endografts accompanying increased operator experience, the need for urgent surgical bail-out maneuvers has become insignificant, and therefore performing EVAR in the cardiac catheterization laboratory, or an angiography suite, with peripheral capabilities and an appropriate sterile environment, is a reasonable alternative.

INTERVENTIONAL TECHNIQUE FOR EVAR

The Basic Setup of the Operation Room

Owing to the improvement in devices and increased experience, acute conversion to open repair is becoming less frequent. However, it is still advisable to sterilize the patient from the nipple down to the upper thigh so that one can perform laparotomy without delay, if needed. Also since endografts are permanent implants and since there have been several reports of endograft infection strict adherence to sterile techniques and use of prophylactic 4 antibiotics is strongly recommended. The operator and first assistant usually stand on the right side of the patient and the screen of the fluoroscope is placed so that it faces the operator. The operating table must be radiolucent, and have the ability to be controlled by the surgeon using a joy-stick or a foot switch. An extension table is attached caudal to the operating table to provide support for the lengthy guidewires and catheters. This extension table may have wheels so that it may simultaneously move with the operating table. Alternatively, a draped Mayo stand placed at the caudal end of the OR table may suffice.

Techniques to Obtain Vascular Access

All currently available devices require surgical exposure and an arteriotomy, owing to the large profiles of the introducer systems. The incision is placed higher (i.e., close to the inguinal ligament) than for a standard femoral-popliteal bypass, and retraction or partial division of the inguinal ligament may be necessary in order to dissect the external iliac artery. This technique is helpful in straightening a tortuous external iliac artery, which is not an uncommon finding in complex AAA cases. In addition, it allows access to the larger section of the iliac artery.

Following arterial exposure, vessel loops are placed around the artery proximal, and distal, to the puncture site. It is not necessary to dissect the origin of the deep femoral artery. An 18-gauge, one-wall needle is used to puncture the artery, and a 0.035″ guidewire is inserted through the needle. The needle is then removed and an introducer sheath (7 Fr to 9 Fr., 10 cm to 25 cm long) is inserted over the guidewire. The same steps are repeated in the contralateral femoral artery.

Alternatively, one may perform EVAR percutaneously (17). Although no closure device is designed for closure of puncture sites as large as that of the EVAR delivery system, by deploying the closure device prior to introduction of the EVG, it may be done with a reasonable success rate. This technique using the Perclose device has been termed the "preclose" technique. Not every patient is a candidate for the percutaneous approach. Patients with small, diseased femoral arteries, with preexisting plaque and calcification, and those with femoral aneurysms, should undergo open access. The advantage of the percutaneous approach includes the fact that one may perform EVAR with minimal or no

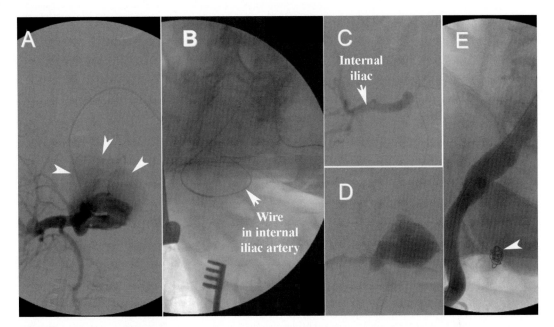

FIGURE 11-6 ● **Coil embolization of a right internal iliac artery. A:** Selective injection shows a large right internal iliac artery aneurysm (*arrowheads*). **B, C:** Selective catheterization of the outflow vessel is performed via the contralateral approach. **D, E:** Coils (*arrowhead*) were placed at the orifice of the outflow vessel to preserve collateral circulation between distal branch vessels and reduce the incidence of buttock claudication.

anticoagulation, in addition to the obvious advantage of avoiding a surgical incision.

Aortogram

A marker pigtail catheter is inserted into the abdominal aorta, for an initial aortogram. This pigtail catheter should be introduced from the common femoral artery, contralateral to the side for which the main endograft deployment is planned. If a pre-operative angiogram has not been obtained, angiographic confirmation of the proximal and distal neck aneurysmal diameters, as well as the length of the required endograft is necessary. As the internal iliac artery takes off from the common iliac artery in a posterior-medial direction, a contralateral oblique perspective may be used to best visualize the orifice of the internal iliac artery.

Coil Embolization of the Internal Iliac Artery

If the common iliac arteries are aneurysmal and lack an adequate landing zone, one may decide to extend the limb into the external iliac artery. It is generally believed that bilateral internal iliac

artery occlusion carries a risk of colonic or pelvic ischemia. However, if this may not be avoided, it may be performed with a relatively low complication rate, with the exception of buttock claudication, which occurs in up to 30 to 40% of patients. Coil embolization may be performed at the time of EVAR or it may be staged. In order to preserve as much collateral flow as possible, the embolization coils are best placed as close to the ostium of the internal iliac artery as possible (Fig. 11-6).

If the external iliac artery is tortuous, selective cannulation of the internal iliac artery, from the ipsilateral approach may be difficult. In such cases, a contralateral approach may be preferred (Fig. 11-6). Achieving immediate and complete cessation of antegrade flow is not mandatory, as antegrade flow will be obstructed by the placement of the endograft limb.

Determining the Side of EVG Introduction

Once the decision to proceed with EVAR is made, a super-stiff wire (i.e., Amplatz super-stiff wire,; Lunderquist wire) is introduced from the side where the endograft is to be deployed. This is

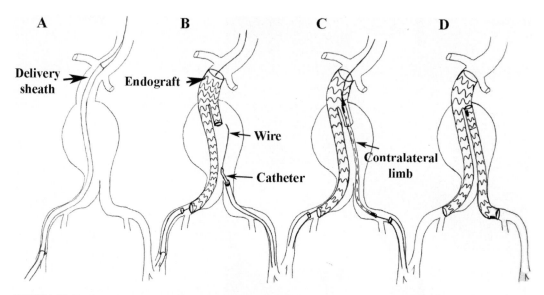

FIGURE 11-7 ● **Deployment of the endograft. A:** Endograft delivery sheath is introduced from the femoral artery. **B:** After confirming that the endograft is in the correct direction (i.e., short limb facing the contralateral iliac) and confirming the location of the lowest renal artery, the endograft is deployed. **C:** Short limb is cannulated from the contralateral side. **D:** Deployment of the contralateral limb completes the procedure.

performed to straighten any tortuosity in the access vessel and to improve the tracking capability of the EVG. The tip of the wire should be carefully placed, under fluoroscopic guidance, across the arch in the ascending aorta. Once the wire is placed in a good position, the location of the caudal end of the wire should be marked on the operating table, for future reference. In choosing the side of EVG insertion, several factors should be considered. These include the size, tortuosity, and degree of calcification of the iliac artery. Using the larger, less tortuous, and less calcified artery is obviously better. If everything is equal, introduction through the right femoral artery is convenient.

Introduction of the EVG

After the proper dosing of intravenous heparin, the ipsilateral femoral artery is clamped, proximally and distally, to the sheath insertion site with a hydrogrip clamp or a vessel loop, and the sheath is then removed (Fig. 11-7).

A horizontal arteriotomy is made with a scalpel, in preparation for the insertion of the large sheath containing the main graft. If the femoral artery is of good quality, one may introduce the device without creating an arteriotomy.

One may encounter difficulties in introducing the device. This may be caused by several factors. First, the iliac artery may be diseased or too small. In such cases, balloon angioplasty of the lesion may be helpful. Stenting should be avoided, as insertion of the endograft may dislodge the stent, and also because the stent may damage the delivery system.

If the difficulty is related to tortuosity, one should use the push-and-pull technique. This is done by simultaneously pulling on the super-stiff wire while introducing the endograft. Having maximum purchase of wire, distally, should help the operator perform this maneuver. Alternatively, one may stabilize the tortuous vessel by applying external pressure onto the access vessel or the aneurysm (Fig. 11-8). If such maneuvers are ineffective, introduction through the contralateral iliac should be attempted. Finally, a limited retroperitoneal exposure of the common iliac artery may be made to bypass the diseased external iliac artery (Fig. 11-9). A temporary conduit may be made by anastomosing a vascular graft to the common iliac artery, or an arteriotomy may be made in the iliac artery, for direct insertion. One should also consider the option of performing a standard, open repair, if difficulties are encountered and if the patient is a reasonable candidate for open surgery.

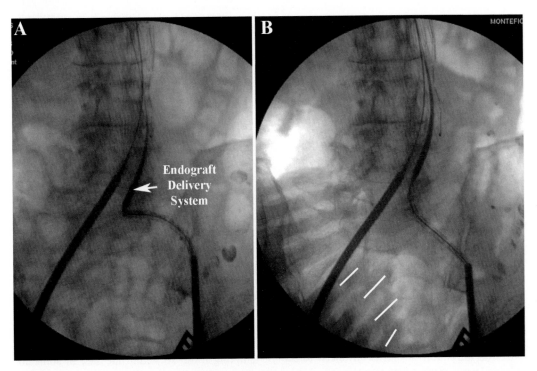

FIGURE 11-8 ● **External compression to facilitate stent graft delivery. A:** Fluoroscopic image shows difficulty of introducing the endograft delivery system through the left iliac artery, owing to vessel tortuosity. **B:** External compression applied on the abdominal wall prevents kinking of the delivery system and facilitates introduction. Note hands compressing the iliac artery (i.e., fingers of right hand are highlighted by straight lines).

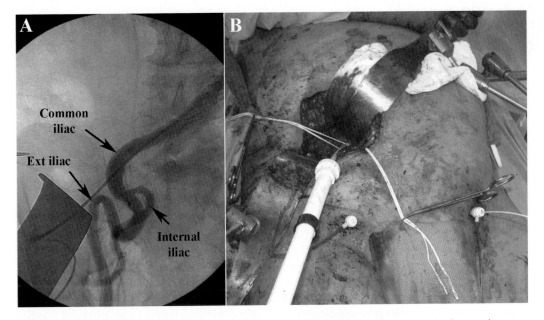

FIGURE 11-9 ● **Iliac access for difficult access from the common femoral artery. A:** Angiogram shows a tortuous right external iliac that made endograft insertion difficult. **B:** Retroperitoneal exposure and direct iliac access facilitates stent delivery.

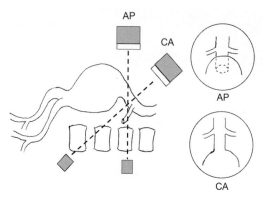

FIGURE 11-10 ● Appropriate image intensifier positioning for an angulated neck in an aneurysm with severe anterior-posterior neck angulation. If the image intensifier is positioned incorrectly (i.e., anteroposterior [AP]), one may not appreciate the length of the true neck. Appropriate cranial angulation (CA) provides best visualization of the neck.

Deployment of the EVG

Once the introducer sheath is advanced to the proximal neck of the AAA, an angiogram is performed via the pigtail catheter inserted from the contralateral side, to identify the location of the lowest renal artery. It is important to magnify the image and also to place the renal artery in the center of the image intensifier, to minimize parallax. Also, if there is any anterior-posterior angulation to the proximal neck, the image intensifier should be positioned appropriately (i.e., perpendicular to the neck) (Fig. 11-10). The position of the sheath containing the stent graft is adjusted, based on this angiogram. Each endograft has a unique deployment mechanism and one should refer to the manufacturers' deployment instructions for individual details.

Deployment of the Contralateral Limb

For modular endografts, it is necessary to deploy the contralateral iliac limb, separately. A 7 Fr sheath should be introduced into the aneurysm sac, in order to straighten the iliac artery, such that the directional catheter may be better controlled. In general, a single-curve catheter, such as a Vertebral or Bernstein catheter, is sufficient. For better torque control as well as maneuverability, an angled Glidewire should be used. The directional catheter should be kept away from the

short limb of the stent graft, and be placed close to the iliac orifice (Figs. 11-7 and 11-11).

By changing the direction and the position of the catheter, as well as by torquing the guidewire, cannulation may be performed in most cases. However, in some cases, this approach may be difficult and time consuming. As it is easy to lose track of time during a procedure, and as overheating the portable C-arm fluoroscope may be encountered, it is a good practice to time this step. The authors attempt an alternative approach if more than 10 minutes is spent during this step. Alternative approaches include the contralateral up-and-over technique, and the brachial approach. With the contralateral approach, a curved catheter such as the SOS-Omni catheter, is placed at the flow divider of the endograft and a Glidewire is introduced into the sac. If it is possible to guide this wire into the contralateral iliac artery, it may be easier to snare the wire in the iliac artery, as opposed to attempting to do so within the sac. In some instances, it is also possible to guide the wire into the contralateral sheath (Fig. 11-11). If one decides to snare the wire inside the sac, the Microvena Snare or the Ensnare retrieval devices are useful.

Once cannulation has been accomplished, it is important to confirm that the guidewire is located within the endograft, and not outside (i.e., in between the proximal stent and the aortic wall). Also one needs to confirm that the wire has not traversed between the stent and the graft material. A pigtail-type catheter is introduced over the guidewire and a "spinning test" is then performed within the proximal stent. If the catheter spins freely without resistance, one may be sure that the catheter is within the endograft.

The next step is to deploy the contralateral limb. A final confirmation of the length as well as diameter should be made with an angiogram. The marker pigtail may be used to measure the distance between the short limb and the internal iliac artery. When obtaining this angiogram, it is important to obtain the contralateral-oblique view, to visualize the orifice of the internal iliac artery. Also, as it is difficult to obtain another angiogram once the delivery system of the limb is inserted, one should obtain this angiogram with both the short stump and the internal iliac artery within the same view. By doing so, and by

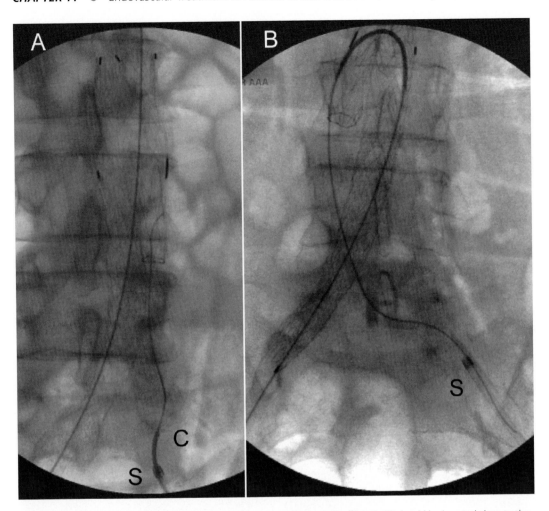

FIGURE 11-11 ● **A:** Cannulation from the contralateral femoral. The sheath (S) should be inserted close to the aortic bifurcation for better control of the directional catheter (C). The directional catheter should also be kept near the iliac artery to have a better chance at cannulation of the short limb of the stent graft. **B:** If short limb cannulation is difficult from the contralateral femoral approach, the up-and-over approach should be performed. The Glidewire may either be introduced into the sheath (S) placed from the contralateral femoral or it may be captured with a snare.

marking the two target sites on the fluoroscopic screen, or using the roadmap function, one may deliver and deploy the contralateral limb at the desired position without the need for moving the table or the image intensifier. In some instances, it may be impossible to cannulate the short limb and deploy the contralateral limb. This may be encountered when the orifice of the short limb is obstructed by a plaque or thrombus, or if the distal aorta is too small. In such cases, use of an aorto-uni-iliac converter, followed by creation of a femoral-femoral bypass and occlusion of the contralateral common iliac artery, should be performed (Fig. 11-12).

In cases where the distal end of the ipsilateral or contralateral limb of the graft is too small and results in an endoleak, one may use the "bell bottom" technique. This is done by deploying an over-sized proximal extension cuff at the distal attachment site. In doing so, one needs to terminate the first limb 3 cm to 4 cm above the landing zone, because the second over-sized stent needs some room for it to flare out (Fig. 11-13).

Touch-up Ballooning of the Endograft

Although all the stents are self-expanding, the authors recommend the performance of

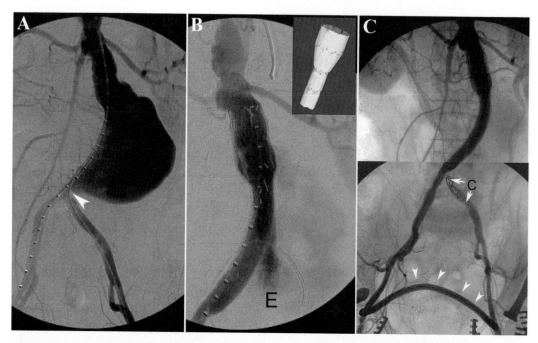

FIGURE 11-12 ● **Aorto-uni-iliac (AUI) converter for failure to access the contralateral limb.**
A: Pre-operative angiogram shows a large AAA with a tight aortic bifurcation (*arrowhead*). **B:** Contralateral limb
cannulation was not possible, owing to lack of space in the aortic bifurcation. Angiogram shows an endoleak (E)
through the short limb. **C:** AUI converter (*inset*) is placed within the endograft. Femoral-femoral bypass (*arrowheads*)
and coil embolization (C) of the common iliac artery completes the procedure.

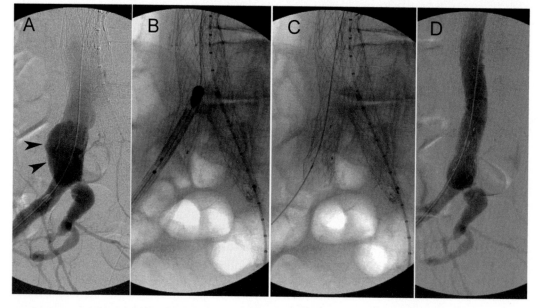

FIGURE 11-13 ● **'Bell bottom' technique to facilitate treatment of large iliac artery. A:** A short main
endograft was chosen so that the distal end will terminate 3 cm above the internal iliac artery. Note the presence of a
distal type 1 endoleak (*arrowheads*). **B, C:** Appropriately sized proximal extension cuff is deployed above the internal
iliac artery. **D:** Completion angiogram shows satisfactory result.

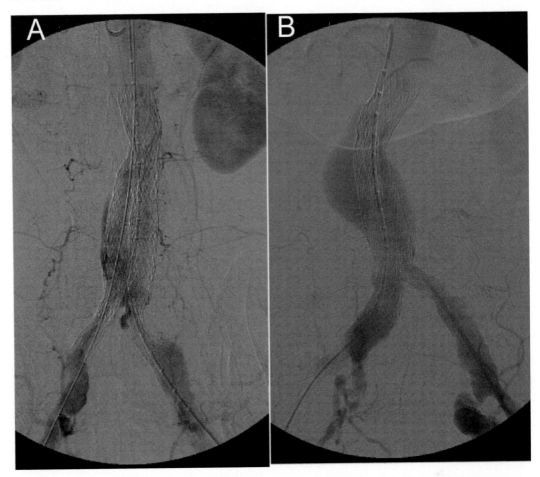

FIGURE 11-14 ● **Delayed phase angiogram at completion of procedure may reveal various endoleaks.**
A: Type 2 endoleak. **B:** Type 4 endoleak.

"touch-up" balloon angioplasty. This maneuver is performed at both the proximal as well as the distal attachment sites. Also, any junction of the modular components should be touched up. It is important to use a compliant balloon and to avoid high-pressure dilation that may damage the endograft. In addition, it is important to introduce the touch-up balloon over a super-stiff wire, and to keep the balloon catheter stationary during inflation. This is performed to prevent downward movement of the balloon as it inflates. This may potentially dislodge (i.e., distally) the previously deployed endograft.

Completion Angiogram

A completion angiogram should be obtained with a power injector. It is important to visualize the early phase, as well as the late phase, where one may detect subtle endoleaks such as small type-1

or type-3 endoleak, or type-2 and type-4 endoleaks (Fig. 11-14). All the sheaths and wires are removed and the femoral arteriotomy is closed with running sutures. In cases where the femoral artery is small or diseased, a patch closure of the arteriotomy may be performed.

TROUBLE SHOOTING

Diagnosis and Management of Endoleaks

Endoleaks have been classified into five different types (20). The types of endoleaks and their management are detailed below, and in Figs. 11-15 and 11-16.

Type 1 Endoleak

A type-1 endoleak arises from the attachment sites and is classified as proximal or distal.

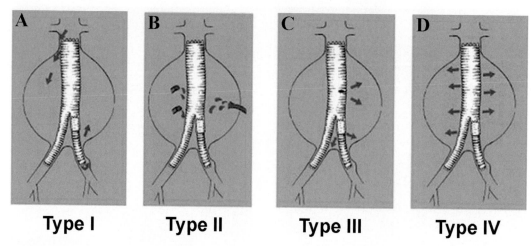

FIGURE 11-15 ● **Various types of endoleaks. A:** Type I endoleak (i.e., peri-prosthetic) occurs at the proximal or distal attachment zones. **B:** Type II endoleak is caused by retrograde flow from patent lumbar or inferior mesenteric arteries. **C:** Type III endoleak arises from a defect in the graft fabric, inadequate seal, or disconnection of modular graft components. **D:** Type IV endoleak is the result of graft fabric porosity, often resulting in a generalized mild blush of contrast within the aneurysm sac. (Reprinted with permission: White GH, et al. Type III and Type IV endoleak: toward a complete definition of blood flow in the sac after endoluminal AAA Repair. *J Endovasc Surg.* 1998:5:305–309)

Causes of type-1 endoleaks include: (1) undersizing the stent, (2) poor fixation, (3) neck dilation, (4) stent fracture or separation, and (5) poor patient selection (i.e., those with short, angulated, or irregular aneurysmal necks). If there is a type-1 endoleak, it is generally agreed that the aneurysm should be considered untreated, and immediate treatment is required. However, there is one exception. If the endoleak channel is small in diameter, and long, one may expect a significant pressure reduction after it thromboses and therefore, it is reasonable to leave it untreated if it is difficult to treat. If the type-1 endoleak arises from low deployment of the EVG, deployment of an additional proximal cuff may be attempted. In doing so, one needs to know the length of the EVG body (Fig. 11-17, Table 11-2) as well as the length of the cuff, as the distal end of the cuff needs to be placed above the flow divider. During this step, it is useful to place a curved catheter on the flow divider, to denote its location and to avoid deploying the distal end of the cuff into one of the iliac limbs (Fig. 11-18).

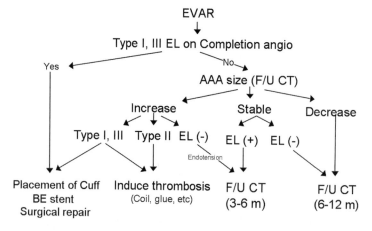

FIGURE 11-16 ● Treatment strategy for various endoleaks. BE, balloon-expandable stent; EL, endoleak.

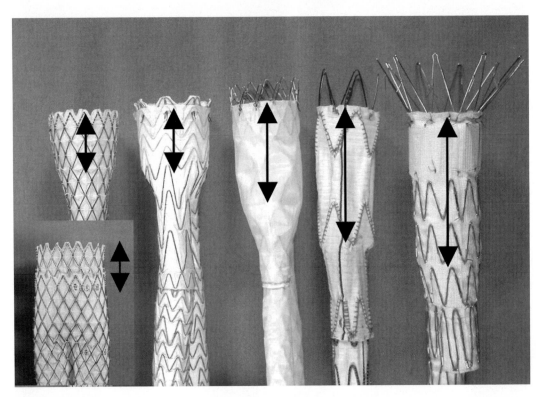

FIGURE 11-17 ● Pitfalls in the deployment of a proximal cuff. Each endograft is available in various body lengths (i.e., above the flow divider). The body length and the length of proximal cuff used should be kept in mind when deploying a proximal cuff in order to avoid deploying the distal end of the cuff within the iliac limb and to avoid covering the renal arteries. Inset shows the protrusion of the AneuRx extension cuff from the AneuRx endograft as the cuff is longer than the body of the endograft.

If the type-1 endoleak is due to deficient apposition of the stent, caused by an angulated or irregular aneurysmal neck, performing additional touch-up balloon angioplasty may be attempted. If this is unsuccessful, deployment of a balloon-expandable stent is usually effective. The authors prefer to use the extra-large Palmaz stent, deployed with a Maxi LD balloon or a Braun balloon. When doing so, it is important to avoid dilation of the iliac limb with the shoulder of the large balloon (Fig. 11-19). As deployment of an extra-large stent in a large-caliber aorta may be difficult, it is highly recommended to test it outside the patient's body and to learn how the stent expands, before insertion. (Figs. 11-20 and 11-21)

Distal type-1 endoleaks may be treated in the same manner as the proximal type-1 leaks, with an appropriately sized stent or a cuff.

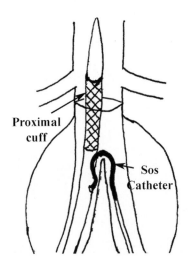

FIGURE 11-18 ● A curved catheter should be placed on the flow divider to denote its location during proximal cuff deployment.

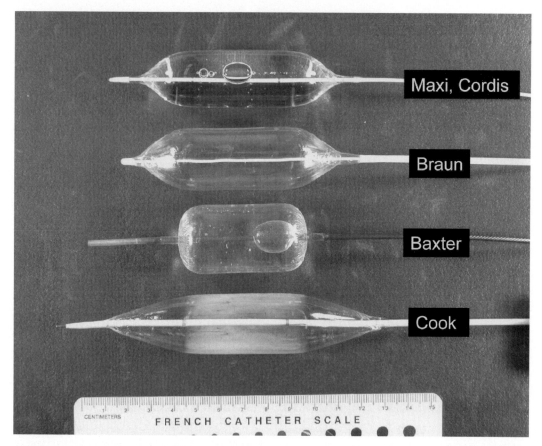

FIGURE 11-19 ● Various over-sized balloons that may be used for large Palmaz stent deployment: The Cordis Maxi LD, the Braun valvuloplasty balloon, the Edwards balloon, and the Cook balloon. Note the difference in the length of the shoulders.

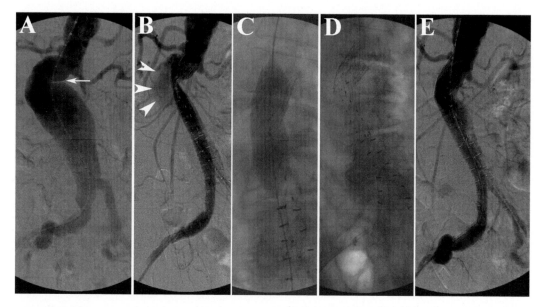

FIGURE 11-20 ● **A:** Pre-operative angiogram shows severe proximal angulation (*arrow*). **B:** Neck angulation may lead to misalignment of the stent and a type 1 endoleak (*arrowheads*). **C, D:** Touch-up balloon angioplasty failed to achieve a seal and a large Palmaz stent was deployed within the proximal stent. **E:** Completion angiogram shows a satisfactory result.

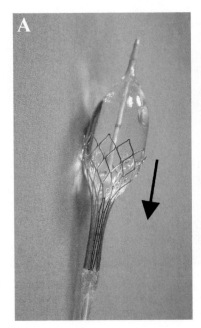

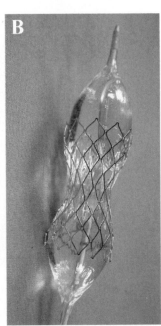

FIGURE 11-21 ●
Deployment of a large balloon-expandable (Palmaz) stent and importance of appropriate mounting. A: If the stent is not mounted properly in the center of the balloon, the stent may migrate proximally or distally during inflation of the balloon. **B:** Appropriate stent deployment.

Type 2 Endoleak

Type 2 endoleaks result from retrograde filling via the lumbar or internal iliac artery, and are more benign, compared with type-1 or type-3 endoleaks (21). Consequently, the indication for treatment is controversial. However, many agree that endoleaks that result in enlargement of the aneurysmal sacs should be treated. Treatment options include transarterial embolization, translumbar embolization, and surgical ligation, via a laparoscopic or open surgical approach. Owing to its high success rate and minimally invasive nature, the translumbar approach is favored.

The translumbar approach is performed by placing the patient in a prone position. Under fluoroscopic guidance, the location of various bony landmarks, such as the lumbar spine, iliac crest, and the endograft, are outlined (marked) on the patient"s skin. The location of the endoleak nidus, relative to these bony landmarks, should further be outlined (Fig. 11-22).

A TLA Needle is used for percutaneous access to the sac. The puncture site should be four finger breadths lateral to the midline, and the needle should be pointed medially, toward the aneurysm sac. If the endoleak nidus may not be accessed with a straight needle, then a sheath should be placed inside the aneurysmal sac, and an appro-priate directional catheter may be used. Multiple Gianturuco coils (i.e., 5 mm to 15 mm) are then placed inside the nidus to interrupt the communication between inflow and outflow vessels (Fig. 11-23). It is not necessary to selectively embolize each feeding vessel.

Type-3 Endoleak

Type-3 endoleaks result from limb separation or fabric wear. Depending on the location of the endoleak, deployment of an additional cuff may be effective. If the leak is located close to the flow divider, this may be difficult, and either surgical conversion or endovascular conversion to an aorto-uni-iliac configuration may be performed.

Type-4 Endoleak

This type of endoleak is the result of the porosity of the fabric material and may be seen following EVAR made from thin-walled Dacron fabric (Fig. 11-14). The treatment of type-4 endoleaks is controversial. Many believe that it will thrombose spontaneously, and does not result in any clinical sequelae. If one decides to treat it, one of the options is the addition of cuffs inside the EVG. If the endoleak is close to the flow divider, it may be impossible to seal it. In this circumstance and if open conversion is needed, it may be better to perform it on a separate occasion, as

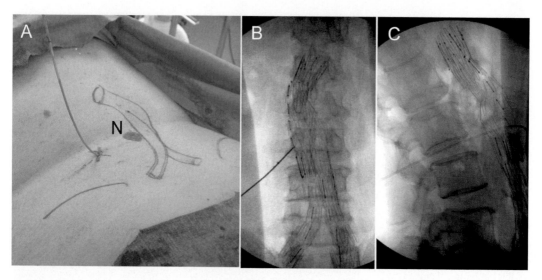

FIGURE 11-22 ● **Translumbar angiogram and embolization for Type II Endoleak. A:** The bony landmarks as well as the location of the endoleak nidus (N) is depicted on the patient's skin to facilitate needle access of the AAA sac and the endoleak nidus. **B, C:** AP and lateral imaging facilitates AAA sac access.

open conversion performed at the time of EVAR carries a higher risk of complications.

Type-5 Endoleak

Endotension (i.e., type-5 endoleak) refers to the circumstance in which the intrasac (i.e., the space between the aortic graft and native aorta) pressure is elevated without a demonstrable endoleak, as seen on a delayed-contrast CT scan. The exact etiology as well as the natural history of endotension is unknown and therefore a treatment strategy has not been established. The possible cause of endotension includes missed endoleak, thrombosed endoleak, hygroma, infection, fluid accumulation caused by hyperosmolarity, and transgraft flow (Fig. 11-24).

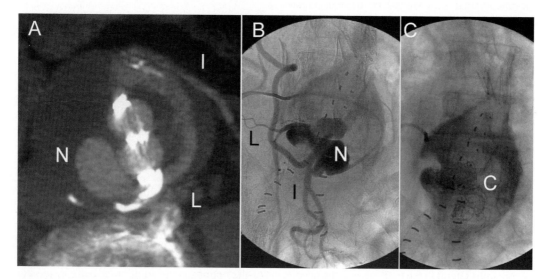

FIGURE 11-23 ● **A:** CT scan shows a type 2 endoleak arising from the IMA (I) and lumbar (L) arteries. A well-defined nidus (N) is seen. **B:** Translumbar angiogram confirms the CT scan finding. Pressure measured within the nidus was identical to systemic pressure. **C:** 40 embolization coils (C) were placed within the nidus. Embolization resulted in stagnant flow within the sac and a decrease of sac pressure to 30 mmHg.

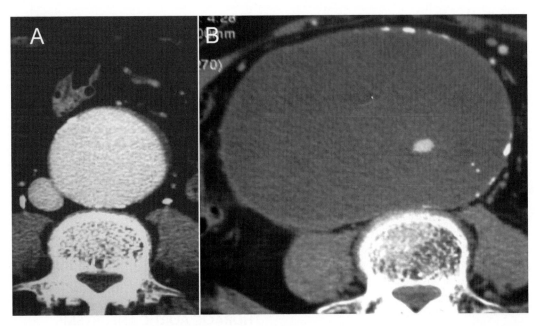

FIGURE 11-24 ● **An example of endotension (i.e., type V endoleak).** The aneurysm diameter measured 5.5 cm, pre-operatively. Three years later, the aneurysm has grown to 16 cm, without a demonstrable endoleak.

Iliac Artery Injury

Dissection and perforation of the access vessel is becoming less frequent, as a result of the development of lower profile, more flexible devices. The treatment is rather straight forward once the diagnosis is made but one may easily overlook this complication. When obtaining the completion angiogram, the femoral vessels are usually clamped and therefore, visualization of the external iliac artery is difficult. Prior to removing the guide wires from the access vessels, placement of a 5 Fr to 7 Fr sheath into the external iliac artery is recommended, to perform a retrograde injection. If dissection is detected, placement of an appropriate self-expanding stent may readily treat this condition, so long as the wire is still in place. For iliac artery perforation, deployment of a covered stent is indicated. Temporarily occluding the perforation site with an appropriately sized balloon is essential, while one prepares the covered stent. Either the Viabahn or the Wallgraft are the preferred covered stents, by virtue of their ease of use, flexibility, and availability of appropriate sizes (Fig. 11-25).

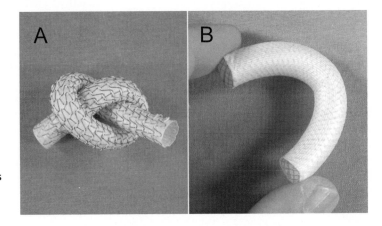

FIGURE 11-25 ● **Examples of covered stents. A:** Viabahn endoprosthesis (WL Gore). **B:** Wallgraft (Boston Scientific Corp).

Embolization

Embolization may take place at any step of the procedure. It most commonly occurs in the lower extremity vessels, but may also be seen in the visceral, renal, and internal iliac arteries. As the treatment of embolization is generally difficult, prevention is of paramount importance. Gentle manipulation of endovascular devices during the procedure, as well as avoiding cases with mural thrombus within the proximal neck or distal thoracic aorta, is advised (Fig. 11-2). Comparing the post-operative with the pre-operative status of the lower extremity pulses is important in the detection of lower extremity embolization. If lower extremity embolization is suspected, one should proceed with lower extremity angiography and perform any treatment required, at the time of EVAR.

KINKING OF ENDOGRAFT LIMBS

Kinking may occur as a result of pre-existing iliac artery tortuosity or stenosis. It also may be caused by the presence of a small, distal aorta. In such cases, deployment of a self-expanding or balloon-expandable stent is indicated. If the kink is the result of a small distal aorta, a kissing-balloon angioplasty should be performed within the graft. In some cases, making the diagnosis of a kinked endograft may be difficult, as the angiogram only provides a single-plane image. In such case, the use of intravascular ultrasound (IVUS) is extremely helpful. Alternatively, one may perform a pull-back pressure-gradient study, after the femoral artery is closed and the outflow is re-established.

LATE FAILURES

EVAR may fail in a number of ways, and success in the acute condition does not always guarantee long-term treatment success (8,14). For this reason, the use of EVAR in low-risk patients who are good candidates for open surgery, has been controversial. Owing to the frequent need for secondary procedures, and the continued risk of rupture, life-long surveillance of these patients has been recommended. Various imaging modalities have been used, including CT scan

with intravenous contrast enhancement, MRA or MRI, kidney-ureters-bladder (KUB) radiograph, duplex ultrasonography, as well as periodic physical examination. If failure is detected, an angiogram may be indicated.

Although late endograft failure and endoleaks have been thought to be the Achilles' heel of EVAR, it is noteworthy that most failures following EVAR may be managed endovascularly, and should not always be considered clinical failures. For example, Arko et al. showed that the overall aneurysm-related death was seven times higher following open surgery, compared with EVAR (22). This is related to the reduced peri-operative mortality as well as the fact that secondary procedures following EVAR are relatively benign.

ENDOVASCULAR TREATMENT OF THORACIC AORTIC ANEURYSMS

Surgical Indication for TAAs

Although TAAs are less common than AAAs, there has recently been a significant increase in their incidence. This could be related to an aging population as well as to improvements in diagnostic modalities. TAAs have a higher tendency to rupture than AAAs, with more than 70% of patients dying within 5 years of diagnosis (23). Until a few years ago, open repair was the only option to prevent rupture and death. Even with refinement of surgical techniques and the improvement in anesthesia and intensive care, open repair still carries significant morbidity and mortality. The operative mortality rates range from 10 to 30%, spinal cord injury from 5 to 15%, respiratory failure from 25 to 45%, myocardial infarction from 7 to 20%, and renal complications from 8 to 30% (22,23).

The size threshold for treatment is not as clearly defined as it is for AAA. Crawford et al. studied a series of 117 ruptured TAAs, and found that 80% of the patients had aneurysms of less than a 10 cm diameter (i.e., 13% were less than 6 cm) (26). They suggested elective reconstruction for aneurysms with a diameter greater than 5 cm. Cambria and colleagues, reporting on 57 patients with TAAs managed medically, showed no rupture for aneurysms with a diameter of less than 5 cm (25). The mean size for rupture was

5.8 cm. COPD and renal failure were strongly associated with an increased risk of rupture, with female gender, and advanced age less strongly associated. The rate of growth was also higher in patients with COPD. Symptomatic patients (i.e., those with chest or back pain) have a significantly higher risk of rupture. The overall consensus is to treat TAAs when the diameter exceeds 6 cm, taking into consideration the aforementioned risk factors.

Benefit of Endovascular Repair of TAA

The study comparing endovascular TAA repair (EVTAR) with traditional open repair was reported in 1998 by Ehrlich et al. (25). EVTAR was clearly superior, with one-third the operative mortality rates (i.e., 10% vs 30%), half the operative time (i.e., 150 vs 320 minutes) and one-third the ICU stays (i.e., 4 vs 13 days), compared to open repairs. Spinal cord ischemia (SCI) was absent in the EVTAR group, while it was observed in 12% of the open-repair patients. However, 20% of patients required repeat stenting for treatment of endoleaks. Fattori reported his series of 70 patients that included both degenerative TAAs as well as type-B aortic dissections, traumatic aneurysms, intramural hemorrhages, penetrating ulcers, and pseudoaneurysms (29). The technical success rate was 97%. Aneurysm-related death and conversion to open repair was observed in 9% of patients. There was no incidence of SCI as noted in the previous study. Endoleaks occurred in 7% of cases.

Additional disadvantages of open surgery include the fact that it may only be performed in specialized centers. This relates to the fact that open TAA repair is a technically demanding procedure requiring tremendous intra-operative and post-operative resources, including surgical intensive care unit and heart-lung bypass pumps. This is not the case for EVTAR, which may be performed readily, even in hospitals with limited resources.

Despite these promising results, at this time there are no FDA-approved endografts for thoracic aortic pathologies. Several devices are currently undergoing clinical trials in the US for FDA approval. These devices include the TAG device, the Talent endograft, and the TX2 endograft. Next generation devices include the NanoEndoluminal Apollo endograft.

General Indications for TAA Repair

The following are indications for TAA Repair:

1. Symptomatic (i.e., chest or back pain)
2. Maximum diameter of the aneurysm sac larger than 6 cm, or more than twice the diameter of the adjacent non-aneurysmal aorta

Indications for Type B Aortic Dissection Repair

The following are indications for repair of type B aortic dissections:

1. Continuing pain despite optimal medical management
2. Evidence or suspicion of visceral (i.e., renal, hepatic, bowel) ischemia
3. Lower extremity ischemia
4. Hemothorax
5. Aneurysm formation (at least 6 cm or more)

Other pathologies that may be treated with EVTAR include intramural hemorrhage and penetrating ulcer of any size.

General Inclusion Criteria for EVTAR

1. The proximal neck (i.e., the distance from the origin of the left subclavian artery [LSA] or the left common carotid artery [LCCA] to the proximal end of the aneurysm) should be at least 15 mm long
2. The distal neck (i.e., the distance from the distal end of the aneurysm to the origin of the celiac artery) should be at least 15 mm long
3. Proximal and distal neck diameter must measure between 18 mm to 42 mm
4. The diameter of the iliac artery should be at least 7 mm or larger. Smaller arteries are encountered in as much as 10 to 15% of patients. A vascular conduit may be sewn to the common iliac artery to provide access in these situations.

There are a significant number of TAAs that extend proximal to the LSA and even proximal to

Zone TAA

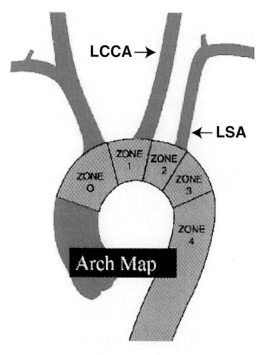

FIGURE 11-26 ● Proximal fixation site for a thoracic endograft. (Reprinted with permission: Criado FJ, McKendrick C; Monaghan K, et al. The Talent thoracic stent graft: a 6-year experience. TAA, thoracic aortic aneurysm; LSA, left subclavian artery; LCCA, Left common carotid artery. *Endovascular Today.* 2003;Nov/Dec(suppl):S6–S9.).

the LCCA. For patients with aneurysms extending into or proximal to the LSA (i.e., zones 2 and 3) (Fig. 11-26), it has been shown that covering the origin of the LSA may be performed safely. Obtaining a pre-operative duplex ultrasound assessment documenting antegrade flow in the contralateral vertebral artery is crucial. This technique is contraindicated for patients who have undergone previous coronary revascularization with the left internal mammary artery.

Pre-operative Work Up

Similar to the work-up evaluation for AAA, computer-enhanced, 3-D reconstruction of the aorta (i.e., CTA or MRA) is the imaging modality of choice. Exact morphometry of the aorta and side branches allows custom endovascular grafts to be constructed or ordered. Endografts need to

be over-sized by 20 to 25%, compared to the adjacent neck. Center-line measurements with 3-D CT are helpful for measurement of the aneurysm length.

Operative Technique (30)

Stent graft placement is ideally performed in the operating room, as the likelihood of creating a surgical conduit in the iliac artery is higher than with EVAR for AAAs. Either general anesthesia, epidural anesthesia, or local anesthesia may be used. A percutaneous puncture is made in the femoral artery that is not going to be used for endograft insertion. If the operator has any questions regarding the findings of the pre-operative CT scan, it may be beneficial to perform a confirmation aortogram prior to performing a surgical cutdown. A unilateral femoral cutdown is performed in a similar manner described in the AAA section. Fifteen percent to 25% of patients may have diseased, small iliac arteries and may require a surgical conduit consisting of a 10 mm polyester graft sewn into the common iliac artery. In addition to the catheter placed from the contralateral femoral artery, it may be beneficial to place an angiographic catheter in either the innominate or the LSA via the left or right brachial artery. This catheter may serve as a useful landmark for endograft deployment in the region of the aortic arch. Also, in cases where there is severe tortuosity in the aortic arch, introduction of the stent graft delivery system around the arch may be difficult. In such cases, a wire placed from the groin exiting from the brachial artery may provide increased stability for device delivery (Fig. 11-27).

Most TAAs are located distal to the left subclavian artery in the proximal descending thoracic aorta. If the aneurysm involves the left subclavian artery, it may either be covered with the endograft, or a carotid-subclavian artery bypass may be performed if perfusion to the left arm or the vertebral artery is a concern (Fig. 11-28).

The LAO projection provides the best visualization of arch morphology and branching. Lateral projections are needed distally, to visualize the orifice of the celiac artery. The patient is given heparin, 100 U/kg of body weight. The device is introduced over a Lunderquist guide wire. Ideally, stent graft coverage should include a

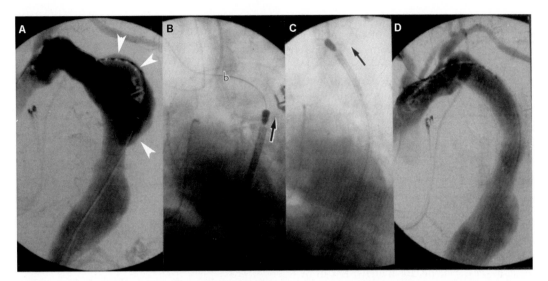

FIGURE 11-27 ● **Use of a through-and-through wire to assist the deployment of a thoracic endograft (EVG) A:** Arch angiogram showing a large thoracic aneurysm (*arrowheads*). Note the unfavorable angle that the EVG needs to negotiate. **B:** Fluoroscopic image showing the insertion of a brachial "through - and - through" wire (b). Without tension, the EVG does not track the course of the superstiff wire. **C:** By applying tension on both ends of the brachial-femoral guidewire, one may navigate the EVG safely to the target site. **D:** Completion angiogram shows complete exclusion of the aneurysm with no signs of an endoleak. (Reprinted with permission: Ohki T. Technical adjuncts to facilitate endovascular repair of various thoracic pathology. *J Card Surg.* 2003;18(4):351–358).

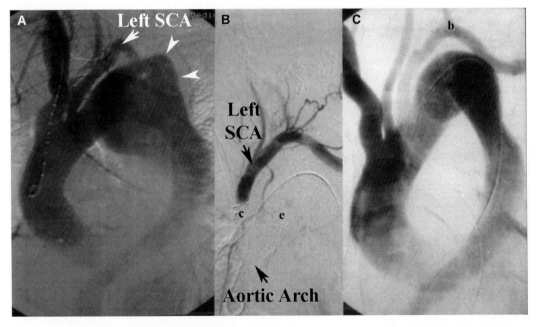

FIGURE 11-28 ● **Technique to manage TAAs that involve the arch vessels. A:** Intraoperative angiogram shows a large thoracic aortic aneurysm (*arrowheads*) adjacent to the left subclavian artery (SCA). **B:** Coil embolization (C) was performed to prevent retrograde filling of the aneurysm. e – endovascular graft (EVG). **C:** Left common carotid to left subclavian artery bypass (b) was performed prior to EVG deployment. Completion angiogram reveals complete exclusion of the aneurysm as well as perfusion of the left subclavian via the bypass graft. (Reprinted with permission: Ohki T. Technical adjuncts to facilitate endovascular repair of various thoracic pathology. *J Card Surg.* 2003;18(4): 351–358).

minimum of 20 mm of disease-free aorta, proximally and distally. This may not be achievable
in some cases. Less then 15 mm coverage might
be associated with higher incidence of endoleak.
It is therefore advisable to cover the thoracic
aorta with as much of the graft length as possible. This strategy reduces the incidence of type-1
endoleak, which probably is the result of continuous neck dilation, aortic remodeling, or inadequate fixation. The risk of clinically significant, spinal cord ischemia (SCI) is less than
5%, and its occurrence has not been correlated
with the length of endograft coverage. However,
one should consider prophylactic placement of
a cerebrospinal fluid (CSF)-drain catheter in patients with a previous infrarenal aortic replacement, as these patients are at higher risk of SCI.
Generous overlapping of modular junctions is
key for reducing type-1 endoleaks. A completion
angiogram is helpful for detecting endoleaks.
Both type 1 and type 3 may be managed with
careful ballooning or the placement of an additional endograft at the area of concern. However, keep in mind that balloon dilation of the
aorta might be more detrimental in the thoracic
arch. EVAR for thoracic pathologies may be performed even with difficult anatomy, and in patients with high-risk factors (i.e., patients who are
not candidates for open repair). The procedure
has, thus far, shown remarkable results with minimal morbidity and mortality. Long-term durability of the devices requires further investigation
and follow-up evaluation. At least three devices
are currently undergoing clinical trials in the US,
for FDA approval. These devices include the
TAG device, the Talent endograft, and the TX2
endograft.

REFERENCES

1. Dubost D, Allary M, Oeconomos NA. Preoperos du treatment des aneurysmes de l'aorta. *Arch Surg.* 1952;64:405–408.
2. Parodi JC, Palmaz JC, Barone HD. Transfemoral intraluminal graft implantation for abdominal aortic aneurysms. *Ann Vasc Surg.* 1991;5:491–499.
3. Mortality results for randomized controlled trial of early elective surgery or ultrasonographic surveillance for small abdominal aortic aneurysms. The UK Small Aneurysm Trial Participants. *Lancet.* 1998;353:1649–1655.
4. Lederle FA, Wilson SE, Johnson GR, et al. Immediate repair compared with surveillance of small abdominal aortic aneurysms. *N Engl J Med.* 2002;346:1437–1444.
5. Brewster DC, Cronenwett JL, Hallett JW, et al. Guidelines for the treatment of abdominal aortic aneurysms report of a subcommittee of the Joint Council of the American Association for Vascular Surgery and Society for Vascular Surgery. *J Vasc Surg.* 2003;37:1106–1117.
6. Sterpetti AV, Cavallaro A, Cavallari N, et al. Factors influencing the rupture of abdominal aortic aneurysms. *Surg Gynecol Obstet.* 1991;173:175–178.
7. Greenhalgh RM, Brown LC, Kwong GP, et al. EVAR trial participants. Comparison of endovascular aneurysm repair with open repair in patients with abdominal aortic aneurysms (EVAR trial 1). *Lancet* 2004;364:843–848.
8. Prinssen M, Verhoeven EL, Buth J, et al. Dutch Randomized Endovascular Aneurysm Management (DREAM) Trial Group. A randomized trial comparing conventional and endovascular repair of abdominal aortic aneurysms. *N Engl J Med* 2004;351:1607–1618.
9. Anderson PL, Arons RR, Moskowitz AJ. A statewide experience with endovascular abdominal aortic aneurysm repair: rapid diffusion with excellent early results. *J Vasc Surg.* 2004;39:10–19.
10. Feigal DW. FDA Public Health Notification: Updated Data on Mortality Associated with Medtronic AVE AneuRx® Stent Graft System. Available at http://www.fda.gov/cdrh/safety/aaa.html Accessed 02-08-2005.
11. Cronenwett JL, Birkmeyer JD, eds. *The Dartmouth Atlas of Vascular Healthcare.* Chicago, Ill: AHA Press; 2000.
12. Johnston KW. Multicenter prospective study of nonruptured abdominal aortic aneurysm. Part II. Variables predicting morbidity and mortality. *J Vasc Surg.* 1989;9:437–447.
13. May J, White GH, Yu W, et al. Concurrent comparison of endoluminal versus open repair in treatment of abdominal aortic aneurysms: analysis of 303 patients by life-table method. *J Vasc Surg.* 1998;27:213–221.
14. Lederle FA, Johnson GR, Wilson SE, et al. Aneurysm detection and management. Veterans Affairs Cooperative Study: quality of life, impotence, and activity level in a randomized trial of immediate repair versus surveillance of small abdominal aortic aneurysm. *J Vasc Surg.* 2003;38:745–752.
15. Harris PL, Vallabhaneni SR, Desgranges P, et al. The EUROSTAR Collaborators. Incidence and risk factors of late rupture, conversion, and death after endovascular repair of infrarenal aortic aneurysms: the EUROSTAR experience. *J Vasc Surg.* 2000;32:739–749.
16. Ohki T, Veith FJ, Shaw P, et al. Increasing incidence of midterm and long-term complications after endovascular graft repair of abdominal aortic aneurysms: a note of caution based on a 9-year experience. *Ann Surg.* 2001;234:323–335.
17. Chaikof EL, Blankensteijn JD, Harris PL. Reporting standards for endovascular aortic aneurysm repair. *J Vasc Surg.* 2002;35:1048–1060.
18. Ahn SS, Rutherford RB, Johnston KW. Reporting standards for infrarenal endovascular abdominal aortic aneurysm repair. *J Vasc Surg.* 1997;25:405–410.
19. Howell M, Villareal R, Krajcer Z. Percutaneous access and closure of femoral artery access sites associated with endoluminal repair of abdominal aortic aneurysms. *J Endovasc Ther.* 2001;8:68–74.
20. White GH, May J, Waugh RC, et al. Type III and Type IV endoleak: toward a complete definition of blood flow in the sac after endoluminal AAA repair. *J Endovasc Surg.* 1998;5(4):305–309.

21. van Marrewijk CJ, Fransen G, Laheij RJ, et al. Is a type II endoleak after EVAR a harbinger of risk? Causes and outcome of open conversion and aneurysm rupture during follow-up. *Eur J Vasc Endovasc Surg*. 2004;27: 128–137.

22. Arko FR, Lee WA, Hill BB. Aneurysm-related death: primary endpoint analysis for comparison of open and endovascular repair. *J Vasc Surg*. 2002;36:297–304.

23. Hill BB, Zarins CK, Fogarty TJ. Endovascular repair of thoracic aortic aneurysms. In: White R, Fogarty T, eds. *Peripheral Endovascular Interventions*. New York, NY: Springer-Verlag,1999: 383–389.

24. Cambria RP, Clouse WD, Davison JK. Thoracoabdominal aneurysm repair: results with 337 operations performed over a 15-year interval. *Ann Surg*. 2002;236: 471–479.

25. Ehrlich M, Grabenwoeger M, Cartes-Zumelzu F. Endovascular stent graft repair for aneurysms on the descending thoracic aorta. *Ann Thorac Surg*. 1998;66: 19–24.

26. Crawford ES, Hess KR, Safi HJ. Ruptured aneurysm of the descending thoracic and thoracoabdominal aorta. *Ann of Surg*. 1991;213:417–426.

27. Cambria RA, Gloviczki P, Stanson A. Outcome and expansion rate of 57 thoracoabdominal aneurysms managed nonoperatively. *Am J Surg*. 1995;170:213–217.

28. Perko MJ, Norgaard M, Herzog TM. Unoperated aortic aneurysm: a survey of 170 patients. *Ann Thorac Surg*. 1995;59:1204–1209.

29. Fattori R, Nazpoli G, Lovato L. Descending thoracic aortic diseases: stent-graft repair. *Radiology*. 2003;229:176–183.

30. Ohki T, Veith FJ. Technical adjuncts to facilitate endovascular repair of various thoracic pathology. *J Card Surg*. 2003;18:351–358.

CHAPTER 12

Aortic, Iliac, and Common Femoral Intervention

Marco Roffi and Giancarlo Biamino

According to the results of the Framingham study, symptomatic peripheral arterial disease (PAD) may be as frequent as cardiac angina, with an annual incidence of 26 per 10,000 in males and 12 per 10,000 in the female population (1). The infrarenal abdominal aorta and iliac arteries are among the most common sites of chronic, obliterative atherosclerosis, accounting for about one-third of all PAD cases.

Aortoiliac artery obstructions have traditionally been treated surgically, mainly with aortofemoral bypass. Axillofemoral bypass has been considered a lower risk, surgical alternative, compared with aortobifemoral bypass, for patients with occlusive disease of the distal abdominal aorta and severe comorbidities. Focal iliac disease has been approached with aortoiliac endarterectomy. Finally, patients with extensive but unilateral iliac disease have been on occasion treated with femorofemoral bypass.

Surgical revascularization of aortoiliac disease generally achieves high rates of long-term patency (more than 80%) (2–4). However, this mode of revascularization is associated with significant morbidity and mortality. For example, a meta-analysis of 23 series, including over 8000 patients undergoing aortobifemoral bypass between 1975 and 1995, reported an operative mortality of 4.6% in early studies (i.e., performed in the 1970s) and 3.3% in late studies (i.e., in the 1990s), and significant morbidity in 13% and 8% of cases, respectively (5). In an effort to reduce the morbidity and mortality associated with sur-

gical aortoiliac revascularization, endovascular techniques were attempted and have been successfully applied in the treatment of the whole spectrum of aortoiliac disease. This chapter summarizes the selection and evaluation of patients considered for percutaneous revascularization of aortoiliac disease, and provides a description of the interventional techniques most commonly employed.

PATIENT SELECTION

Patients with aortoiliac occlusive disease present most frequently with lifestyle-limiting claudication. Whereas calf pain on exertion is the leading symptom in femoropopliteal arterial disease, patients with aortoiliac involvement may have less suggestive symptoms, such as ambulatory pain in the thigh, hip, back, or buttock. These conditions are frequently misinterpreted as lower back or hip affections, delaying the diagnosis for many years. Since the chronic, progressive nature of the disease allows for the development of a collateral circulation, associated critical limb ischemia is rare, even in the presence of distal aortic occlusion (i.e., Leriche Syndrome).

Routine diagnostic work-up evaluation of patients with aortoiliac disease includes peripheral pulse-volume recording (PVR), and standardized treadmill test, as well as an assessment of the ankle-brachial index (ABI) at rest and during exercise. Doppler ultrasound plays a minor role in assessing disease in this vascular bed, since the technique does not allow for adequate assessment of the collateral circulation. Spiral computed tomography (CT) imaging and magnetic resonance angiography (MRA) are particularly helpful if aortoiliac occlusion is suspected; they may provide important information, such as the length and the location of the occlusion, the presence of collateral circulation, the degree of vessel calcification, and the presence of thrombus.

A stenosis is generally considered hemodynamically significant if the diameter of the vessel, by angiography, is reduced by 50 to 60%. In borderline cases, assessment of the translesional gradient may be helpful. Although clearcut pressure-gradient thresholds to define the hemodynamic relevance have not been identified, a systolic gradient of at least 10 mmHg is generally considered significant. Appropriate patient selection takes into consideration the clinical status of the patient, the location, morphology and physiologic significance of the aortoiliac lesion, as well as operator's experience, all of which are key factors for a successful endovascular procedure.

The Transatlantic Intersociety Consensus (TASC) Working Group published a comprehensive review of the management of PAD, which included classification and management guidelines for iliac disease (Table 12-1) (4).

There was a consensus that percutaneous revascularization was the therapy of choice for simple stenosis (i.e., TASC type A lesions), and that surgery should be preferred for very complex stenosis/occlusion (i.e., TASC type D lesions). However, no agreement was reached on how to manage moderately severe aortoiliac occlusive disease (i.e., TASC type B and C lesions). The lack of randomized data, and the continuous evolution in revascularization techniques and equipment, make comparisons between surgery and PTA difficult.

ANATOMY

The iliac vessels originate from the distal abdominal aorta. The common iliac artery (CIA) subsequently divides into the internal iliac artery (IIA) supplying the pelvic organs, and the external iliac artery (EIA), which continues as the common femoral artery (CFA). The diameter of the common iliac and the external iliac arteries

TABLE 12-1

Transatlantic Inter-Society Consensus (TASC) Morphologic Stratification of Iliac Lesions (4)

Lesion Type	Description
A	Single stenosis of CIA or EIA <3 cm long (unilateral or bilateral)
B	Single stenosis 3–10 cm long, not extending into CFA
	Two stenoses of CIA or EIA <5 cm long, not involving CFA
	Unilateral CIA occlusion
C	Bilateral stenosis of CIA and/or EIA 5–10 cm long, not involving CFA
	Unilateral EIA occlusion not involving CFA
	Unilateral EIA stenosis extending into CFA
	Bilateral CIA occlusion
D	Diffuse stenosis of the entire CIA, EIA, and CFA >10 cm long
	Unilateral occlusion of CIA and EIA
	Bilateral EIA occlusion
	Iliac stenosis adjacent to aortic or iliac aneurysm

CIA = common iliac artery; EIA = external iliac artery; CFA = common femoral artery

TABLE 12-2

Atherosclerotic Involvement of the Iliac Vasculature

Disease Type	Prevalence	Vascular Beds Involved
Type I	5 to 10%	Infrarenal aorta
		Common iliac arteries
Type II	35%	Infrarenal aorta
		Common and external iliac arteries
		Common femoral arteries
Type III	55 to 60%	Infrarenal aorta
		Common and iliac arteries
		Common and superficial femoral arteries
		Popliteal and infrapopliteal circulation

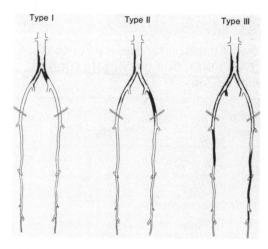

FIGURE 12-1 ● Pattern of atherosclerotic involvement of the infrarenal aorta and the iliac vessels, as described also in Table 12-2. Reproduced with permission (6).

ranges from 7 mm to 10 mm, and from 5 mm to 7 mm, respectively.

Three distinct patterns of atherosclerotic involvement of the infrarenal aorta and the iliac vessels have been described (Table 12-2 and Fig. 12-1) (6).

Type I atherosclerosis affects exclusively the distal abdominal aorta and the CIA. This form is present in about 5 to 10% of patients with PAD, and is more frequently encountered among women. Type II atherosclerosis involves the infrarenal aorta, CIA and EIA, and may extend into the CFA. This pattern may be observed in 35% of patients with PAD. Type III atherosclerosis is the most common form and involves the infrarenal aorta, iliac, femoral, and popliteal arteries as well as the infrapopliteal circulation.

DIAGNOSTIC ANGIOGRAPHY

Access

As a general rule, angiography of the lower extremities is performed accessing, in a retrograde manner, the CFA contralateral to the limb that is more symptomatic or is demonstrating a worse ABI/PVR. If imaging studies have defined the location of the obstruction, then access will be chosen based on the planned intervention. The location of the lesion is the single most important factor determining access strategy for inter-

vention. On occasion, access may differ, in the presence of a stenosis or a total occlusion.

Views

Excessive tortuosity of the iliac arteries and eccentricity of atherosclerotic involvement is frequent. Therefore, if significant stenosis is suspected, angulated views (i.e., RAO and LAO) should be obtained, in addition to the standard posteroanterior (AP) projection. Additional imaging of the CIA is best obtained with a contralateral, angulated (30° to 45°) view. Conversely, the same degree of ipsilateral angulation is preferred to delineate pathologies of the EIA and CFA.

Catheters

In most cases, diagnostic angiography may be performed, using a 4-Fr or 5-Fr pigtail catheter. Imaging of the infrarenal aorta, aortic bifurcation, and pelvic arteries may be obtained with mechanical injection of 20 mL to 25 mL of contrast media, at a flow of approximately 15 mL per second, using digital subtraction angiography (DSA). No anticoagulation is needed. Following manual compression to the arteriotomy site and the application of a pressure dressing for a few hours, the non-anticoagulated patient may be rapidly mobilized and discharged. Same-session endovascular intervention should be considered in the absence of severe renal insufficiency or heart failure.

INTERVENTION

Antiplatelet Agents and Anticoagulants

Ideally, patients should be on aspirin for a minimum of 48 hours prior to the procedure. Routinely, 5.000 units to 10.000 units of unfractionated heparin are administered after interventional sheath insertion. The optimal level of anticoagulation for peripheral interventions has not been defined. Most investigators feel comfortable at an activated clotting time (ACT) of about 250 seconds. Other operators administer fixed doses of heparin without checking an ACT. Alternative anticoagulation strategies have been used,

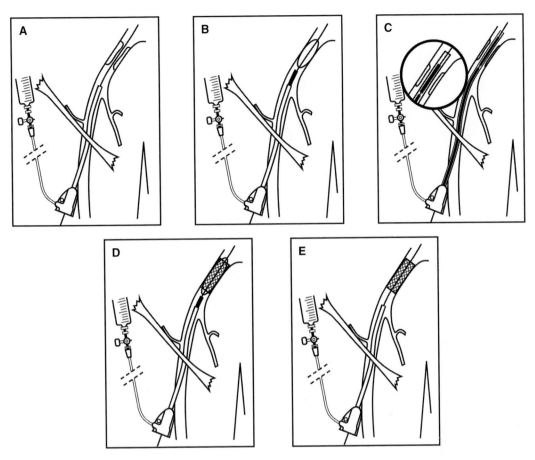

FIGURE 12-2 ● PTA and stent deployment of a right common iliac artery stenosis using an ipsilateral retrograde femoral approach. Reproduced with permission (27).

although they are not FDA approved for this indication, and include direct thrombin inhibitors (i.e., bivalirudin) or low molecular-weight heparin.

Following stenting, clopidogrel 300 mg, as an oral loading dose, is recommended and a maintenance dose of 75 mg per day is continued for at least 1 month, in addition to lifelong aspirin therapy. This management is borrowed from the coronary experience and has not been validated in studies on the peripheral vasculature. Platelet glycoprotein (GP) IIb/IIIa-receptor inhibitors have not been tested in aortoiliac intervention and may not be currently recommended.

Access

Retrograde CFA access should be considered the standard approach for aortoiliac percutaneous revascularization and may be obtained ipsilateral (Fig. 12-2) or contralateral (Fig. 12-3) to the lesion site.

With either approach, the CFA is punctured more than 2 cm below the inguinal ligament. Punctures above the inguinal ligament should be avoided because there is an increased hemorrhagic risk, and in particular, the risk of retroperitoneal hematoma. Similarly, access below the femoral bifurcation is associated with higher rates of vascular complications, such as arteriovenous fistula, pseudoaneurysm, or acute occlusion.

When access is obtained in the contralateral CFA, a cross-over technique must be employed to delivery the interventional sheath proximal to the lesion. This is achieved by placing a 5-Fr diagnostic catheter (e.g., Judkins right coronary catheter, internal mammary artery, Cobra, Hook,

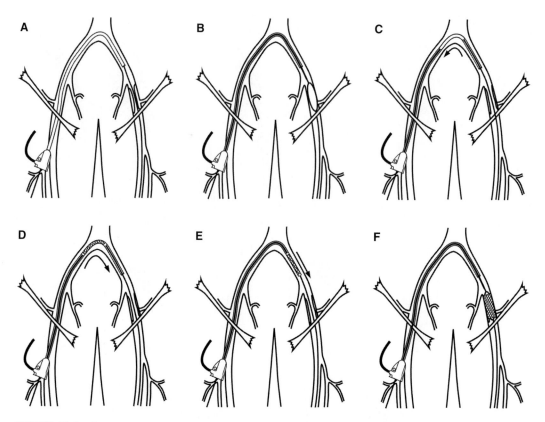

FIGURE 12-3 ● PTA and stent deployment of a left external iliac artery stenosis using a contralateral retrograde femoral access with crossover technique. The figure is described in detail in the text. Reproduced with permission (27).

pigtail) at the level of the aortic bifurcation, and advancing a 0.035″ directionally controlled wire into the common femoral artery or, if possible, into the superficial femoral artery. If the bifurcation angle is greater than 45° and the iliac vessels are straight, either nonhydrophilic directionally controlled wires (e.g., Magic Torque, Wholey) or hydrophilic wires (e.g., angled GlideWire) may be used. In contrast, if the bifurcation angle is less than 45° or there is severe iliac tortuosity, a stiff hydrophilic wire (e.g., stiff-angled GlideWire) will usually be required. Once the wire is advanced into the superficial femoral artery, it is often helpful to exchange it for a 0.035″ superstiff, nonhydrophilic wire (e.g., stiff Amplatz wire or Hi-Torque Supracore) over a 5-Fr catheter, in order to open the angle of the aortic bifurcation, thus facilitating the advancement of the cross-over sheath. Subsequently, a 7-Fr 40-cm cross-over sheath with its dilator (i.e.,

to prevent kinking) (e.g., Flexor Balkin, Super Arrow-Flex) is advanced just proximal to the lesion.

The choice of access strategy (i.e., ipsilateral retrograde CFA [Fig. 2] or contralateral retrograde CFA with cross-over placement of interventional sheath [Fig. 3], is largely determined by the anatomic location of the lesion, and the nature of the target lesion (i.e., stenotic or occlusive) as outlined below.

Ostial Common Iliac Artery and Aortic Bifurcation Disease

Ostial lesions of the common iliac artery are best approached using an ipsilateral, retrograde CFA access. Where reconstruction of the aortic bifurcation is planned, using a kissing angioplasty/stenting technique, bilateral retrograde-femoral access is required. This strategy, using simultaneous balloon inflation at the level of the

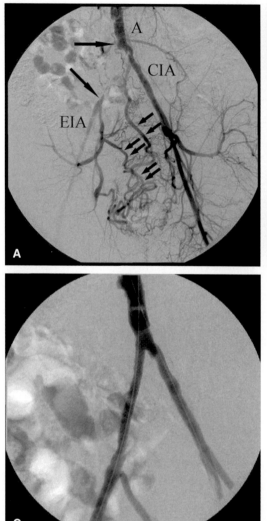

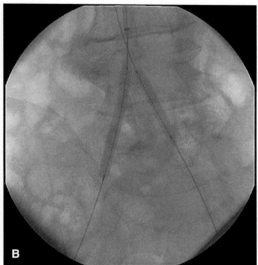

FIGURE 12-4 ● **A:** Aortoiliac bifurcation disease with ostial total occlusion of the right common iliac artery (large arrows) and ostial stenosis of the left common iliac artery (CIA). Angiography is performed using a left brachial approach. A = abdominal aorta, EIA = right external iliac artery. Small arrows demonstrate collateral circulation with filling of the right internal iliac artery and subsequently of the right EIA. The right common iliac occlusion was recanalized using a left brachial approach (note the tip of the 90-cm sheath at the aortic bifurcation), while the stenosis of the left common iliac was passed using a retrograde femoral approach. **B:** Kissing PTA/stenting of aortic bifurcation. **C:** Excellent angiographic result after kissing stenting.

aortic bifurcation, was developed to prevent contralateral flow impairment arising from plaque shift, in patients with severe, bilateral ostial iliac disease. Frequently, the procedure is followed by kissing stenting, which is performed with balloon-expandable stents (Fig. 12-4).

Kissing angioplasty/stenting may also be useful in the presence of single iliac ostial involvement, in order to prevent compromise of the contralateral site by plaque shift.

To this purpose, a 7-Fr or 8-Fr, 25-cm to 30-cm sheath (e.g., Brite Tip, Flexor) is introduced in a retrograde manner, bilaterally. Kissing balloon angioplasty and stenting may be performed over an 0.018″ or 0.035″ wire. In order to prevent plaque protrusion at the level of the bifurcation, stents should extend slightly (i.e., 2 mm to 5 mm) into the distal aorta. Importantly, reconstruction of the aortic bifurcation may compromise future lower-limb access from the contralateral site. Therefore, it is crucial to minimize the amount of iliac stent protrusion into the distal aorta. The use of balloon-expandable stents is strongly recommended for ostial iliac lesions. In the presence of associated severe disease of the distal aorta, the deployment of a large balloon-expandable stent in the distal aorta, as described later in this chapter, should precede iliac kissing stenting.

Common Iliac and Proximal External Iliac Artery Disease

These lesions are usually approached using an ipsilateral CFA access. An 0.035″ guidewire with directional control (e.g., Magic Torque, Wholey) is advanced into the abdominal aorta, and a 25-cm to 30-cm, 7-Fr or 8-Fr sheath is placed just distal to the lesion (Fig. 12-2).

If balloon angioplasty, only, is planned, a balloon (e.g., Opta Pro or Ultra Thin Diamond) that is either the same diameter as, or slightly larger than, the estimated size of the vessel is typically used. The usual sizes of the common iliac and the external iliac arteries are 7 mm to 10 mm and 5 mm to 7 mm, respectively. Typical balloon lengths are 20 mm to 40 mm. Stenting should be considered in the presence of a flow-limiting dissection, a residual translesional mean gradient of more than 10 mmHg, or in the presence of heavy calcification.

If stenting is planned, balloon predilation with an undersized balloon is recommended. Following angioplasty, the sheath is advanced over the deflated PTA balloon and the lesion is traversed with the sheath (Fig 12-2c). The stent is positioned within the sheath, the sheath withdrawn, and the stent deployed. This method minimizes the risk of dislodging the stent from the balloon delivery system during stent placement. It is generally not advisable to perform primary stenting in the iliac vessels, except for straightforward, noncalcified lesions. Self-expanding, stainless steel (e.g., Wallstent) or nitinol stents (e.g., SMART) are suitable for non-ostial, common iliac and external iliac lesions.

Distal External Iliac or Common Femoral Artery Disease

In the presence of a stenosis located in the distal portion of the external iliac artery, the retrograde approach may not be used, owing to the immediate proximity between the access site and the lesion. Therefore, access should be gained using a cross-over technique, from the contralateral CFA. An 0.035″ wire is passed, in an antegrade manner, across the lesion, followed by angioplasty and stenting as described above (Figs. 12-3 and 12-5).

Owing to the stiffness of the Balkin sheath, the authors advise against crossing the lesion with this sheath to facilitate stent positioning. Self-expandable stents should be used in the distal external iliac vessel, as this vessel approaches the anatomical flexion point at the level of the hips.

For lesions of the common femoral artery, surgery should be considered the therapy of

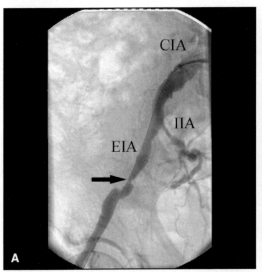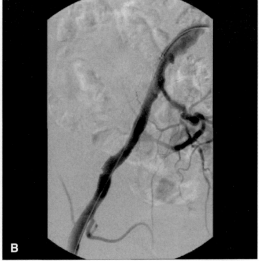

FIGURE 12-5 ● **A:** Stenosis (arrow) of the right external iliac artery (EIA) accessed with a crossover approach. CIA = common iliac artery; IIA = internal iliac artery. **B:** Final results following deployment of a self-expanding stent and post-inflation of the stent.

choice, as it may be performed using local anesthesia, may yield superior results, and does not jeopardize future access. If a percutaneous intervention is performed, the cross-over approach is mandatory. Balloon angioplasty is preferred in this setting. Should stenting be required, then a self-expanding nitinol stent should be used to avoid stent crushing associated with hip flexion.

Iliac Total Occlusions

Whenever feasible, the cross-over approach is recommended for iliac total occlusions, as it minimizes the risks of extensive dissections involving the distal aorta. This technique may not be used in the presence of ostial iliac occlusion, as there is usually insufficient support to allow successful crossing of the occlusion.

The first step of the technique is a retrograde puncture of the contralateral femoral site, with the introduction of a short 7-Fr or 8-Fr sheath (Fig. 12-6). Over a stiff 0.035″ hydrophilic wire (e.g., stiff-angled Glide Wire) a 5-Fr guiding catheter (e.g., Hook, or Shepherd-Hook) is positioned at the aortic bifurcation. Subsequently the occlusion is passed with the stiff hydrophilic wire, which is then positioned in the CFA. Using the wire as a marker, the ipsilateral CFA is punctured under fluoroscopic guidance, and a 7-Fr or 8-Fr short sheath is introduced. Using an angled, shaped, wire loop introduced through the ipsilateral sheath, the tip of the wire is snared and retrieved out of the sheath. At this point, the

procedure may be continued as described above, using the ipsilateral retrograde technique. The retrograde approach provides superior support for stent delivery and allows more precise stent placement.

Alternatively, and in particular, in the absence of a very proximal or ostial occlusion of the common iliac artery, once the lesion is passed with a stiff hydrophilic wire and is positioned in the superficial femoral artery, a 5-Fr, hydrophilic, angled catheter (e.g., angled Glide Catheter) may be passed through the lesion and then positioned in the common femoral artery. Intraluminal position may be ascertained by dye injection through the catheter. Subsequently, the hydrophilic wire may be exchanged for a stiffer 0.035″ wire (e.g., Amplatz Superstiff). Then, a 7-Fr, 40-cm crossover sheath (e.g., Flexor Balkin, Super Arrow-Flex) may be advanced just proximal to the occlusion.

A third way to approach iliac total occlusions is using brachial access (Fig. 12-4). This approach is challenging and should be practiced only by experienced interventionalists. The left brachial access is preferred because it allows for a more direct access to the descending aorta, and at the same time, it minimizes the risk of cerebral embolization while crossing the aortic arch. The brachial artery should be punctured in its distal part, above the antecubital fossa, where effective compression may be achieved against the humerus to obtain hemostasis. After introducing

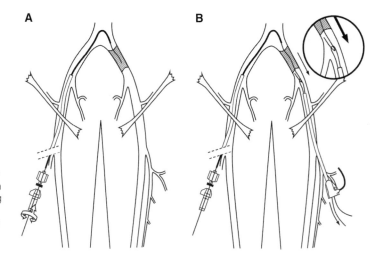

A   **B**

FIGURE 12-6 ●
Recanalization of a left common iliac artery occlusion using initially a contralateral crossover approach **(A)**, followed by ipsilateral snaring of the wire **(B).** Subsequently, the procedure is terminated using the ipsilateral retrograde approach. Reproduced with permission (27).

A
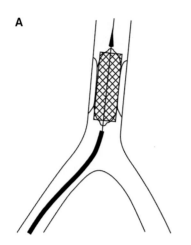

B
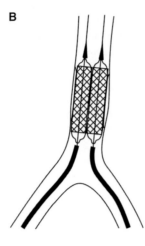

FIGURE 12-7 ● A stenosis of the distal aorta is treated with large balloon-expandable stent using a retrograde common femoral approach **(A).** After contralateral retrograde access is gained, optimal stent expansion is achieved with double-balloon postinflation **(B).** Reproduced with permission (27).

a 5-Fr short sheath, a 300-cm 0.035″ wire (e.g., Magic Torque, Wholey) is advanced under fluoroscopy into the distal aorta. Subsequently, the 5-Fr sheath is exchanged for a 90-cm long, 7-Fr sheath (e.g., Shuttle). The requirement for this large sheath size increases the risk of forearm or hand ischemia. Additional contralateral CFA access is needed if kissing PTA or stenting is planned. At the end of the procedure, the long brachial sheath is exchanged for a short one that is then removed as soon as the level of anticoagulation allows, at which point manual compression is applied.

Distal Abdominal Aorta Disease

Access is usually gained using a single retrograde CFA approach. On occasion, bilateral retrograde CFA access may be used if balloon dilation or stent expansion is performed with a double-balloon technique. Following arterial puncture, a 9-Fr to 12-Fr short sheath is inserted and a; pre-procedural angiogram is obtained. The aortic stenosis is crossed with a 0.035″ guidewire with directional control, either nonhydrophilic (e.g., Magic Torque, Wholey) or hydrophilic (e.g., angled Glide Wire). If a balloon-expandable stent is chosen (e.g., Palmaz XL, which may be expanded between 14 mm and 25 mm), and is crimped on a 12-mm to 18-mm balloon (e.g., XXL, with diameters ranging between 12 mm and 18 mm; or MAXI LD, with diameters ranging between 14 mm and 25 mm). Since large, aortic balloons with diameters between 20 mm and 25 mm may allow for only low-pressure inflations

(i.e., 2 to 4 atmospheres [atm]), post-inflation using 2 balloons (e.g., 8 mm to 12 mm in diameter) should be performed to achieve optimal stent expansion in this location (Fig. 12-7).

For the purpose of double-balloon inflation, the contralateral CFA is accessed and the aortic lesion is crossed with the same equipment as described above. Conventional, self-expanding stents reach lower maximal expansion (e.g., 16 mm for the Easy Wallstent or 14 mm for the large SMART) and always require a postinflation. Self-expanding stents should be sized 1 mm to 2 mm larger than the vessel diameter.

Stents in Iliac Intervention

The first series on the use of stents in the iliac circulation was published in 1988 (7). The Palmaz 308 stent gained FDA approval in 1991, for iliac interventions in which there was suboptimal results following PTA due to extensive dissection or residual pressure gradient, and for primary treatment of total occlusions or restenosis after PTA. In clinical practice, the use of these scaffolding devices is far more liberal and stents are used widely for ostial, long, or severely calcified lesions (Table 12-3). Frequently, stent placement is considered the primary treatment for iliac disease.

Two additional devices have subsequently gained FDA approval, namely the self-expandable stainless-steel Wallstent, and the self-expandable nitinol SMART stent. Nevertheless, numerous other devices that are FDA

TABLE 12-3

Indications for Stenting in Aortoiliac Disease

Indications

- Provisional stenting for suboptimal result of PTA
  - ○ Extensive dissection
  - ○ Residual translesional pressure gradient ≥10 mmHg
- Total occlusion
- Recurrence after PTA
- Ostial location
- Severe calcification
- Alternatively, primary treatment for all aortoiliac lesions

approved for biliary or tracheobronchial applications have been used in an off-label manner in the iliac circulation.

The value of balloon pre-dilation prior to planned stenting in aortoiliac interventions remains controversial. While some investigators routinely perform balloon pre-dilation, others frequently proceed to direct stenting. Pre-dilation with a slightly undersized balloon may be particularly helpful in ostial or severely calcified lesions, as it may facilitate stent placement and expansion. In addition, balloon inflation may convey important information, such as lesion length, vessel size, and lesion characteristics, for use in making the proper stent choice. A theoretic advantage of direct stenting, although never demonstrated, may be the reduction of the incidence of dissection or distal embolization.

Balloon-Expandable Stents

The slotted-tube, stainless-steel Palmaz stent is the prototype for balloon-expandable stents. These devices have several advantages in the aortoiliac circulation, compared with self-expanding stents. Their high radial force makes them suitable for use in heavily calcified lesions. Minimal foreshortening at deployment and good visibility allow for precise placement in ostial lesions. Finally, balloon-expandable stents may be further expanded after initial deployment by using larger balloons, until the desired diameter is achieved.

Currently, most stents are premounted on a balloon. This feature makes them more user-friendly than previous device generations that needed to be mounted, manually, on the balloon. In addition, stent flexibility has improved, allowing for stent delivery using the cross-over technique. One of the potential disadvantages of balloon-expandable stents in the iliac circulation is the propensity to create edge dissections, particularly in heavily calcified vessels or if the stent diameter is oversized. Additionally, balloon-expandable stents lack elastic deformation properties, potentially leading to stent crushing in the presence of extensive compressive forces. Therefore, these devices should not be placed in the common femoral artery. Since currently available, peripheral balloon-expandable stents are made of stainless steel, they all cause artifacts (i.e., signal loss) on magnetic resonance imaging (MRI).

Self-Expanding Stents

The most distinguishing features of self-expanding stents are elasticity and flexibility. These devices self expand to their nominal diameter when released from a constrained state within the delivery system. Typically, a slightly oversized stent is chosen to allow for optimal vessel wall apposition. This flexibility facilitates stent delivery using the cross-over technique, and allows for excellent tracking and conforming capability in tortuous iliac vessels. After stent release, post-dilation is usually performed to achieve a good angiographic result.

Disadvantages of self-expanding stents include suboptimal radial strength and foreshortening at deployment. Therefore, this stent type is less suitable for ostial lesions. Self-expanding stents should be considered for non-ostial lesions of the common iliac artery and all external iliac artery lesions. These devices should be sized 1 mm to 2 mm larger than the vessel diameter.

In the common femoral artery, stent placement should be avoided whenever possible and surgery should be considered the preferred treatment. Nevertheless, if stent placement is needed, then a self-expandable device should be chosen to avoid the stent crushing associated with hip flexion. While the prototype of this stent class (i.e., Wallstent) is made of stainless steel, newer generations (e.g., SMART, Dynalink) are composed of nitinol, an alloy of nickel and titanium. Compared with their stainless steel counterparts, nitinol stents allow for increased radial strength and minimal foreshortening at deployment. In addition, the superior conforming capability is precious in vascular segments with abrupt vessel-diameter changes, as might be encountered between the common and external iliac artery. Accordingly, the segmental expansion of nitinol stents may prevent incomplete stent apposition. A further advantage of nitinol over stainless steel stents is their magnetic resonance compatibility, achieved at the cost of reduced x-ray visibility.

The literature shows only one head-to-head comparison between stents used in the iliac circulation, thus far. In the years between 1998 and 2001, the CRISP (i.e., Cordis Randomized Iliac Stent Project) trial randomized a total of 203 patients with symptomatic iliac disease and suboptimal results following angioplasty, to a nitinol stent (SMART) or a stainless steel stent (Wallstent) (8). Acute procedural success was significantly higher with the nitinol stent, compared with the stainless steel stent (98% versus 87%, respectively). Primary vessel patency at 12 months was comparable (95% and 91%, respectively).

Covered Stents

Covered stents are composite devices consisting of a metallic skeleton covered with synthetic graft material. Because of the bulky graft material, these devices require larger delivery systems. They are currently not FDA approved for use in iliac occlusive disease. Nevertheless, covered stents have been used in this vascular bed, mainly for the treatment of aneurysms but also for arterial ruptures or arteriovenous fistulas. Isolated aneurysms of the iliac arteries are relatively uncommon, accounting for 2 to 7% of all intra-abdominal aneurysms (9). The two most popular devices are the Jostent Stent Graft and the Wallgraft. The Jostent consists of a PTFE graft material sandwiched between two stainless steel stents. Although peripheral and coronary versions of the stent are manufactured, the peripheral stent graft is not available in the US. The Wallgraft consists of a Wallstent covered with polyethylene terephthalate. The stent should be oversized by 1 mm to 2 mm to the vessel

diameter, to allow for optimal vessel wall apposition. The Wallgraft is approved in the US for tracheobronchial use, and requires a 9-Fr to 11-Fr introducer sheath. In a series of 48 patients, percutaneous exclusion of aneurysmal lesions of the iliac arteries, using this stent, was associated with high technical success rates (98%) and the 1-year, 2-year, 3-year, and 4-year patency rates were 100%, 98%, 95%, and 88%, respectively (10). No secondary leaks and no deaths, either periprocedurally or at follow-up evaluation, were observed. The results compare well with the surgical approach, which has been associated with a mortality rate in elective cases of up to 13% (11,12). Recently, a PTFE/nitinol self-expanding, stent graft has been developed. This stent graft is unique in that the metal stent is external to the graft material.

RESULTS OF ILIAC INTERVENTION

Aortoiliac PTA/Stenting

The largest series of PTA-only iliac interventions included 200 patients and documented a technical success rate of 93%. The peri-procedural complication rate was 10% and included major hematoma (2.0%), CFA thrombosis (1.5%), iliac artery rupture (0.5%) and distal embolization (1.5%). The projected, cumulative, primary-patency rate at 7.5 years was 85%. Importantly, only a minority of patients (3%) in this series had total occlusions. Therefore, in a favorable subset of patients, PTA alone, appears to yield good results.

A recent meta-analysis summarized the results of endovascular intervention for aortoiliac-occlusive disease stratified for stent use (13). This analysis included six angioplasty studies enrolling a total of 1300 patients, and eight stent series for a total of 816 patients. No difference was observed in terms of technical success between PTA or stenting (91% and 96%, respectively). Although the success rate was inferior for total occlusions compared with stenosis, only a minority of studies reported the results separately. Overall, the systemic complications rate was 1% (i.e., ranging from 0 to 3.5%), the local complications rate 9% (i.e., ranging from 2.7 to 17.8%), and the rate of major complications necessitating treatment was 4% (i.e., ranging from

1.6 to 10.8%). In-hospital mortality ranged from 0 to 2.7%. The two groups had comparable ABI at baseline. Yet, mean post-procedural ABI was significantly greater in the stent group, compared with the PTA group (0.87 and 0.76, respectively). Among patients treated for claudication, the 4-year, primary patency rate following treatment of stenotic lesions was 65% in the PTA group and 77% in the stent group. Corresponding patency rates for the treatment of total occlusions were 54% and 61%, respectively. Among patients presenting with critical limb ischemia, the 4-year patency rate following treatment of stenotic lesions was 53% for PTA and 67% for stent placement. Corresponding patency rates for patients with total occlusions were 44% and 53%, respectively. Despite the limitations of pooling results of series that greatly differ in the patient populations enrolled, endovascular techniques used, and outcome assessment methods, this analysis suggests that stenting may be superior to PTA in terms of acute success and long-term patency.

Thus far, only the Dutch Iliac Stent Trial (DIST) (14), enrolling 279 patients with intermittent claudication, compared in a prospective randomized manner, a strategy of routine stenting for aortoiliac lesions with angioplasty and provisional stent use (i.e., in the presence of a suboptimal result following PTA). In the PTA group stenting was performed in 43% of cases according to a predefined criterion of residual mean-pressure gradient of more than 10 mmHg across the treated site following angioplasty. Initial success and complications did not differ among the groups. Two-year, cumulative patency rate (i.e., 71% in the routine stent group versus 70% in the provisional stent group) and re-intervention rate (i.e., 7% versus 4%) were similar. These data demonstrate that PTA, alone, is unable to deliver an optimal hemodynamic result in the aortoiliac vasculature in a significant proportion of patients. Nevertheless, in the absence of a post-procedural gradient or evidence of complications following angioplasty, PTA alone seems a valid alternative to routine stenting.

A European multicenter trial addressed the value of stenting with a flexible balloon-expandable device (i.e., Perflex) in the iliac circulation in 126 consecutive patients who demonstrated an unsatisfactory angioplasty result (i.e., post-dilation gradient of at least 10 mmHg) or

had a primary occluded lesion (15). Primary stent patency was 94% at 6 months and 89% at 12 months, supporting the notion that stents are an effective device in the treatment of iliac artery obstructive disease.

A recent US series including 365 patients, for a total of 505 aortoiliac lesions, gives additional information on the short- and long-term results of stenting (16). Periprocedural success, defined as mean pressure gradient of no more than 5 mm Hg, was achieved in 98% of patients. Major complications (e.g., stent thrombosis, distal embolization, arterial rupture, or acute renal failure) were observed in 7% of cases, with 2% of cases requiring surgery. The 30-day mortality rate was 0.5%. At a mean observation time of almost 3 years, the need for bypass at follow-up evaluation was 6% and an additional 1% of patients underwent ipsilateral lower limb amputation. At 8 years, the primary and secondary patency rates were 74% and 84%, respectively.

No study has randomized patients with aortoiliac obstructive disease to surgery or endovascular intervention. Whereas there is general agreement that simple lesions should be treated percutaneously, it remains a source of debate as to what is the best approach for more complex disease. A single-center, retrospective analysis addressed the outcomes of stenting (n = 136) and surgery (n = 52) for complex aortoiliac lesions (i.e., TASC type B and C) (17). Primary patency rates at 1, 3, and 5 years were 85%, 72%, and 64% after iliac stenting, and 89%, 86%, and 86% after surgical reconstruction, respectively. Although, no conclusive recommendation may be made in complex lesions, it may be reasonable to attempt percutaneous treatment first, so long as the lesion appears amenable and the operator has the necessary expertise. Should this approach fail, then the patient should be referred for vascular surgery.

Total Occlusions

The treatment of total occlusions remains a limitation of percutaneous intervention. In a series reporting PTA of 82 iliac, chronic total occlusions, the success rate was 76% (18). After exclusion of the initial failures, the patency rate at 3 years was 59%. Another report involving 59 patients reported a technical success rate of 92%

and a primary patency rate at 2 years of 73% (19). Major procedural complications occurred in 6% and included four episodes of distal embolization and one massive bleeding event. Late complications occurred in 12% and included nine stent total occlusions and one severe restenosis.

A recent single-center experience addressed the results of a strategy based on Excimer-laser debulking, prior to PTA/stent, among 212 consecutive patients with iliac occlusion (20). The rate of major complications was 1.4% and included one arterial rupture and two embolic events. Technical success was achieved in 90% of cases. Primary patency rates were 84% at 1 year, 81% at 2 years, 78% at 3 years, and 76% at 4 years. Secondary patency rates were 88% at 1 year, 88% at 2 years, 86% at 3 years, and 85% at 4 years. Overall, stent-supported angioplasty appears to be an effective treatment for iliac artery occlusion, with less morbidity and mortality compared with surgery. However, reported long-term patency rates after bypass surgery are generally greater than those observed with interventional treatment.

Aortoiliac Bifurcation

Three recent series on the use of kissing stenting for the reconstruction of the iliac bifurcation have been published. A series from Germany documented, among 48 patients, a technical success rate of 100% in the absence of major procedure-related complications, and a primary patency rate of 87% at 2 years (21). Noteworthy, about half of the patients were treated for total occlusion. An Austrian single-center series, including 25 patients, reported a technical success rate of 86% and a 2-year primary patency of 65% (22). Peri-procedural complications occurred in 20% of cases and included two dissections of the distal aorta that were managed conservatively and three cases of common femoral artery pseudoaneurysm. No deaths occurred within 30 days of the procedure. A group in Milwaukee described a technical success rate of 100% and a primary patency rate at 20 months of 92%, among 50 patients treated with this technique (23). Acute complications occurred in 4% of cases and were all related to distal embolization. One patient required surgery. Amputation-free survival at follow-up evaluation was 100% and

92% of patients were free of lifestyle-limiting claudication. No periprocedural deaths occurred. Overall, percutaneous reconstruction of the aortic bifurcation appears to be associated with low periprocedural morbidity/mortality and satisfactory mid-term results.

Stenosis of the Infrarenal Aorta

Localized stenosis of the infrarenal abdominal aorta is relatively infrequent and occurs predominantly in young females with a significant smoking history (24). Until the early 1980s, distal abdominal aortic stenosis was treated surgically with endarterectomy or bypass grafting. Currently, percutaneous transluminal aortic angioplasty (PTAA) with or without stenting has become the treatment of choice for short abdominal aortic stenosis in the absence of significant iliac disease. Failures of PTAA may be the result of elastic recoil, obstructive intimal dissection, or late restenosis. In a series of 102 patients, the main portion of whom had isolated distal aortic disease treated with angioplasty, technical success (i.e., defined as residual stenosis of less than 50% or residual mean pressure gradient lower than 10 mmHg) was achieved in only 76% (25). Stents were placed in a minority of patients (i.e, 12%) for suboptimal PTAA results. No major complications were reported. After 10 years, primary clinical (i.e., absence or improvement of symptoms) and hemodynamic patency (i.e., normal Doppler waveforms in the common femoral arteries) were achieved in 72% and 46% of cases, respectively.

A recent series addressed the use of provisional stenting of the distal aorta, for failures of angioplasty (26). Outcomes were compared between 55 patients who underwent successful PTAA, and 19 patients who underwent aortic stenting, for angioplasty failure. Three-year clinical and hemodynamic patency rates, respectively, were 85% and 79% for PTAA and 69% and 43% for stenting. No morbidity or mortality was reported. The significant difference in outcomes in the univariate analysis disappeared following multivariate modeling, suggesting that stenting is a valuable option even in patients with poor results following PTAA. Nevertheless, the authors described surprise at the low patency rates achieved with stenting, since the immediate angiographic and hemodynamic results in this group of patients had been optimal. No prospective study has addressed routine versus provisional stenting in the distal aorta. The use of primary stenting has been advocated for the treatment of complex lesions (e.g., irregular, eccentric, ulcerated, or calcified) and occlusions. Although not proved clinically, covering the lesion with a stent before balloon dilation may, theoretically, minimize the risk of distal embolization by trapping the atheroma between the stent and the vessel wall, and similarly reduce the risk of vessel rupture by distributing the dilating forces against the arterial wall more evenly.

It remains a source of debate whether balloon-expandable (e.g., Palmaz) or self-expandable stents (e.g., Wallstent) are the devices of choice for the distal aorta. The advantage of balloon-expandable stents includes more accurate positioning and achievement of larger diameters. Self-expanding stents may achieve further gradual expansion because of intrinsic radial force, thus allowing the use of smaller balloons, and minimizing the risk of acute vessel trauma. In addition, owing to the smaller stent struts, a self-expandable device like the Wallstent may trap atheroembolic material more efficaciously at the time of deployment, potentially decreasing the risk of distal embolization.

COMPLICATIONS

Potential complications of aortoiliac interventions include dissections, vessel occlusions, perforations, and distal embolization. The specific risks according to the type of procedure employed have been described earlier in the chapter. On a broader perspective, the incidence of complications is greater during recanalization of total occlusions, compared with the treatment of nonocclusive lesions. Extensive iliac dissection usually may be treated with self-expanding stents. In the presence of vessel rupture, immediate balloon occlusion proximal to the perforation, followed by reversal of heparin with protamine, and placement of a covered stent, is indicated. In the mean time, blood should be typed and cross-matched and the vascular-surgery specialist notified. If distal embolization is suspected, immediate angiography should be performed and further treatment (e.g., prolonged heparinization,

intra-arterial lytic therapy, endovascular clot extraction, surgery) should be guided by the angiographic and clinical findings. Since angiography has not been routinely performed following aortoiliac intervention in a large prospective study, the exact incidence of restenosis is unknown. Nevertheless, its incidence is far less than that of the infrainguinal circulation, as demonstrated by non-invasive studies and by the lower rate of repeat revascularization. Drug-eluting stents have not been tested in aortoiliac disease.

LONG-TERM FOLLOW-UP MONITORING

All patients should receive life-long aspirin therapy. Clopidogrel is recommended for at least 4 weeks following stent implantation. The efficacy and safety of prolonged combined therapy with aspirin and clopidogrel, in high-risk individuals and among them patients with PAD, is currently being addressed in the CHARISMA trial. In addition to life-style changes, secondary pharmacologic, cardiovascular preventive measures, such as statins are critical in all patients with PAD. An ABI should be obtained following the procedure and yearly, thereafter, or earlier if symptoms recur.

KEY PRINCIPLES

The indications for endovascular therapy in the aortoiliac circulation have gradually expanded over the last two decades. While discrete iliac stenosis may be amenable to PTA, the treatment of long iliac total occlusion or advanced disease of the aortic bifurcation remains challenging. Depending on the localization and type of the lesion, as well as the anatomy of the aortic bifurcation, different access techniques may be chosen. The retrograde CFA approach is the easiest and least traumatic, and leads to success in the majority of patients with isolated iliac stenosis. In the presence of total occlusions or involvement of the distal external iliac artery, crossover access may be necessary. Severe disease of the aortoiliac bifurcation is usually treated with kissing balloon/stenting, using a bilateral retrograde femoral approach. The more challenging brachial approach may be required in a minority of aortoiliac interventions.

For discrete, noncalcified, nonostial stenosis, with a good angiographic and hemodynamic result following PTA, stenting may not be necessary. Stenting is recommended for the treatment of long or ostial lesions, total occlusions, and for suboptimal (e.g., residual stenosis and/or pressure gradient, dissection) PTA results. Some investigators consider stenting the primary treatment for iliac disease, irrespective of the lesion characteristics. Regarding stent type selection, the high radial strength of balloon-expandable stents and the lack of foreshortening make them suitable, in particular, for ostial or severely calcified lesions. The greater flexibility and conformability of self-expanding stents make them suitable for treating long lesions in tortuous segments. Based on the low incidence of major complications, as well as good long-term results, percutaneous revascularization has replaced surgery for most aortoiliac occlusive conditions.

REFERENCES

1. Kannel WB, Skinner JJ, Jr., Schwartz MJ, et al. Intermittent claudication. Incidence in the Framingham Study. *Circulation.* 1970;41:875–883.
2. Vitale GF, Inahara T. Extraperitoneal endarterectomy for iliofemoral occlusive disease. *J Vasc Surg.* 1990;12:409–413; discussion 414–415.
3. van den Dungen JJ, Boontje AH, Kropveld A. Unilateral iliofemoral occlusive disease: long-term results of the semi-closed endarterectomy with the ring-stripper. *J Vasc Surg.* 1991;14:673–677.
4. Management of peripheral arterial disease (PAD). TASC Working Group. TransAtlantic Inter-Society Consensus (TASC). *J Vasc Surg.* 2000;31:S1–S296.
5. de Vries SO, Hunink MG. Results of aortic bifurcation grafts for aortoiliac occlusive disease: a meta-analysis. *J Vasc Surg.* 1997;26:558–569.
6. Brewster DC. Clinical and anatomical considerations for surgery in aortoiliac disease and results of surgical treatment. *Circulation.* 1991;83:I42–I52.
7. Palmaz JC, Richter GM, Noeldge G, et al. Intraluminal stents in atherosclerotic iliac artery stenosis: preliminary report of a multicenter study. *Radiology.* 1988;168:727–731.
8. Pontec et al. CRISP (Cordis Randomized Iliac Stent Project) Presented at the SIR Annual Scientific Meeting SLC, March, 2003.
9. Nachbur BH, Inderbitzi RG, Bar W. Isolated iliac aneurysms. *Eur J Vasc Surg.* 1991;5:375–381.
10. Scheinert D, Schroder M, Steinkamp H, et al. Treatment of iliac artery aneurysms by percutaneous implantation of stent grafts. *Circulation.* 2000;102:III253–III258.
11. Schroeder RA, Flanagan TL, Kron IL, et al. A safe approach to the treatment of iliac artery aneurysms. Aortobifemoral bypass grafting with exclusion of the aneurysm. *Am Surg.* 1991;57:624–626.
12. Richardson JW, Greenfield LJ. Natural history and management of iliac aneurysms. *J Vasc Surg.* 1988;8:165–171.
13. Bosch JL, Hunink MG. Meta-analysis of the results of percutaneous transluminal angioplasty and stent placement for aortoiliac occlusive disease. *Radiology.* 1997;204:87–96.
14. Tetteroo E, van der Graaf Y, Bosch JL, et al. Randomised comparison of primary stent placement versus primary angioplasty followed by selective stent placement in patients with iliac-artery occlusive disease. Dutch Iliac Stent Trial Study Group. *Lancet.* 1998;351:1153–1159.
15. Reekers JA, Vorwerk D, Rousseau H, et al. Results of a European multicentre iliac stent trial with a flexible balloon expandable stent. *Eur J Vasc Endovasc Surg.* 2002;24:511–515.
16. Murphy TP, Ariaratnam NS, Carney WI, Jr.,et al. Aortoiliac insufficiency: long-term experience with stent placement for treatment. *Radiology.* 2004;231:243–249.
17. Timaran CH, Prault TL, Stevens SL, et al. Iliac artery stenting versus surgical reconstruction for TASC (TransAtlantic Inter-Society Consensus) type B and type C iliac lesions. *J Vasc Surg.* 2003;38:272–278.
18. Johnston KW. Iliac arteries: reanalysis of results of balloon angioplasty. *Radiology.* 1993;186:207–212.
19. Reyes R, Maynar M, Lopera J, et al. Treatment of chronic iliac artery occlusions with guide wire recanalization and primary stent placement. *J Vasc Interv Radiol.* 1997;8:1049–1055.
20. Scheinert D, Schroder M, Ludwig J, et al. Stent-supported recanalization of chronic iliac artery occlusions. *Am J Med.* 2001;110:708–715.
21. Scheinert D, Schroder M, Balzer JO, et al. Stent-supported reconstruction of the aortoiliac bifurcation with the kissing balloon technique. *Circulation.* 1999;100:II295–II300.
22. Greiner A, Dessl A, Klein-Weigel P, et al. Kissing stents for treatment of complex aortoiliac disease. *Eur J Vasc Endovasc Surg.* 2003;26:161–165.
23. Mouanoutoua M, Maddikunta R, Allaqaband S, et al. Endovascular intervention of aortoiliac occlusive disease in high-risk patients using the kissing stents technique: long-term results. *Catheter Cardiovasc Interv.* 2003;60:320–326.
24. Jernigan WR, Fallat ME, Hatfield DR. Hypoplastic aortoiliac syndrome: An entity peculiar to women. *Surgery.* 1983;94:752–757.
25. Audet P, Therasse E, Oliva VL, et al. Infrarenal aortic stenosis: long-term clinical and hemodynamic results of percutaneous transluminal angioplasty. *Radiology.* 1998;209:357–363.
26. Therasse E, Cote G, Oliva VL, et al. Infrarenal aortic stenosis: value of stent placement after percutaneous transluminal angioplasty failure. *Radiology.* 2001;219: 655–662.
27. Scheinert D, Braunlich S, Biamino G. Recanalization of pelvic arteries. In: Ed. J. Marco. *The Paris Course on Revascularization Book 14:* Europa Edition. 2003;497–509.

CHAPTER 13

Endovascular Therapy for Superficial Femoral Arterial Disease

Jeffrey A. Goldstein, Ivan P. Casserly, and
Krishna Rocha-Singh

ndovascular revascularization of the superficial femoral artery (SFA) is one of the most commonly performed peripheral endovascular procedures. The ability to replace a surgical revascularization, limited by significant morbidity and mortality, with a same-day outpatient percutaneous procedure underlies the popularity of the endovascular approach. However, endovascular recanalization of the SFA faces a number of unique challenges; specifically, the SFA is the longest artery in the body, with two major flexion points at the hip, proximally, and knee joint, distally. It courses through the muscular portion of the thigh, and is therefore subject to significant torsion, flexion, and extension forces. Finally, the atherosclerotic disease process in the SFA is typically diffuse with a high incidence of occlusive and calcific disease.

Over the last decade, advances and refinements in intervention techniques and equipment have occurred to meet these unique challenges, such that progressively more complex disease may be safely and successfully treated using the endovascular approach. This chapter provides an overview of the approach to the interventional management of SFA disease, including a description of the most promising, newer technologies available for use in treatment, and a summary of the published outcomes following SFA intervention.

ANATOMIC CONSIDERATIONS

The SFA represents the direct continuation of the common femoral artery (CFA) following the origin of the profunda femoral branch (PFA) in the femoral triangle (Figs. 13-1 and 13-2).

This transition from CFA to SFA usually occurs at the level of the inferior margin of the femoral head. At its origin, the SFA lies medial, and anterior, to the PFA. Proximally it courses through the femoral triangle to reach the adductor canal. In the adductor canal, the SFA is surrounded by the muscles of the thigh: the adductor longus and magnus muscles posteriorly, the sartorius muscle anteriorly, and the vastus medialis muscle, medially. The SFA exits the adductor canal through the tendinous opening in the adductor magnus muscle (i.e., adductor hiatus) to reach the popliteal fossa, located in the distal portion of the posterior surface of the femur. At this point, the SFA changes its name to the popliteal artery.

One of the distinguishing features of the SFA is the absence of significant branches throughout its course. This explains the constant diameter of this vessel, typically about 6–7 mm. A number of small, muscular branches may be seen. In addition, the SFA gives off the descending genicular branch, just above the adductor canal, which contributes to the collateral circulation at the knee.

A brief description of the anatomy of the PFA is also pertinent in a discussion of SFA intervention, since it makes an important contribution to collateral flow in the presence of SFA disease, and also impacts decision-making during intervention to the ostium of the SFA. The PFA arises from the lateral aspect of the CFA and runs posteriorly, and laterally, to the SFA.

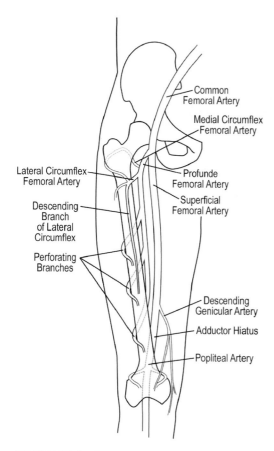

FIGURE 13-1 ● Schematic illustration of anatomy of superficial femoral artery (right leg).

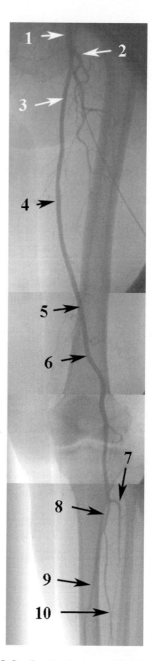

FIGURE 13-2 ● **Angiogram of left lower extremity. 1.** Common femoral artery. **2.** Profunda femoral artery. **3.** Superficial femoral artery in femoral triangle. **4.** Superficial femoral artery in adductor canal. **5.** Adductor hiatus. **6.** Popliteal artery. **7.** Anterior tibial artery. **8.** Tibioperoneal trunk. **9.** Posterior tibial artery. **10.** Peroneal artery.

It gives off two major branches, proximally, the medial and lateral circumflex femoral branches. One or both of these branches may occasionally (i.e., about 15 to 20%) arise directly from the CFA. In its mid- and distal portion, the PFA typically gives off three perforating branches to the muscles of the thigh. Proximally, the medial and lateral circumflex branches and the first perforating branch have connections with branches of the internal iliac artery (i.e., superior and inferior gluteal, and obturator branches). Distally, the lateral-circumflex artery and the perforating branches have important connections with the collateral network at the knee joint, which connect with the popliteal and tibial vessels. Through these proximal and distal connections, the PFA provides an important source of collateral flow to the leg and foot, in patients with significant SFA stenoses or occlusion.

NONINVASIVE EVALUATION

All of the details regarding the noninvasive evaluation of patients with lower extremity ischemia are outlined in Chapter 2.

CLASSIFICATION OF SUPERFICIAL FEMORAL ARTERY ATHEROSCLEROTIC DISEASE

The TransAtlantic Inter-Society Consensus (TASC) has classified SFA disease into four types (i.e., A–D) based on lesion length, the number of lesions, and the presence of stenosis or occlusion (Fig. 13-3) (1).

This classification has been developed in an attempt to reach consensus regarding the optimal approaches to the revascularization of various lesions, and is useful when performing and comparing investigational studies of SFA intervention.

INDICATIONS

Revascularization of the SFA has traditionally been reserved for only a subset of patients with symptomatic disease, including those with severe lifestyle-limiting claudication, ischemic resting pain, or ischemic tissue loss (1). These indications reflect the approach adopted by vascular surgeons who appropriately balanced the high risk of surgical revascularization in a population with significant comorbidities, with the potential benefit to the patient. For example, the operative mortality rate for femoral-popliteal bypass ranged from 1.3 to 6%, with a perioperative risk of myocardial infarction of 1.9 to 3.4%, and a wound complication rate of 10 to 30%. The conservative approach to surgical revascularization was also supported by the recognition that 75% of patients with symptomatic peripheral vascular disease experience stabilization or improvement of their symptoms, and that conservative measures such as exercise therapy, pharmacologic therapy, and risk factor modification may provide significant improvements in walking distances and symptoms.

With the advent of endovascular techniques, the safety of SFA revascularization, even in high-risk patients was dramatically transformed, with a major complication rate with the endovascular approach of less than 1%. This has led to a major shift toward percutaneous revascularization as the therapy of choice for the indications outlined above. The superior safety of the endovascular approach has overridden the continued controversy regarding the long-term efficacy of endovascular versus surgical revascularization.

Understandably, the shift in the risk-versus-benefit ratio provided by percutaneous revascularization of the SFA has resulted in a broader population of patients, with less severe symptomatic SFA disease, being treated. This practice is supported by nonrandomized data from this population showing that revascularization is associated with improved functional capacity, leg symptoms, and quality of life compared with medical therapy (2). However, randomized data would provide more reassuring evidence of the appropriateness of the broader application of SFA intervention in less severely symptomatic SFA disease.

SUPERFICIAL FEMORAL ARTERY INTERVENTION

Diagnostic Angiography

Quality angiography of the lower extremity is an important component of the evaluation of

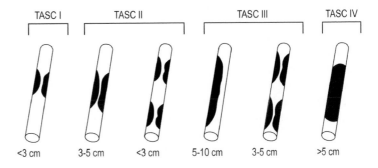

FIGURE 13-3 ● TASC classification of superficial femoral artery disease.

TASC I   TASC II   TASC III   TASC IV

<3 cm   3-5 cm   <3 cm   5-10 cm   3-5 cm   >5 cm

patients with suspected SFA disease. Assessment of the inflow and outflow from the SFA determine the suitability of the patient for SFA intervention and the most appropriate interventional strategy. With modern noninvasive angiographic techniques (i.e., computed tomography [CT] or magnetic resonance [MR] angiography), invasive angiography is no longer required to make this assessment.

If these noninvasive techniques are not available, or are suboptimal, invasive angiography remains essential. For diagnostic studies, the most common access site chosen is the CFA contralateral to the leg with the greatest symptoms, since this allows subsequent contralateral CFA access if an intervention is required. A pigtail catheter is advanced over a wire and placed in the distal abdominal aorta, and a static pelvic angiogram spanning the aortic bifurcation to the CFA is performed (i.e., power injector settings: 15 mL per second for a total of 30 mL). If there is a suspicion of iliac disease at the aortic or common iliac bifurcation that is not well visualized, contralateral oblique views are indicated. If the CFA bifurcation is not clearly visualized, ipsilateral oblique views are usually helpful in displaying the origins of the SFA and PFA.

At this point, visualization of the infrainguinal arteries may be performed using one of two methods: (1) sequential static overlapping digital subtraction angiography (DSA) at multiple levels. The authors perform this method by placing a side-holed diagnostic catheter (e.g., multipurpose) in the ipsilateral and contralateral common femoral artery. The arteries of each limb are then visualized sequentially from proximal to distal, with hand injections of contrast medium (i.e., about 10 mL) from the catheter in the CFA ipsilateral to the leg of interest; and (2) the bolus-chase technique. With this technique, a contrast bolus is injected and continually imaged as it progresses distally. Both limbs may be visualized with a pigtail catheter placed in the distal abdominal aorta (i.e., power injector settings: 15 mL per second for a total of 90 mL), or an individual limb may be visualized with a side-holed, multipurpose catheter in the ipsilateral CFA (i.e., power injector settings: 15 mL per second for a total of 45 mL). A 15″ image intensifier is required for bilateral leg run-off visualization. With smaller image intensifiers, each leg must be visualized separately.

The quality of lower extremity angiography is enhanced by a number of simple techniques. The feet should be held close together with tape to avoid patient movement. A central wedge filter placed between the legs and two lateral wedge filters placed lateral to each leg results in a more even penetration of x-rays through the field of view, providing superior imaging. Finally, utilization of a radio-opaque ruler, placed under the patient in the midline, provides a useful landmark for analysis of lesion lengths and positioning of equipment during endovascular procedures.

Pharmacology

The adjunctive pharmacologic therapies administered during SFA intervention are similar to those used in most other peripheral vascular procedures. In clinical practice, patients receive aspirin pre-procedurally. Unfractionated heparin is the anticoagulant of choice, with a target activated clotting time (ACT) of approximately 250 seconds. Low molecular-weight heparins or direct thrombin-inhibitors may be used in specific circumstances, but there are no data to support their routine use. Most operators reserve glycoprotein (GP) IIb/IIIa inhibitors for cases complicated by thrombosis.

Access for Intervention

The success and ease with which any endovascular procedure may be performed relies on the platform constructed to perform the procedure (Fig. 13-4). This begins with the choice of arterial access (Table 13-1).

Contralateral CFA Retrograde Access

When approaching an SFA lesion, the most commonly chosen and technically simple access is the contralateral CFA, approached in a retrograde manner. The modified Seldinger technique is used to gain access in the contralateral CFA (Fig. 13-5).

A catheter (Simmons, cross-over, or IMA) is then advanced over a wire into the distal aorta and used to selectively engage the ostium of the contralateral common iliac artery. A stiff-angled Terumo Glide Wire is then advanced with care into the CFA and the diagnostic catheter is then

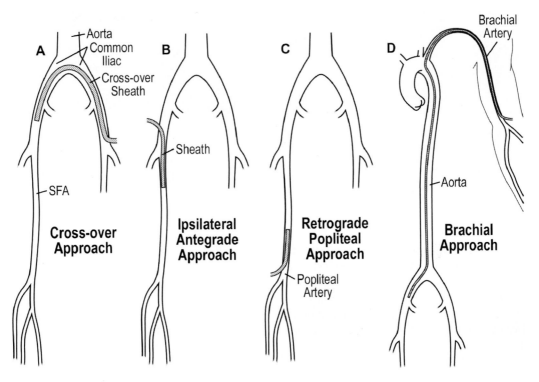

FIGURE 13-4 ● Illustration of array of access site strategies for superficial femoral artery intervention.

TABLE 13-1

Access Sites Used for Superficial Femoral Artery Intervention and Factors Influencing the Choice of Access Site

Access site	Comments
Contralateral CFA - retrograde	• Most common and technically feasible approach
Ipsilateral CFA - antegrade	• Indicated in patients with: 　• Acute angulation of aortic bifurcation 　• Significant iliac tortuosity or disease • Unsuitable for ostial or proximal SFA disease
Popliteal - retrograde	• Should consider in patients with contraindication to both contralateral or ipsilateral CFA approach • Useful in SFA occlusions with failure to cross proximal margin of occlusion and definable stump at inferior margin of occlusion
Brachial - retrograde	• Should consider in patients with contraindication to contralateral or ipsilateral CFA approach • Only suitable for treatment of proximal or mid-SFA disease

CFA - common femoral artery; SFA- Superficial femoral artery.

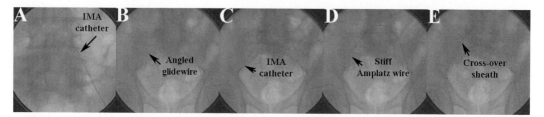

FIGURE 13-5 ● **Technique used to deliver cross-over sheath from left common femoral artery (CFA) to right CFA. A:** Internal mammary (IMA) catheter at origin of right common iliac artery. **B:** Angled glidewire advanced into right CFA. **C:** IMA catheter advanced over wire to right CFA. **D:** Angled glidewire exchanged for 1cm tipped stiff Amplatz wire. Note the change in shape of the aortic bifurcation caused by the stiff Amplatz wire. **E:** Cross-over sheath delivered over stiff Amplatz wire.

advanced over the wire into the CFA. The glide wire is then exchanged for a 1-cm tipped, stiff Amplatz wire. The catheter and sheath are then removed over the stiff wire and a long kink-resistant sheath approximately 40 cm in length (e.g., Balkan Contralateral, Termumo Pinnacle Destination, Crossover, Arrow) is advanced into the contralateral CFA. The sheath should always be advanced in combination with a dilator, to avoid dissection.

Ipsilateral CFA Antegrade Access

An antegrade, ipsilateral CFA access may be desirable in patients with specific anatomic issues involving the iliac arteries, including: severe tortuosity or disease in either iliac, or acute angulation of the native or reconstructed (i.e., surgical or percutaneous) aortoiliac bifurcation (Fig. 13-6).

Although antegrade access provides for improved back-up support, compared with the contralateral CFA approach, this is rarely a significant issue during SFA intervention. In patients with ostial or proximal SFA disease, the antegrade approach may be contraindicated, owing to insufficient room in the CFA to allow a sufficient length of sheath for stable sheath placement (Fig. 13-7).

Particular caution should be exercised in using the antegrade CFA approach in obese patients, and this approach is relatively contraindicated in the morbidly obese, owing to the increased risk of bleeding.

The technical aspects of obtaining antegrade CFA access are outlined in Chapter 3. In brief, right and left-handed operators should stand on the right and left side of the catheterization table, respectively. A 4-Fr or 5-Fr micropuncture set

should be used routinely, and the CFA punctured under fluoroscopic guidance, using the head of the femur to guide the anticipated location of the CFA bifurcation. This will result in a skin-puncture site that is significantly higher than that used for the retrograde approach. Once the needle is in the CFA, the 0.018″ wire is advanced into the SFA and a standard short sheath placed.

Ipsilateral Popliteal Retrograde Access

The ipsilateral popliteal retrograde approach is rarely used for SFA intervention. However, in situations in which both the contralateral CFA and ipsilateral CFA approaches are contraindicated (e.g., severe iliac tortuosity and ostial SFA lesion), it may be used. A further indication for the popliteal approach is the presence of an SFA occlusion that may not be crossed from its proximal margin. This is usually caused by the presence of a bridging collateral or branch vessel adjacent to the proximal stump. If there is a definable stump, inferiorly, that is sufficiently proximal to the popliteal artery to allow safe placement of a sheath, then a retrograde popliteal approach is indicated.

The technical aspects of popliteal artery access are outlined in Chapter 3. In brief, the popliteal artery is accessed as it courses through the popliteal fossa enclosed in a common sheath with the popliteal vein and tibial nerve. The degree of overlap of the vessels is minimal at a point approximately 6.5 cm above the level of the femorotibial joint space, which serves as a useful target during arterial puncture.

While the patient is in a supine position, access should be obtained from either the ipsilateral or contralateral CFA. After securing sheath

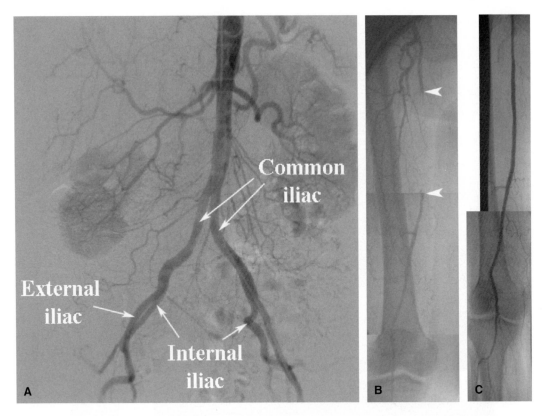

FIGURE 13-6 ● **Influence of anatomy of iliac vessels and aortic bifurcation, and superficial femoral artery (SFA) lesion on access strategy for SFA intervention. A:** Pelvic angiogram showing acute angulation of aortic bifurcation and significant tortuosity of the right external iliac artery. **B:** Angiogram of the right SFA showing long occlusion (margins denoted by white arrowheads) in the mid-portion of the vessel. There is a sufficient length of normal vessel in the proximal SFA to allow placement of a sheath placed antegrade in the ipsilateral common femoral artery. The occlusion was crossed with a 0.035″ wire, dilated with a 5.0 × 100-mm balloon, and stented with a 7.0 × 120-mm nitinol self-expanding stent that was postdilated with a 6.0 × 60-mm balloon. **C:** Final angiography following angioplasty and stenting.

placement at this site, the patient is placed in a prone position and the popliteal fossa is prepped and draped. The level of the femorotibial joint space is determined fluoroscopically. The skin (i.e., approximately 3 cm superior to the joint space) is anesthetized. Using the CFA access (i.e., direct injection of contrast medium through the ipsilateral CFA sheath, or injection through a diagnostic catheter placed in the distal aorta or ipsilateral iliac artery from the contralateral CFA), the popliteal artery is visualized. Using the road-map function, the popliteal artery is then punctured under fluoroscopy, using a 4-Fr to 5-Fr micropuncture needle, the 0.018″ wire is advanced, and the artery is sheathed with a standard short sheath. Most popliteal arteries are large enough to accommodate a 6-Fr sheath.

Brachial Retrograde Approach

Brachial artery access may also be used in patients with a contraindication to contralateral or ipsilateral CFA access. Current limitations in the length of the delivery systems of interventional equipment only allows treatment of proximal and mid-SFA lesions, in normal-sized individuals, from the brachial approach. The authors also rarely use more than a 6-Fr sheath size from the brachial artery, which may limit the types of interventional devices that may be delivered to the SFA.

Interventional Technique

Before proceeding with an intervention in the SFA, one should be certain that the access sheath

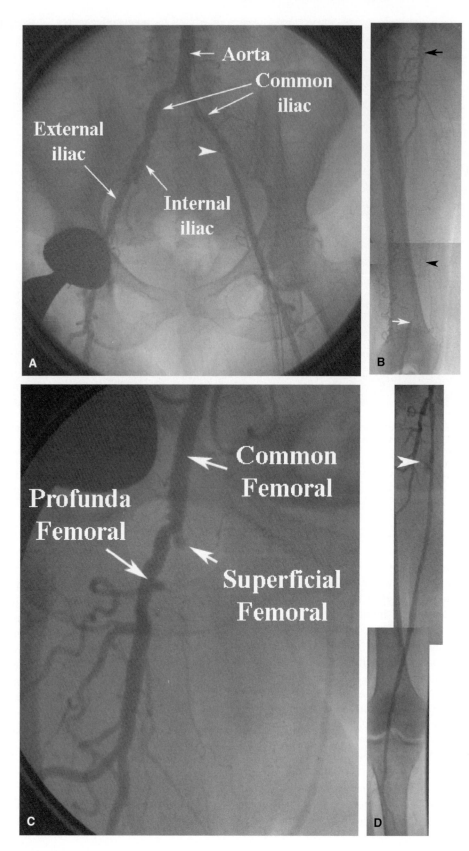

size chosen accommodates the interventional equipment required to treat the lesion. In general, when using the contralateral CFA approach, the authors use a 7-Fr sheath, as this will accommodate the angioplasty balloons and stents that are appropriate for SFA intervention, regardless of type. When using the antegrade approach, every effort should be made to minimize the sheath size because there is the risk of access-site bleeding; the authors most commonly use a 6-Fr sheath, and select stents with lower profiles if these are required (e.g., Zilver 518). One should also check the compatibility of the sheath size chosen, with that of newer interventional devices, if their use is anticipated.

Treatment of Stenosis

Having obtained arterial access, the treatment of SFA stenosis is generally straight forward (Fig. 13-8). A soft-tipped, 0.035″ wire (e.g., Magic Torque or Wholey wire) either alone, or supported by an angled glide catheter (e.g., Terumo GlideCath), is usually successful in crossing the lesion. The tip of the wire should be parked in the distal popliteal artery to provide sufficient support to deliver interventional equipment. Avoid allowing the wire to pass into the tibial vessels, so as to eliminate the risk of trauma to these vessels. A more easily torqued hydrophilic wire (e.g., floppy glidewire, stiff-angled glidewire) may occasionally be required. It is important to exchange this wire immediately for a soft-tipped nonhydrophilic wire having successfully crossed the lesion, as its routine use is associated with an increased risk of arterial injury.

The angioplasty balloon size and length is matched to the size (i.e., usually about 6 mm) and lesion length of the SFA. The inflation should be performed with the minimum pressure that releases the constriction and provides for the appropriate balloon-to-artery ratio. If the diameter of the vessel is in question, it is prudent to choose an under-sized balloon and progressively increase the diameter. Improved angiographic results may be accomplished with prolonged inflations lasting several minutes.

After angioplasty, the lesion must be carefully examined for the presence of flow-limiting dissections. Owing to the heavy calcification of atheroma in the SFA, dissections are commonly seen, but are not usually flow limiting. Digital subtraction angiography tends to underestimate the severity of dissection, which emphasizes the importance of carefully examining the fluoroscopic images. Evaluating the lesion for the presence of hemodynamically significant gradient is a crucial part of evaluating the lesion after angioplasty. Despite the angiographic appearance, if the lesion is not associated with a residual gradient, consideration should be given to accepting the angioplasty, alone, result.

There remains considerable controversy regarding the utility of adjunctive stenting in the SFA. Based on the poor outcomes achieved with balloon-expandable Palmaz stents and self-expandable stainless steel Wallstents, current recommendations are that intravascular stenting be reserved for salvage of patients with angioplasty failures or complications. However, newer data with self-expanding nitinol stents and self-expanding PTFE stent grafts have challenged this paradigm. In practice, there is a relatively low threshold for using self-expanding nitinol stents in the SFA location, sizing the stent about 1 mm greater than the diameter of the SFA

FIGURE 13-7 ● **Treatment of complicated right superficial femoral artery (SFA) occlusion. A:** Pelvic angiogram showing benign aortic bifurcation and iliac vessels allowing contralateral access and cross-over technique. **B:** Angiogram of SFA showing long occlusion of the right SFA extending from the origin to the mid-popliteal artery *(arrows)*. Note the previously placed stent in the distal SFA *(arrowhead)*. The extension of the occlusion into the mid-popliteal artery makes access to the true lumen just distal to the occlusion critical. **C:** RAO oblique view of the common femoral artery (CFA) bifurcation clearly delineating the stump of the SFA. Access was obtained in the left CFA, and a cross-over sheath was placed in the right CFA. The occlusion was crossed with a stiff angled glidewire dissected through the subintimal place. Access to the true lumen distally was obtained using the Pioneer catheter. Angioplasty of the occlusion was performed using a 6.0 × 10-mm balloon, and the entire occlusion sequentially stented using 7.0 mm diameter nitinol self-expanding stents. The stents were postdilated with the 6.0 mm diameter balloon. **D:** Angiogram following angioplasty and stenting shows perforation in the proximal SFA that was treated by prolonged balloon inflation and reversal of anticoagulation.

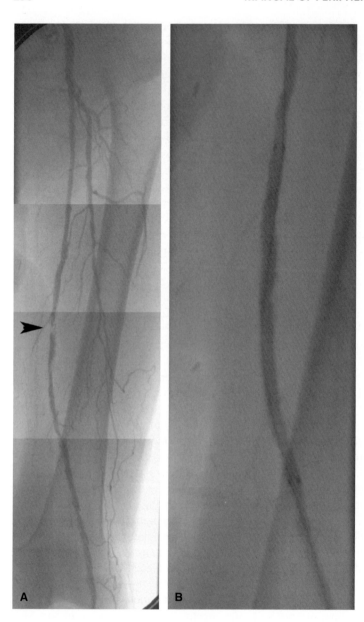

FIGURE 13-8 ● **Treatment of a superficial femoral artery stenosis. A:** Angiogram of the left superficial femoral artery shows a focal severe lesion in the mid-portion of the vessel *(arrowhead)*, with moderate diffuse disease proximal and distal to the lesion. The focal lesion was dilated with a 4.0 × 40 mm balloon, and the treatment site stented with a 7.0 × 100 mm nitinol self-expanding stent that was post dilated with a 5.0 × 80 mm balloon. **B:** Final angiogram of the treatment site following intervention.

(i.e., usual stent diameter is approximately 7 mm) and typically, postdilating with a 6.0-mm diameter balloon.

Treatment of Occlusions

SFA occlusions represent a significantly greater technical challenge. These occlusions are typically very long, beginning in the proximal third of the SFA and extending to the level of the adductor hiatus (Fig. 13-7). In crossing these occlusions, a 0.035″ stiff glidewire, supported by a diagnostic catheter (e.g., Terumo Glidecath) or balloon catheter, is almost always required. It is typical for the wire to enter the subintimal space inadvertently, during a significant portion of the length of the occlusion. Indeed, the authors increasingly perform purposeful, subintimal angioplasty for the treatment of long SFA occlusions. This is achieved by first passing the wire through the proximal margin of the occlusion and finding the subintimal space. This is recognized by the wire coursing in a spiral fashion, with a

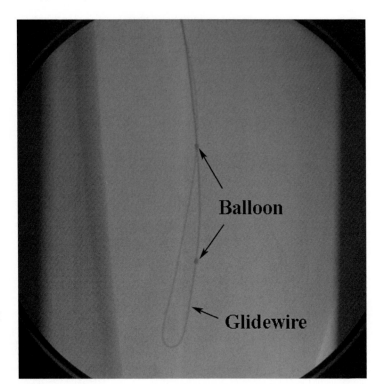

FIGURE 13-9 ● Subintimal angioplasty technique. Note that the stiff wire is looped such that the stiff portion of the wire is advancing through the subintimal space.

circumference that is greater than the diameter of the vessel lumen. At this point, the glide wire is prolapsed to create a large-enough loop that the stiff part of the wire leads the path through the subintimal space (Fig. 13-9).

The wire is supported throughout its course by the diagnostic or balloon catheter. This technique is very effective and usually straight forward, which may be explained by the fact that in an occluded vessel, the subintimal space is less vital and more vulnerable to dissection. At the distal end of the occlusion, the angled glide wire should be advanced until the wire dissects into the subintimal space, just distal to the point where the artery reconstitutes via collaterals. The major challenge of the technique is regaining access from this point, back into the true lumen, while minimizing any further dissection of the subintimal space. In heavily calcified vessels, this may be extremely difficult.

Prior to the recent availability of novel technologies (see below), the operator patiently probed, using varying combinations of straight or angled glide wires, and straight or angled supporting catheters, in an effort to direct from the subintimal space into the true lumen. In some cases, the use of stiff, nonhydrophilic, 0.014″ coronary wires that are more directionally controlled is successful (e.g., Cross-IT, Asahi Confienza). When the occlusion extends into the popliteal artery, the operator should be extremely careful not to extend the subintimal dissection plane during these maneuvers, as this increases the risk of the need for stent placement, at the flexion point of the knee. The success of this technique is approximately 80%.

For the remaining cases, and in those cases in which it is critical not to extend the subintimal space beyond the distal margin of the occlusion, two novel devices are available that facilitate reentry from the subintimal space to the true lumen: the Pioneer catheter and the Outback® catheter.

The Pioneer catheter (i.e., formerly the Cross-Point TransAccess catheter) is a 6.2-Fr catheter with a 64-element, phased-array, intravascular ultrasound (IVUS) probe just proximal to its tip, and a 0.014″ lumen needle just proximal to the IVUS that may be advanced 1 mm to 7 mm, radially (Fig. 13-10[A,B]) (3).

In order to use this device, one must appreciate that the catheter has two lumens: (1) one that runs

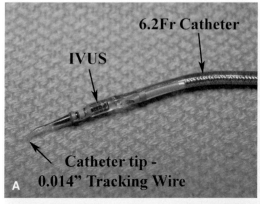

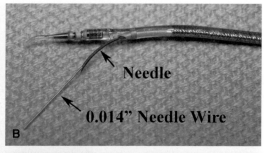

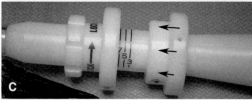

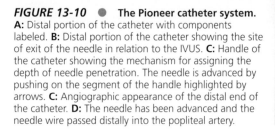

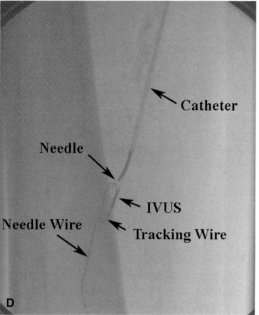

FIGURE 13-10 ● **The Pioneer catheter system.**
A: Distal portion of the catheter with components
labeled. **B:** Distal portion of the catheter showing the site
of exit of the needle in relation to the IVUS. **C:** Handle of
the catheter showing the mechanism for assigning the
depth of needle penetration. The needle is advanced by
pushing on the segment of the handle highlighted by
arrows. **C:** Angiographic appearance of the distal end of
the catheter. **D:** The needle has been advanced and the
needle wire passed distally into the popliteal artery.

the length of the catheter, from the depth gauge
at the proximal end through the needle tip (needle lumen for needle wire), and (2) another that
extends from the catheter tip to the distal shaft of
the catheter in a monorail configuration, and allows delivery of the catheter (i.e., delivery lumen
for tracking wire). Both lumens accommodate a
0.014″ wire.

Once a 0.035″ wire has been advanced within
the subintimal space, to a level approximately
2 cm distal to the point of vessel reconstitution,
the subintimal space is dilated with a 4-mm to
5-mm diameter balloon to facilitate delivery of
the catheter. The 0.035″ wire is then exchanged
for a 190-cm, heavy-support 0.014″ wire (e.g.,
Ironman, Balance Heavy Weight). This serves as
the tracking wire for delivery of the catheter to
the distal end of the tracking wire.

Having connected the IVUS catheter with a
JOMED IVUS console, an IVUS picture of the
true lumen is obtained with the aid of Chro-
moFlo imaging (i.e., similar to color Doppler
imaging). The injection of agitated saline, mixed
with blood, through the femoral sheath dramatically enhances the ability to visualize flow within
the true lumen. The catheter is then rotated until the true lumen is positioned at 12 o'clock in
the IVUS picture. A direct measurement of the
depth between the false lumen and the center of
the true lumen is made, which determines the
needle depth that is set using the depth gauge
(Fig. 13-10[C]). This measurement is usually
around 4 mm to 5 mm. The needle is then advanced into the true lumen, and a second 300-cm,
0.014″ wire is advanced through the needle lumen to exit the needle.

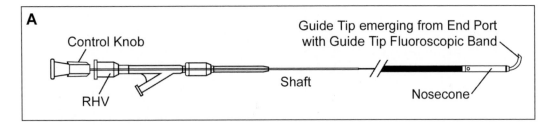

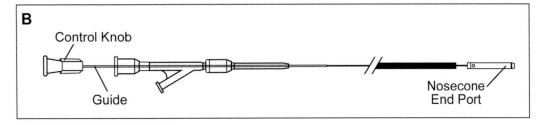

FIGURE 13-11 ● **The Outback catheter system. A:** Catheter system with needle advanced. **B:** Catheter system with needle in nosecone.

If the true lumen has been successfully punctured, the needle wire passes easily and distally into the popliteal and tibial vessels (Fig. 13-10[D]). The needle is then retracted, the tracking wire removed, and the catheter exchanged over the needle wire for a glide or balloon catheter that is passed into the popliteal artery. The 0.014″ wire is then exchanged for a soft-tipped, 0.035″ wire and the operator may proceed with angioplasty. Occasionally it is necessary to dilate the reentry site with a coronary balloon to facilitate exchange, using a diagnostic or balloon catheter.

The Outback catheter is remarkably similar to the Pioneer catheter, except that it lacks ultrasound guidance (Fig. 13-11).

It consists of a single-lumen, 4.8-Fr catheter that is compatible with 0.014″ and 0.018″ wires. At its distal tip, there is a nose cone that houses a curved nitinol needle, activated by a control knob at the proximal end of the catheter. Similarly to the method described above, the Outback catheter is tracked over a wire whose tip is in the subintimal space adjacent to the true lumen, just distal to the inferior margin of the occlusion. The wire is then withdrawn proximally. By torque manipulation of the catheter, the tip of the device is pointed toward the true lumen, using orthogonal angiographic views for guidance. The needle is then advanced into the true lumen and the wire follows, distally, into the tibial vessels. Finally

the needle is withdrawn, the catheter removed, and the 0.014″ or 0.018″ wire is exchanged for a 0.035″ wire, and the remainder of the procedure completed.

Once the lesion is successfully crossed, the length of the occlusion is dilated with an angioplasty balloon. All of the comments regarding angioplasty in the setting of the treatment of SFA stenosis are applicable in the treatment of SFA occlusions. In addition, for long occlusions, it is best to use 10-cm long balloons, in the interest of time efficiency. Careful attention should be paid to patient discomfort during subintimal angioplasty. Excessive dilation in this circumstance may result in an increased risk of vessel perforation (Fig. 13-7). Regarding stenting in the treatment of SFA occlusion, the authors typically stent the inflow and outflow of the occlusion. If there is an adequate angioplasty result in the intervening portion of the occlusion (i.e., no flow-limiting dissection, no pressure gradient), no further stenting is performed.

Ostial SFA lesions

Ostial SFA lesions deserve special mention. These lesions are difficult to treat because of the proximity of the PFA, and its importance in the arterial supply to the thigh. The risks of treatment in this location include plaque shift into the ostium of the PFA. In addition, with longer, self-expanding stents, it may be extremely

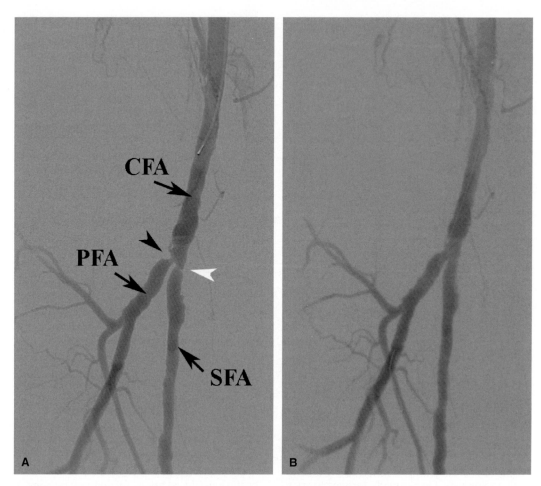

FIGURE 13-12 ● **Treatment of ostial superficial femoral artery disease. A:** Angiogram of the right common femoral artery demonstrating critical ostial disease of the superficial and profunda femoral arteries. **B:** The ostia of both arteries was treated with the Foxhollow atherectomy catheter producing an excellent angiographic result and no compromise of the profunda ostium.

difficult to place the proximal end of the stent at the SFA ostium, precisely, thereby avoiding inadvertent coverage of the PFA ostium. A helpful approach is to use a short, 20-mm length stent to treat the ostial disease, since the degree of stent shortening at this stent length is minimal. If the risk of plaque shift is viewed to be prohibitive, atherectomy (see below) may be a reasonable option, either as stand-alone therapy or as an adjunct to angioplasty (Fig. 13-12).

SFA Intervention—Clinical Efficacy Outcomes

The interpretation of outcomes following SFA intervention is complicated by a lack of randomized trials evaluating the various therapeutic modalities. Much of the literature consists of case series involving heterogenous patient populations, with varied indications for intervention, and varied complexity of disease. Therefore, it is very difficult to compare the patency rates for the different treatment modalities reliably. In addition, many of the studies involve antiquated devices that do not reflect the outcomes achieved with contemporary technology. Within the limitations of the current data, Dorrucci has performed a useful analysis of the outcomes of all the studies of SFA revascularization using surgical techniques and the various percutaneous treatment modalities (summarized in Table 13-2) (4).

The gold standard for revascularization of the SFA remains surgical bypass, using a venous

TABLE 13-2

Summary of Primary and Secondary Patency Rates Achieved with Various Surgical and Endovascular Interventions for the Treatment of Superficial Femoral Artery Disease

Revascularization Method	Patency Rates (%)									
	6 mo		1 year		2 years		3 years		4 years	
	1°	2°	1°	2°	1°	2°	1°	2°	1°	2°
Above-knee vein conduit	87	90	81	89	77	86	71	82	70	81
Above-knee prosthetic conduit	85	91	77	86	66	73	59	68	51	61
Covered stents*	62	79	54	75	—	—	—	—	—	—
Hemobahn endoprosthesis	81	89	74	85	73	84	64	80	—	—
Bare metal stents[†]	81	84	65	75	55	60	55	50	37	52
Nitinol stents	93	96	85	93	—	—	—	—	—	—
Angioplasty	73	80	58	69	51	63	47	53	40	53
Subintimal angioplasty	55	—	46	—	36	—	—	—	—	—

*Excluding Hemobahn endoprosthesis, [†]balloon-expandable stents
1° primary patency, 2° secondary patency.

or prosthetic (e.g., PTFE) graft conduit. For an above-the-knee vein graft using either type of conduit, the primary patency rates at 1 and 4 years are 81% and 70%, respectively. In analyses of outcomes by individual graft, there does appear to be a benefit in favor of the venous conduit (i.e., 5-year patency of 75% vs. 60%). With below-the-knee grafts, the difference is more dramatic (i.e., 5-year patency of 75% vs. 30%). Based on these data, it is generally recommended to use a venous conduit for both above- and below-the-knee bypass surgery. However, the use of a venous conduit is complicated by prolonged operative times, an increased risk of wound complications, and the removal of veins that may be subsequently required for other revascularization procedures (e.g., coronary artery bypass surgery). For these reasons, many operators continue to use prosthetic conduits, particularly for above-the-knee bypass surgery, where the potential benefit of the venous conduit on long-term patency is less dramatic.

The patency data for surgical bypass serve as a useful reference for assessing the efficacy of endovascular therapies. However, it should be emphasized that in making the clinical decision to treat by surgical or percutaneous techniques,

consideration of these data, together with an assessment of the potential morbidity and mortality from either procedure, should be considered.

Angioplasty, alone, is associated with excellent results in patients with focal SFA disease, with patency rates at 1 and 5 years of more than 80% and 70%, respectively (5–7). With the use of hemodynamic assessments of pressure gradients across the lesion to guide optimal angioplasty, these results may be improved upon. However, angioplasty performs poorly for patients with diffuse disease and poor vessel run off (8). Inclusion of this population of patients in the review by Dorrucci explains the overall 1- and 4-year patency rates for angioplasty of about 58% and 40%, respectively (4).

Initial studies using balloon-expandable stents in the SFA demonstrated poor outcomes, with no benefit over angioplasty alone (9,10). These types of stents appear particularly unsuited in the SFA location, where they generate an exaggerated intimal hyperplastic response and are prone to compression from external forces. This led to the use of the stainless-steel self-expanding stents (e.g., WallStent). Early results with this type of stent were similarly disappointing, suggesting no benefit over angioplasty alone (11). In retrospect, studies using these stents have been criticized on the basis of poor interventional technique and suboptimal periprocedural pharmacotherapy (12). It is unclear if modern techniques and current advances in periprocedural anticoagulant and antiplatelet regimens would significantly improve the outcomes achieved in these studies.

Contemporary stenting of the SFA is achieved using nitinol self-expanding stents, and to a lesser extent, using endovascular stent grafts. The IntraCoil stent is the only nitinol self-expanding stent that is FDA approved for use in the femoral-popliteal arteries (13). However, this stent has a number of limitations: it is high profile, the absence of a sheath covering the stent makes it difficult to deliver through calcified lesions (i.e., making predilation mandatory), and precise placement is difficult as a result of the deployment mechanism. For these reasons, the authors reserve the use of this stent to the treatment of lesions at flexion points, when stenting is required. The remaining self-expanding nitinol stents currently used in the SFA received their FDA approval for use in the biliary system (Table 13-3).

The Gore Hemobahn Endoprosthesis® is the dominant stent graft used in the SFA, and is composed of a PTFE graft supported by an outer nitinol frame. This type of stent graft is distinct from older stent grafts that were constructed from vascular grafts and balloon-expandable stents, and were associated with high complication and restenosis rates when used in the SFA location (4). The primary patency rates at 1 year with contemporary stent designs are in the 75 to 85% range. Accepting the limitation of an unadjusted analysis, patency rates with contemporary stenting represent a significant improvement over angioplasty alone, and approach the rates achieved with surgery. Longer term follow-up evaluation with these stents is clearly required.

Reported outcomes for patients in whom the strategy of subintimal angioplasty was used have generally been poor, with 1- and 2-year patency rates of 46% and 36%, respectively (4,14). Patients undergoing subintimal angioplasty generally have diffuse disease with long SFA occlusions, and this likely explains the outcomes observed. Despite the low patency rates, this technique remains useful in patients with critical

TABLE 13-3

Self-Expanding Nitinol Stents Used for Superficial Femoral Artery Intervention

Name	Manufacturer	Stent Diameter (mm)	Stent Length (mm)	Sheath Size (Fr)	Guidewire (Inch)
Zilver 518	Cook	4, 5, 6, 7, 8, 9, 10	20, 30, 40, 50, 60	5	0.018
Zilver	Cook	6, 7, 8, 9, 10, 12, 14	40, 60, 80	7	0.035
Symphony	Boston Scientific	6, 7, 8, 10, 12, 14	20, 22, 23, 40, 60	7	0.035
Luminexx	Bard	6, 7, 8, 9, 10, 12	20, 30, 40, 50, 60, 80, 100, 120	6	0.035
Wallstent	Boston Scientific	5, 6, 7, 8, 10, 12, 14, 16, 18, 20	20, 40, 55, 45, 60, 80, 90, 94	6	0.035
SMART	Cordis	6–14	20, 40, 60, 80	7	0.035
PRECISE	Cordis	5–10	20, 30, 40	6	0.018
DYNALINK	Guidant	5–10	28, 38, 56, 80, 100	6	0.018 and 0.035
ABSOLUTE	Guidant	5–10	20, 30, 40, 60, 80, 100	6	0.035
Protégé	ev3	6, 7, 8, 9	20, 30, 40, 60, 80	6	0.018 and 0.035
				7	0.035
IntraCoil	ev3	4, 5, 6, 7, 8	40	7–9	0.035

limb ischemia who are nonsurgical candidates, and in whom conventional endovascular therapies are unsuccessful. In such patients, restoration of improved antegrade flow, even in the short term, will maximize the chances of tissue healing. The recent trend of using adjunctive stenting with self-expanding nitinol stents will likely improve long-term patency rates, but large data sets using this strategy have not been reported.

Novel Technologies/Devices in SFA Intervention

Cryoplasty

The PolarCath peripheral balloon catheter is a new system that simultaneously dilates and cools the plaque and vessel wall in the area of treatment. The specifications of the system are summarized in Table 13-4.

A nitrous-oxide cartridge is loaded into an inflation unit that is connected to the balloon catheter. Using an automated mechanism, the balloon is inflated with liquid nitrous oxide. Evaporation of the nitrous oxide cools the balloon to $-10°C$ temperatures, resulting in both angioplasty and cooling of the plaque. The manufacturer argues that cooling induces apoptosis, rather than necrosis, in smooth-muscle cells, thus limiting smooth-muscle cell proliferation and reducing the risk of restenosis (15). The automated mechanism of balloon inflation removes the typical control afforded the operator using conventional balloons. Therefore, we typically predilate the lesion using conventional balloons, prior to

cryoplasty, to minimize the risk of balloon slippage during activation of the cryoplasty balloon.

Preliminary data from a multi-center registry using the PolarCath to treat SFA stenosis or occlusions shorter than 10 cm (PVD-CHILL) have been presented. Acute procedural success was achieved in 96% of cases, with a very low rate of significant dissection (7%) and need for stent placement (9%). Among a subset of the registry with 1-year follow-up evaluation (n = 45), the patency rate was 85%, which certainly compares favorably with historic controls (16). Comparative data between this therapy and either angioplasty or stenting of the SFA will ultimately be required to provide more robust evidence of the efficacy of this mode of therapy.

Atherectomy

Two distinctly different atherectomy devices are used, to a limited degree, during SFA interventions. The first is an excimer-laser catheter (i.e., CliRpath Extreme catheter) that has laser fibers arranged concentrically around the central-guide lumen (Fig. 13-13) (17). This catheter is used in combination with the CVX-300 laser system, which allows delivery of intense bursts of ultraviolet energy in short-pulse durations (120 nanoseconds), through the laser fibers (Table 13-5).

The ultraviolet energy delivered through the catheter has a direct lytic action on tissue, explaining its effectiveness in recanalizing total occlusions. Currently, this device is used to treat

TABLE 13-4

Specifications of the Available Catheters Using the PolarCath System

Specification	
Catheter lengths (cm)	80, 120
Balloon diameters (mm)	4.0, 5.0, 6.0, 7.0
Balloon lengths (mm)	20, 40, 60
Sheath compatibility	6Fr–balloon diameters 4.0, 5.0 7Fr–balloon diameters 6.0, 7.0
Wire compatibility	0.035″ wire

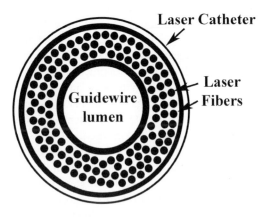

FIGURE 13-13 ● Schematic of an over-the-wire excimer laser catheter showing the laser fibers concentrically arranged around the guidewire lumen.

TABLE 13-5

Specification of the Over-the-Wire Extreme Laser Catheters Used for Superficial Femoral Artery Intervention

Specification	Diameter (mm)		
	2.0	2.3	3.0
Working length	135	120	100
Sheath compatibility	7Fr	7Fr	8Fr
Guidewire compatibility	0.018	0.035	0.035
Energy (mJ/mm^2) range	30–60	30–60	30–50
Pulse rep. rate (Hz) range	25–40	25–40	25–40
Laser activation sequence	10 seconds on – 5 seconds off		

long SFA occlusions in patients with critical limb ischemia, in whom conventional interventional techniques have failed. The catheter is delivered over a wire to the proximal stump of the occlusion. Having confirmed the position of the catheter, and thoroughly flushing it with saline solution to remove all of the contrast medium, the laser system is activated and the catheter advanced through the occlusion. An attempt is usually made to cross the terminal 0.5 cm to 1 cm of the occlusion with a guidewire, to minimize the risk of dissection or perforation of the distal vessel. Having successfully crossed the occlusion, the catheter is removed and angioplasty performed.

The Peripheral Excimer Laser Atherectomy (PELA) Trial randomized 251 patients with claudication and long occlusions (i.e., longer than 10 cm) to excimer laser-assisted angioplasty or angioplasty alone. The acute procedural success and long-term patency rates were similar in both groups. Perforation rates were higher in the laser group (i.e., 8.9% vs. 3.4%), while stent usage was lower (i.e., 42% vs. 59%). Subsequent registries continue to demonstrate the feasibility of the technique, but the data are not capable of demonstrating the superiority of this strategy over angioplasty alone, by virtue of the absence of a comparison group (18). The technique certainly has a role for patients in whom it is impossible to cross the occlusion with a wire. However, with

the recent popularity of subintimal angioplasty techniques, and access to reentry devices (see above), this represents a very small fraction of the SFA-intervention population.

The SilverHawk atherectomy catheter is a directional atherectomy device that is gaining increasing popularity in SFA interventions (Fig. 13-14). This device represents a significant advance over the profile, flexibility, torque capability, and ease-of-use of older, directional atherectomy devices (19). The catheter has a monorail design and an outer diameter of 6 Fr, making it compatible with 7-Fr sheath. It is advanced over a wire just proximal to the lesion of interest. A mechanism in the handle at the proximal end of the catheter activates the device by opening an articulation between the cylindrical housing and shaft (Fig. 13-14). This brings the cutter in contact with the plaque. The catheter is then advanced distally, removing a thin sliver of plaque. Having reached the distal end of the lesion, the device is deactivated, withdrawn proximally, rotated 90°, activated, and then advanced distally to remove further plaque. This process is repeated several times, to achieve optimal debulking of the plaque. There are no published data to support the use of this device in the SFA. It is entirely unclear if restenosis rates are favorably altered by its use, or if any difference in outcome exists between a strategy of atherectomy alone or atherectomy with adjunctive angioplasty. Until these data become available, it seems reasonable to restrict the use of this device to the treatment of disease in locations where the operator wishes to avoid stenting (i.e., ostium of the SFA, common femoral artery, and popliteal artery) (Fig. 13-12). Further, the manufacturer recommends the device not be used for the treatment of in-stent restenosis, since there is a risk that the cutter may catch on a stent strut. Despite this recommendation, some operators have used the device for this off-label indication.

Brachytherapy

Following the publication of reports of disappointing restenosis rates with SFA stenting using stainless steel, balloon-expandable stents and the stainless steel self-expanding Wallstent, significant energies were directed toward the use of brachytherapy, as an adjunct to angioplasty, in

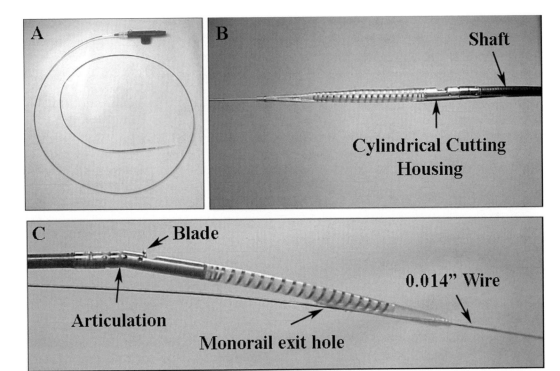

FIGURE 13-14 ● **Fox Hollow atherectomy catheter. A:** Low magnification view of the catheter. **B:** Magnified view of the distal portion of the catheter with the distal shaft and housing in the nondeflected position. **C:** Magnified view of the distal portion of the catheter with the distal shaft and housing in deflected position bringing the blade into contact with the vessel wall. The monorail design of the catheter is shown. Reproduced with modification from Orlic et al, *Catheter Cardiovasc Interv.* 2003;60:159–166.

the prophylaxis of restenosis following SFA angioplasty. This enthusiasm was founded on the promising results achieved in the coronary circulation for the treatment of in-stent restenosis. However, the pathologies of in-stent restenosis and restenosis following angioplasty are distinct. Whereas in-stent restenosis is caused entirely by intimal hyperplasia, restenosis following successful angioplasty is secondary to the combination of elastic recoil, constrictive remodeling, and intimal hyperplasia.

Several clinical studies have been performed to evaluate brachytherapy as an adjunct to angioplasty in the prophylaxis of SFA restenosis and the treatment of restenosis following angioplasty (20,21). The Vienna-2 Study enrolled 117 patients with claudication or critical leg ischemia, with *de novo* SFA stenosis or occlusion of more than 5 cm in length, and SFA restenosis following angioplasty (regardless of length). IR-192 was delivered using a noncentered delivery system with 10-mm safety margins. At

6-months follow-up evaluation, restenosis was observed in 54% of the PTA group and 28% of the PTA and brachytherapy group. At 1-year follow-up evaluation, the restenosis rate was 61% and 36%, respectively. Significant benefit was also demonstrated for restenotic lesions and long (i.e., longer than 10 cm) lesions.

Like the Vienna-2 trial, the Peripheral Artery Radiation Investigational Study (PARIS) attempted to investigate the effectiveness of IR-192 using a centered catheter for the prevention of SFA restenosis (22). Patients included in the trial had stenoses between 5 cm and 15 cm in length or occlusions up to 5 cm. Similarly, 10-mm safety margins were applied. The feasibility arm of the trial demonstrated an increase in rest and exercise ABIs from 0.67 and 0.51, to 0.89 and 0.72 at 1-year follow-up evaluation, respectively. Maximal walking time increased from 3.4 to 4.4 minutes at 30 days, and 4 minutes at 1 year. The binary restenosis rate at 6 months was 17.2%, and the clinical restenosis rate at

TABLE 13-6

Summary of SIROCCO I and II Trials

	SIROCCO I		SIROCCO II	
Number of patients	36		57	
Enrollment criteria	• ≥70% stenosis, 7–20 cm in length		• ≥70% stenosis, 7–14.5 cm in length	
	• total occlusion, 4–20 cm in length		• total occlusion, 4–14.5 cm in length	
Maximum number of stents used	3		2	
Outcome	Drug-Eluting Stent	Bare Metal Stent	Drug-Eluting Stent	Bare Metal Stent
6 mo angiographic restenosis				
In-stent (%)	0	17.6	—	—
In-lesion (%)	0	23.5	0	7.7
Stent strut fracture (%)	8	8	6	

1 year was 13.3%, which certainly compares favorably with historic controls. Unfortunately, the randomized portion of the trial was terminated early as a result of poor enrollment. An assessment of the randomized cohort enrolled revealed no benefit for brachytherapy with adjunctive angioplasty versus angioplasty alone.

Although the data for endovascular radiation for the treatment of SFA stenosis appears promising, its widespread use has been limited. This is based on the perceived improvement in outcomes achieved with nitinol self-expanding stents. An increased incidence of vessel ectasia, together with delayed reendothelialization from brachytherapy, resulting in an increased risk of late thrombosis, have also raised significant safety concerns regarding this therapy. Finally, the practical challenges of administering gamma radiation to long SFA lesions is considerable, and has contributed to the failure of application of this therapy.

Drug-Eluting Stents

The success of drug-eluting stents (DES) in preventing restenosis in coronary arteries provided the impetus to test the concept in the treatment of peripheral vascular disease. Given the high restenosis rates associated with SFA intervention, this seemed like a suitable starting point for this endeavor.

Two separate trials (SIROCCO 1 and 2) evaluated the efficacy of the sirolimus-coated SMART nitinol self-expandable stent compared to an uncoated version of the same stent for the treatment of obstructive SFA disease (Table 13-6) (23).

The SIROCCO 1 trial was a feasibility study involving 36 patients with chronic limb ischemia and either femoral artery occlusions or stenoses. There was a trend toward a decrease in the primary end point in the DES arm, with a 6-month mean percent diameter stenosis of 22.6% in the DES arm and 30.9% in the bare-metal stent group. The binary restenosis rate in the DES arm was 0% versus 23.5% in the bare-metal stent arm. Because of the small numbers of patients, and the lower than expected restenosis rate in the bare-metal stent arm, this difference was not statistically significant. Strut fractures in the stent were reported in about 8% of patients.

Building on the results of the SIROCCO 1 trial, the SIRROCCO 2 trial randomized 57 patients to treatment of SFA disease with a modified sirolimus SMART stent, with modifications in both the stent design (i.e., to reduce the rate of strut fracture) and rate of drug elution (i.e., to reduce the rate of restenosis), versus uncoated SMART stents. The lesions were shorter and a maximum of two stents were allowed. At 6-month follow-up evaluation, the angiographic restenosis rate in the DES arm was 0% versus 7.7% for the bare-metal arm ($P = 0.49$).

Surprisingly, at 9-month follow-up evaluation using duplex ultrasound, the in-lesion binary restenosis rate in the DES arm was higher (not significantly) than in the bare-metal arm (23.1% versus 17.4%, $P = 0.73$).

These results highlight the challenges faced by the use of drug-eluting stents in the SFA location. It is probably true that newer nitinol self-expanding stents perform better than expected, making it harder for drug-eluting stents to provide an incremental benefit. In addition, the properties required of an effective DES in this location may be very different from our current assumption, based on experience in the coronary circulation. Further investigation in this area is clearly warranted.

COMPLICATIONS OF SFA INTERVENTION

In the realm of peripheral vascular intervention, SFA intervention is a relatively safe procedure. Complication rates are heavily influenced by the clinical characteristics of the patient population, the clinical indication for the procedure, the complexity of the treated lesion (e.g., stenosis versus occlusion, short versus long occlusion, non-ostial versus ostial location, atherothrombotic versus atherosclerotic lesions), the interventional technique, and operator experience. These factors explain the wide range of complication rates reported from various series. Access site complications are the most frequently observed adverse events (see Chapter 19, Management of Complications) and include: bleeding, hematoma, and pseudoaneurysm and arteriovenous-fistula formation. Some of the cross-over sheaths (e.g. Balkan sheath) are particularly stiff and iliac dissection frequently occurs during introduction of the sheath in diseased or tortuous iliac vessels (Fig. 13-15).

Clinically significant distal embolization during SFA intervention is uncommon, occurring in about 1 to 2% of cases. Patients with poor distal run off are at increased risk from this complication, highlighting the importance of

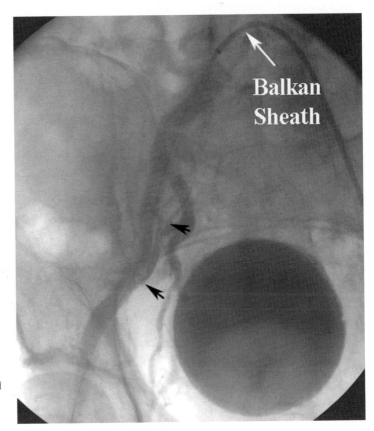

FIGURE 13-15 ●
Angiogram of the right common and external iliac systems following right superficial femoral artery intervention. Note the dissection in the right external iliac artery (*margins shown by arrows*) created by the Balkhan sheath during delivery to the right common femoral artery.

meticulous interventional technique in patients with this anatomy. Treatment of distal embolization includes pharmacologic thrombolysis or thrombectomy techniques (see Chapters 4 and 5). The former is better suited for treatment of embolization to the smaller tibial vessels, while the latter is favored for the treatment of embolization to the distal SFA or PFA.

Dissection at the treatment site is a frequent event, but rarely is it flow limiting. Axial extension of the dissection plane may breach the media of the vessel causing vessel perforation. If the adventitia is not breached, the result is a 'contained' perforation. Extension beyond the adventitia results in a 'free' perforation. There are two distinct forms of free perforation of the SFA: (1) free perforation into the muscle compartment of the thigh; this requires immediate treatment with balloon inflation and placement of a covered stent to prevent the development of compartment syndrome (Fig. 19-6); and (2) free perforation from the SFA to the adjacent deep vein (see Fig. 19-7[B], Chapter 19, Management of Complications: Surgical and Endovascular). This is a relatively benign complication. It is seen during interventions in the SFA, as it courses through the adductor canal, where the vessel is enclosed in a sheath with the deep femoral vein. This perforation is well tolerated because there is no extravasation of blood into the muscle compartment of the thigh and thus no risk of a compartment syndrome. In our experience, placement of a bare metal, self-expanding stent is usually effective in sealing this type of perforation.

Fractures of the stent struts appear to be a particularly unique and common problem with the use of self-expanding stents in the SFA location (24). In some reports, they may occur in up to 20% of cases, and various analyses suggest that excessive stent overlap may predict this event. In general, strut fracture is clinically asymptomatic. The long-term clinical consequence of these fractures is unknown.

Follow-up Evaluation

Aggressive follow-up evaluation of patients following SFA intervention is an important part of patient management. It is our practice to obtain an ABI at rest and following exercise, and duplex ultrasound of the treated vessel, shortly after endovascular therapy. These studies serve as a baseline for future comparisons in the event of recurrence of claudication.

Patients are routinely seen at 6 weeks, 6 months, and at yearly intervals thereafter. At each time point, the patient is questioned about the presence of recurrent claudication, and an ABI and duplex ultrasound of the SFA is performed. Duplex ultrasound is more sensitive than either clinical symptoms or ABI in detecting restenosis. A peak systolic flow velocity greater than 200 cm per second at the site of the lesion or less than 45 cm per second distal to the lesion are indicative of a stenosis of more than 50%. Using contemporary techniques and devices for reintervention after the aggressive use of these monitoring strategies may help achieve secondary patency rates of about 90%. However, there are no data to demonstrate that this confers a measurable clinical benefit to the patient (e.g., reduced rate of clinical restenosis or limb loss).

Medical therapy following SFA intervention is largely empiric. The authors treat with aspirin and clopidogrel for a minimum of 1 month following intervention. Longer term dual antiplatelet therapy may be indicated in patients with poor distal run off or diffuse severe SFA disease, where the risk of stent thrombosis is likely increased. Aggressive secondary risk modification is also indicated in this group at high risk for cardiovascular events.

REFERENCES

1. Dormandy JA, Rutherford RB. Management of peripheral arterial disease (PAD). TASC Working Group. TransAtlantic Inter-Society Consensus (TASC). *J Vasc Surg.* 2000;31:S1–S296.
2. Feinglass J, McCarthy WJ, Slavensky R, et al. Functional status and walking ability after lower extremity bypass grafting or angioplasty for intermittent claudication: results from a prospective outcomes study. *J Vasc Surg.* 2000;31:93–103.
3. Casserly IP, Sachar R, Bajzer C, et al. Utility of IVUS-guided transaccess catheter in the treatment of long chronic total occlusion of the superficial femoral artery. *Catheter Cardiovasc Interv.* 2004;62:237–243.
4. Dorrucci V. Treatment of superficial femoral artery occlusive disease. *J Cardiovasc Surg (Torino).* 2004;45: 193–201.
5. Grimm J, Muller-Hulsbeck S, Jahnke T, et al. Randomized study to compare PTA alone versus PTA with

Palmaz stent placement for femoropopliteal lesions. *J Vasc Interv Radiol.* 2001;12:935–942.

6. Hunink MG, Wong JB, Donaldson MC, et al. Revascularization for femoropopliteal disease. A decision and cost-effectiveness analysis. *JAMA.* 1995;274:165–171.

7. Johnston KW. Femoral and popliteal arteries: reanalysis of results of balloon angioplasty. *Radiology.* 1992;183:767–771.

8. Capek P, McLean GK, Berkowitz HD. Femoropopliteal angioplasty. Factors influencing long-term success. *Circulation.* 1991;83:I70–I80.

9. Chatelard P, Guibourt C. Long-term results with a Palmaz stent in the femoropopliteal arteries. *J Cardiovasc Surg (Torino).* 1996;37:67–72.

10. Rosenfield K, Schainfeld R, Pieczek A, et al. Restenosis of endovascular stents from stent compression. *J Am Coll Cardiol.* 1997;29:328–338.

11. Martin EC, Katzen BT, Benenati JF, et al. Multicenter trial of the Wallstent in the iliac and femoral arteries. *J Vasc Interv Radiol.* 1995;6:843–849.

12. Silver MJ, Ansel GM. Femoropopliteal occlusive disease: diagnosis, indications for treatment, and results of interventional therapy. *Catheter Cardiovasc Interv.* 2002;56:555–561.

13. Ansel GM, Botti CF, Jr., George BS, et al. Clinical results for the training-phase roll-in patients in the Intracoil femoral-popliteal stent trial. *Catheter Cardiovasc Interv.* 2002;56:443–449.

14. Yilmaz S, Sindel T, Yegin A, et al. Subintimal angioplasty of long superficial femoral artery occlusions. *J Vasc Interv Radiol.* 2003;14:997–1010.

15. Laird JR. A new approach to treating SFA disease. *Endovascular Today.* 2003;May/June:38–40.

16. Laird JR, Biamino G. Results of the cryovascular peripheral balloon catheter safety registry. In: *Transcatheter Cardiovascular Therapeutics.* Washington DC; 2003.

17. Laird JR Jr, Reiser C, Biamino G, et al. Excimer laser assisted angioplasty for the treatment of critical limb ischemia. *J Cardiovasc Surg (Torino).* 2004;45:239–248.

18. Boccalandro F, Muench A, Sdringola S, et al. Wireless laser-assisted angioplasty of the superficial femoral artery in patients with critical limb ischemia who have failed conventional percutaneous revascularization. *Catheter Cardiovasc Interv.* 2004;63:7–12.

19. Orlic D, Reimers B, Stankovic G, et al. Initial experience with a new 8 French-compatible directional atherectomy catheter: immediate and mid-term results. *Catheter Cardiovasc Interv.* 2003;60:159–166.

20. Pokrajac B, Potter R, Maca T, et al. Intraarterial (192)Ir high-dose-rate brachytherapy for prophylaxis of restenosis after femoropopliteal percutaneous transluminal angioplasty: the prospective randomized Vienna-2-trial radiotherapy parameters and risk factors analysis. *Int J Radiat Oncol Biol Phys.* 2000;48:923–931.

21. Minar E, Pokrajac B, Maca T, et al. Endovascular brachytherapy for prophylaxis of restenosis after femoropopliteal angioplasty: results of a prospective randomized study. *Circulation.* 2000;102:2694–2699.

22. Waksman R, Laird JR, Jurkovitz CT, et al. Intravascular radiation therapy after balloon angioplasty of narrowed femoropopliteal arteries to prevent restenosis: results of the PARIS feasibility clinical trial. *J Vasc Interv Radiol.* 2001;12:915–921.

23. Duda SH, Pusich B, Richter G, et al. Sirolimus-eluting stents for the treatment of obstructive superficial femoral artery disease: six-month results. *Circulation.* 2002;106:1505–1509.

24. Rocha-Singh KJ, Scheer K, Rutherford J. Nitinol stent fractures in the superficial femoral artery: Incidence and clinical significance. *J Am Coll Cardiol.* 2003;41 (suppl 1):79–80.

CHAPTER 14

Infrapopliteal Intervention

Mitchell J. Silver and Gary M. Ansel

The advancing field of percutaneous endovascular therapy has led to a significant increase in options available for the treatment of patients with symptomatic peripheral vascular disease. Previous reticence of using these procedures in the infrapopliteal arterial bed is slowly giving way, as technologic improvements and operator experience have led to high technical success rates with low complications.

INDICATIONS FOR INTERVENTION

The therapeutic selection decision process for distal vascular disease is multifaceted. Considerations include such limb variables as number of diseased vascular levels involved, patency of the plantar arch, level of tissue destruction, presence of infection, need for debridement or skin grafting, and type of available conduit. General patient variables that play a significant role in the decision process include, the presence of comorbidities such as cardiopulmonary disease, diabetes and renal insufficiency. It should also be recognized that the primary goal of treatment of significant distal-limb ischemia is not necessarily hemodynamic, but is that of safe avoidance of amputation, and salvage of a functioning limb.

The treatment of infrapopliteal vascular disease is complex, whether the treatment is medical, surgical, or endovascular. Critical limb ischemia, manifest as ischemic rest pain or tissue loss, is the most common clinical indication, and presents a significant risk for amputation in that individual (1). In the elderly, who are most at risk, the probability of loss of independence and reduced quality of life from an amputation is significant (2). Currently it appears that whatever treatment successfully prevents major amputation will be cost effective, with benefit to the individual as well as society (3).

Historically, reconstructive femoral-to-tibial bypass surgery using venous conduit has been successful in preserving limb viability. However, unless adequate venous conduit is available, results are universally dismal. Thus, prosthetic grafts are rarely used to the tibial vessels (4,5). Although individual centers may give excellent results, similar results may not be possible in many centers, when audited (6). The problem of postoperative wound infection, necessitating weeks of intensive care occurs commonly (i.e., 10 to 30%), but rarely is mentioned (7). Interestingly, as seen in distal angioplasty, the patency rates of surgical-bypass grafts may lag behind the limb-salvage rates. Similar to restenosis, graft closure after wound healing may not always lead to significant ischemia (8).

The published experience for endovascular intervention of the infrapopliteal arteries began with the advent of balloon angioplasty but even today, it is still limited. In contrast to early data, current reports have documented endovascular revascularization to be highly efficacious at very low risk (9,10). Widespread application is still debated, primarily on the basis of poor long-term, hemodynamic outcome and lack of comparative trials (11,12). However, use of endovascular techniques continues to grow rapidly because these procedures are repeatable, may be accomplished quickly, and are safely completed in patients with multiple comorbidities. Whereas restenosis is a major consideration for endovascular procedures performed above the knee (i.e., performed usually for claudication), it should not be a major limiting factor in below-the-knee intervention (i.e., performed usually for limb salvage).

The tissue in patients with nonhealing ulcers, or gangrene, requires high levels of oxygen and nutrition for tissue repair. This level of oxygenation is usually only adequately supplied by uninterrupted, straight-line arterial flow by at least one of the tibial vessels (i.e., with an intact pedal arch). Once wound healing has occurred, the oxygen requirements are decreased. Thus, if vascular occlusion returns after wound healing, most patients will function satisfactorily. Long-term healing will be particularly successful if patients are instructed in proper foot care, and in the avoidance of foot trauma and infection.

Most of the literature evaluating infrapopliteal endovascular techniques has been reported from studies with populations with limb-threatening ischemia. It should be noted, that except in diabetics, limb threat is usually produced by multilevel, vascular obstruction. Even though this may be treated traditionally by surgical revascularization, it has been the authors' experience that multilevel, endovascular intervention may treat these patients successfully, as well (13). There are also those who advocate that distal intervention should be used to extend the durability of femoral-popliteal angioplasty (14).

ANATOMY

The anterior tibial artery descends against the interosseous membrane, giving off branches to the surrounding muscles, and also small branches that penetrate the membrane to help supply the deep muscles of the posterior side of the leg (Fig. 14-1). As it crosses the ankle joint, its name is changed to dorsalis pedis. In about 3.5% of limbs, the anterior tibial artery either fails to reach the foot, or is reduced to a very slender vessel.

A short segment of vessel, known as the tibioperoneal trunk, arises distal to the anterior

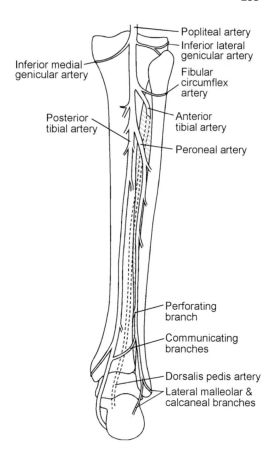

FIGURE 14-1 ● Diagram of the arteries of the leg. Posterior view.

tibial artery, and gives rise to the peroneal and posterior tibial artery. The posterior tibial artery continues downward on the tibialis posterior muscle. When it reaches the plantar surface of the foot, it terminates, as the medial and lateral plantar branches. The peroneal artery passes laterally, across the surface of the tibialis posterior muscle, to lie between the interosseous membrane and the fibula. The peroneal artery gives off branches that pass through the interosseous membrane to help supply anterior muscles.

ACCESS

Access from the contralateral common femoral artery is used to approach most infrapopliteal stenotic disease. A 5-Fr or 6-Fr cross-over sheath may be placed into the ipsilateral, distal external iliac artery from the contralateral common femoral artery (Figure 14-2[A]).

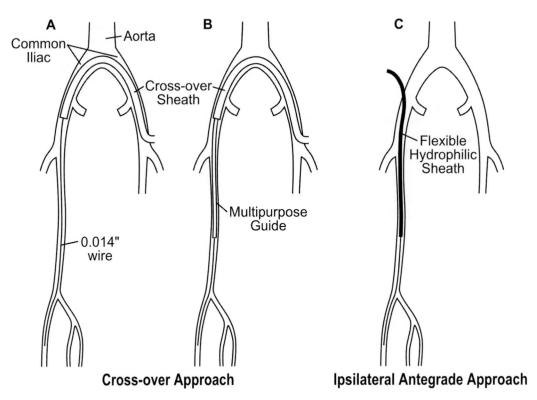

FIGURE 14-2 ● Illustration of the access strategy techniques used for infrapopliteal endovascular procedures. See text for details.

Infrapopliteal intervention may be performed with these short, cross-over sheaths as guides, but this may make intervention somewhat cumbersome, owing to the distance of the cross-over sheath tip to the infrapopliteal location. In addition, more contrast medium will be needed to opacify the distal circulation adequately. To maximize control, a 6-Fr multipurpose, coronary guide catheter may be advanced to the ipsilateral, distal, superficial femoral artery or mid-popliteal artery (Fig. 14-2[B]). This 6-Fr coronary guide catheter will then allow for most intervention modalities to be used. Alternatively, long, flexible, hydrophilic 5-Fr or 6-Fr guide sheaths have recently been introduced, which also may be advanced from the contralateral, common femoral artery to the distal ipsilateral SFA or mid-popliteal artery, to allow for similar control.

Antegrade access from the ipsilateral, common femoral artery is preferred to treat complex infrapopliteal occlusions or severe diffuse dis-

ease (Fig. 14-2[C]). This approach will allow for many options of intervention modalities. A 5-Fr or 6-Fr, flexible, 30-cm sheath is placed into the distal superficial femoral or proximal popliteal artery, using fluoroscopic guidance.

DIAGNOSTIC ANGIOGRAPHY

The infrapopliteal circulation is best viewed from a selective catheter in the ipsilateral, distal, superficial femoral artery or ipsilateral mid-popliteal artery. Injections of contrast agent from a catheter located in the ipsilateral distal external iliac artery, or ipsilateral common femoral artery, do not adequately fill the infrapopliteal bifurcations where atherosclerotic changes are commonly found. A 4-Fr or 5-Fr, straight, angiographic catheter, or multipurpose diagnostic catheter, may be placed into the ipsilateral distal superficial femoral artery or ipsilateral popliteal artery, safely, for contrast injections to view the infrapopliteal circulation.

A straight anteroposterior (AP) view will demonstrate the infrapopliteal vasculature in the majority of patients. If the origin of the anterior tibial artery is not well seen, or the cortex of the fibula or tibia is obstructing visualization, then a 30°, ipsilateral oblique image will usually display the infrapopliteal trifurcation. A true lateral view will also help visualize the very distal aspect of the popliteal artery.

Ideally, a low-osmolar, nonionic contrast solution is used, to maximize patient comfort during peripheral angiography. Alternatively, gadolinium is a contrast agent commonly used during magnetic resonance imaging (MRI) that also may be used for infrapopliteal angiography. Gadolinium has little nephrotoxicity, and when selectively injected from the mid-popliteal artery, provides an adequate image of the infrapopliteal circulation.

INTERVENTION

General Strategy

Infrapopliteal intervention is usually reserved for the patient with ischemic rest pain or tissue loss. There are rare patients that have true, life-style limiting, intermittent claudication from isolated infrapopliteal disease. Obtaining a careful history is essential to determine the duration of symptoms, as thrombolytic therapy may be the initial intervention in the patient with an acute change in clinical status. A meticulous physical examination of the area of tissue loss is necessary to elicit any signs of infection or underlying osteomyelitis, either of which may adversely affect the success of any intervention therapy. Nuclear scanning or MRI may be important additional diagnostic modalities to characterize the presence of osteomyelitis.

The initial diagnostic angiogram will be obtained from the contralateral, common femoral-artery, or brachial artery access. After demonstrating the infrapopliteal anatomy, the decision regarding approach and interventional modality may be made. For proximal, focal, stenotic disease, usually a contralateral, common femoral-artery access will suffice. For long occlusions, severe calcification, or distal disease (i.e., below

mid-calf), an antegrade approach will be preferable.

In general, to resolve ischemic rest pain or heal an ischemic ulcer, one continuous, patent, infrapopliteal vessel to the foot will be necessary. In this regard, a target infrapopliteal vessel may be chosen from the diagnostic angiogram as the vessel that may appear to have the least amount of distal disease, and the vessel that is continuous to the foot. At times, two vessels may be recanalized without too much more time, difficulty, or risk to the patient. In patients with a nonintact plantar arch vessel, the infrapopliteal vessel that would likely perfuse the area of tissue damage should be the target vessel for interventional therapy.

Anticoagulation/Antithrombotics

The pattern of infrapopliteal disease (i.e., focal stenotic, or diffuse) will dictate the intensity of anticoagulation and antiplatelet therapy. In addition, the clinical presentation (i.e., acute or chronic presentation) will play a role in what pharmacologic adjuncts will be used.

In regard to antiplatelet therapy, the patient should be taking the combination of aspirin and an ADP-receptor inhibitor (e.g., ticlopidine or clopidogrel) prior to coming to the angiographic suite. For patients with diffuse infrapopliteal disease that may be scheduled to undergo rotational atherectomy or excimer laser therapy, intravenous glycoprotein (GP) IIb/IIIa inhibitor use may, theoretically, be useful in preventing platelet aggregation and development of the no-reflow phenomenon. In addition, in the limb-salvage situation where there is tissue loss, those patients undergoing stand-alone angioplasty for long-segment, serial, stenotic disease may also be considered candidates for use of a GP IIb/IIIa inhibitor. As the patient with infrapopliteal disease likely has multivascular bed atherosclerosis, a consideration for chronic combination therapy with aspirin and ADP-receptor inhibitor administration, following infrapopliteal intervention, should be made.

Unfractionated heparin has been used most often, as an antithrombotic during infrapopliteal intervention. Patients receive 50 U/kg to 70 U/kg, intravenously, as a bolus at the start of the procedure, with a goal activated clotting time (ACT) of 250 to 300 seconds. There is limited experience using low molecular-weight heparin during infrapopliteal intervention, although a comfort level is certainly being established for its application during coronary intervention. The use of low molecular-weight heparin during peripheral intervention is currently the subject of ongoing clinical trials. In regard to direct thrombin inhibitors for infrapopliteal intervention, the use of bivalirudin is currently being studied as part of the Angiomax Peripheral Procedure Registry of Vascular Events (APPROVE) study (15).

Guide

If intervention is being performed from the contralateral, common femoral artery (i.e., crossing over the aortic bifurcation), the cross-over sheath, itself, may be used as a guide, especially if treating proximal focal stenotic disease. Flexible 5-Fr or 6-Fr cross-over sheaths (i.e., nonkinking) are now available from a number of vendors. The distal portion of the sheath should be advanced to the distal, ipsilateral, external iliac artery or mid-common femoral artery. For more complex disease being approached from the contralateral common femoral artery, a long, 5-Fr sheath, or a 6-Fr multipurpose coronary guide catheter, may be advanced to the level of the distal, superficial femoral artery (SFA) or mid-popliteal artery. If there is significant SFA disease precluding safe passage of the 6-Fr multipurpose coronary guide, the SFA disease should be treated first.

If the infrapopliteal intervention is being performed from an antegrade approach, a flexible, hydrophilic, 5-Fr or 6-Fr, 30-cm to 55-cm sheath, placed to the level of the distal SFA or mid-popliteal artery will be sufficient for a guide. The antegrade approach is preferred when treating more complex, total occlusions or long, segmental, diffuse disease.

Wires

The interventional treatment of infrapopliteal disease most commonly uses coronary modalities (e.g., balloons, rotational atherectomy, stents, laser) on a 0.014″ guide-wire platform.

The selection of which 0.014″ guide wire to use will be driven by the type of disease being treated (i.e., stenotic, occlusive, focal, diffuse). For focal stenotic disease, any commonly used, floppy, 0.014″ coronary guide wire may be used. The guide wire is most easily manipulated if it is inside a 0.014″ coronary balloon catheter, or a 0.018″ Spectranetic support catheter. For more diffuse or calcific stenotic disease, a more supportive 0.014″ coronary guide wire would be recommended. For total occlusions, a hydrophilic-coated, 0.035″ or 0.018″ guide wire may give the best chance for successful crossing. The authors have had success using an 0.018″ angled glide-wire gold inside of an 0.018″ Spectranetic support catheter, for crossing total occlusions. After successful crossing, the 0.018″ angled glide-wire gold is then exchanged for a supportive, 0.014″ coronary guide wire, as a platform to perform intervention.

When dealing with total occlusions that may not be crossed from the antegrade approach, Dorros et al. (16) have described their use of a surgical cut-down procedure on the tibial vessel, to achieve retrograde access in 2 cases. In similar cases, the authors have successfully entered the distal tibial vessel, using a micropuncture technique for advancement of an 0.018″, hydrophilic wire through the occlusion, in a retrograde pedal fashion (17). The wire was then snared at the popliteal artery, and externalized through an antegrade femoral sheath. The endovascular procedure was then completed from the antegrade access (Figs. 14-3 and 14-4).

PTA

Standard 0.014″ coronary balloon catheters, ranging from 2.5 mm in diameter, may be used in the majority of interventions for focal stenoses, when attempting stand-alone angioplasty for infrapopliteal disease. At experienced centers, the acute technical success of angioplasty in primarily focal infrapopliteal stenoses is excellent, at approximately 98%. The success in treating total occlusions appears to decrease to approximately 77%. Clinical results are likewise favorable. When defined by a pain-free extremity and limb salvage, success is reported in up to 84% at 2 to 5 years, in patients treated with angioplasty

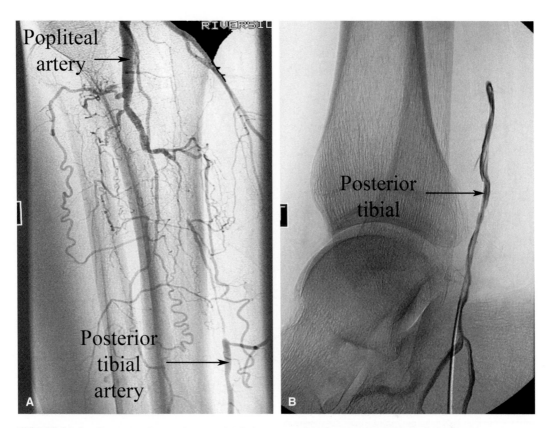

FIGURE 14-3 ● **A:** Baseline angiogram of right lower extremity (i.e., RAO 30 projection) demonstrating an infrapopliteal occlusion with retrograde collateral filling of the posterior tibial artery. **B:** Percutaneous puncture of the right posterior tibial artery, at right ankle, lateral view.

(18,19). More diffuse, long-segment, diseased tibial vessels appear to have a lower clinical success rate when treated with stand-alone balloon angioplasty (i.e., 57% at 3 years) (20). It must be noted that this literature is colored by the lack of secondary, percutaneous intervention, or the failure to convert quickly to surgical bypass. The accurate limb-salvage, and periprocedural and long-term mortality rates, using aggressive techniques and routine surveillance, have not yet been determined.

Recently, the authors have begun to use coronary cutting balloons for complex, infrapopliteal stenoses, such as at vessel bifurcations (Fig. 14-5).

The authors have evaluated the hemodynamic results with 0.014″ pressure wires and have found the early results to be excellent. Long-term evaluation to 1 year has documented an 89.5% limb-salvage rate (21).

Again, it should be noted that for predictable clinical benefit, the goal of therapy should be straight-line flow of one of the tibial vessels to the foot. Merely improving inflow to collaterals usually will not be adequate for tissue healing.

Stents

Data on the adjunctive use of stents in the infrapopliteal arterial bed are limited. The successful stenting of flow-compromising dissection has been reported (22). Currently, until more conclusive data become available, the authors limit stents to a bail-out use. This limits the use in treating significant dissection, or hemodynamically significant, elastic-vessel recoil. Abrupt closure of distal stents has not been evident and this approach has allowed the treatment of large numbers of patients, without the need for any patient to be sent to emergent surgery. The authors use

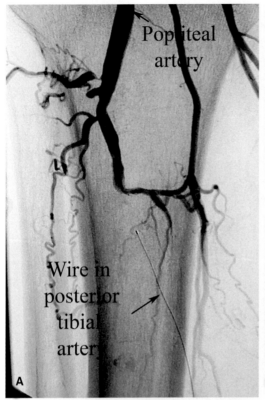

Popliteal artery

Wire in posterior tibial artery

A

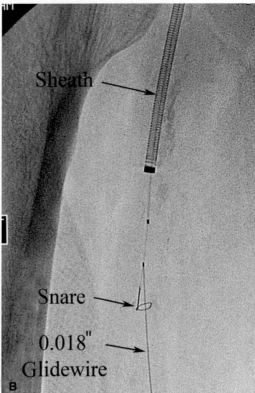

Sheath

Snare

0.018" Glidewire

B

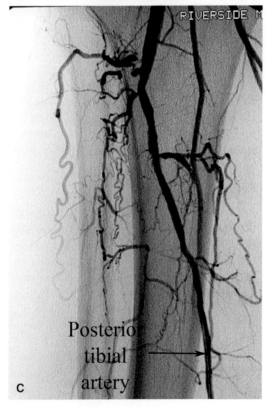

RIVERSIDE M

Posterior tibial artery

C

FIGURE 14-4 ● Posterior tibial artery intervention in patient shown in Figure 14-3. **A:** Right lower extremity AP projection angiogram demonstrating retrograde passage of 0.18″ glide wire into proximal posterior tibial artery. **B:** Snaring the retrograde wire from the femoral access at the level of proximal right SFA. **C:** Result after rotational atherectomy and balloon dilation of right posterior tibial artery, AP projection.

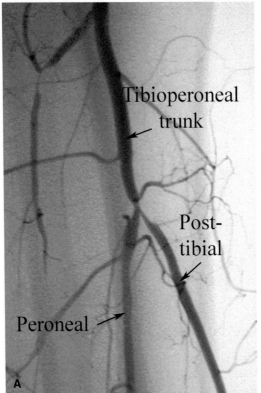

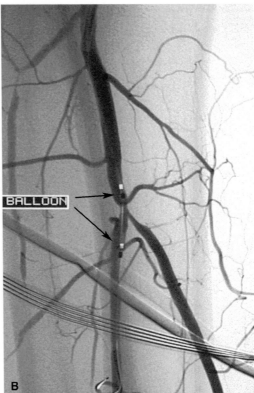

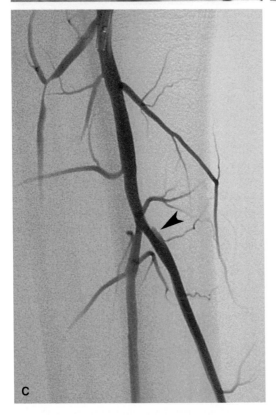

FIGURE 14-5 ● Cutting balloon angioplasty of tibioperoneal bifurcation. **A:** Preprocedure angiogram of severe stenosis at right tibioperoneal bifurcation, AP projection. **B:** Cutting balloon dilation of right tibioperoneal bifurcation with cutting balloon into right peroneal artery, AP projection. **C:** Final angiogram of right tibioperoneal trunk bifurcation after cutting balloon treatment, AP projection. The presence of a non-flow limiting dissection in the proximal portion of the posterior tibial branch is noted (*arrowhead*).

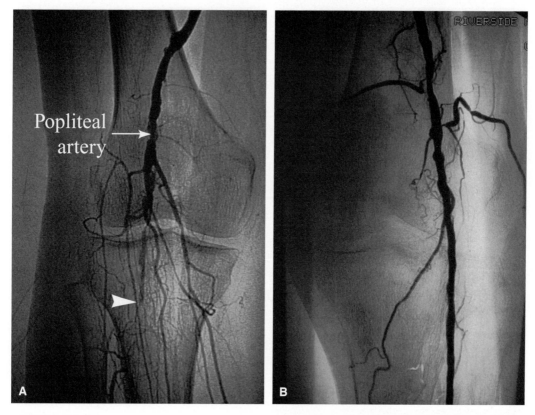

FIGURE 14-6 ● **A:** Angiograms of right distal popliteal and tibioperoneal trunk total occlusion (*arrowhead*), before treatment, AP projection. **B:** Angiogram right popliteal artery post rotational atherectomy, lateral view.

available coronary approved stents empirically, for this use. Self-expanding stents (e.g., Radius) are often used at perceived crush points, such as the segment of anterior tibial artery that has entered the anterior leg compartment, although crushing has not been reported to date.

The introduction of drug-eluting stents has certainly made a paradigm shift in the selection of patients for coronary artery stenting, including high-risk groups such as diabetics with diffuse disease, and patients with multivessel disease who, otherwise, would have had surgical revascularization. Clinical trials to evaluate the appropriateness and durability of drug-eluting stents for the treatment of infrapopliteal disease certainly will address the utility of this technology for limb-salvage situations.

Rotational Atherectomy with Abciximab

The use of rotational atherectomy very early after its introduction was associated with poor re-

sults. Coronary data have shown improved results when this device is combined with platelet inhibition, using the GP IIb/IIIa inhibitor, abciximab. The authors have since reported its use in 15 consecutive patients with total occlusions, diffuse tibial disease, and limb-threatening ischemia (23) (Fig. 14-6). Only one amputation has occurred at an average of 1-year follow-up evaluation. Using abciximab with rotational atherectomy appeared to prevent significant embolization and poor reflow. Further investigation appears warranted.

Laser Angioplasty

Recently, excimer laser recanalization began being studied systematically in a multicenter trial (Laser Angioplasty for Critical Leg Ischemia; LACI 2) (24) (Fig. 14-7). Reports from LACI 2, with a tibial artery intervention strategy that used excimer laser followed by balloon angioplasty, have shown promising results.

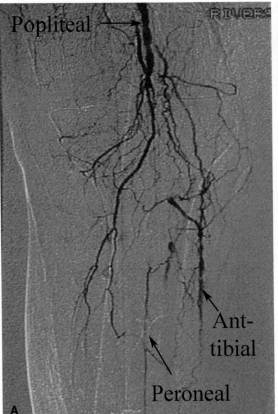

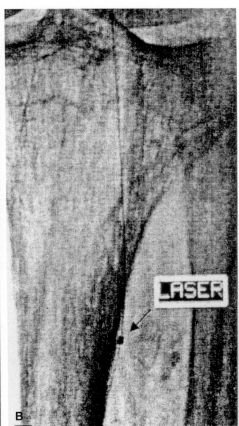

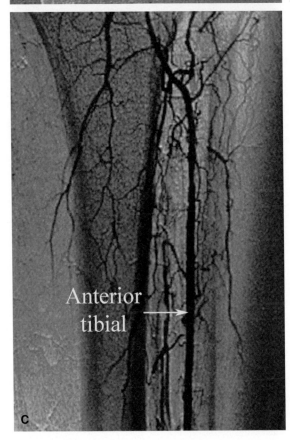

FIGURE 14-7 ● **A:** Pre-procedure angiogram of the left lower extremity demonstrating total occlusion of all infrapopliteal vessels, AP projection. **B:** Concentric 2.0 Excimer laser of proximal left anterior tibial artery, AP projection. **C:** Final angiogram post laser treatment demonstrating patent left anterior tibial artery, AP projection.

In LACI 2, 6-month limb survival was over 90%, with only 16% stent usage in the tibial vessels. Patients in LACI 2 were, by definition, poor surgical candidates.

PROCEDURAL COMPLICATIONS

Vasospasm

The liberal use of intra-arterial nitrates and calcium channel antagonists administered up stream, prior to guide-wire passage, may be useful in preventing vasospasm. Certainly, if vasospasm occurs, intra-arterial nitrates or calcium channel antagonists may be successful in treating vasospasm. Doses of 100 mcg to 200 mcg, given intra-arterially (e.g., nitroglycerin, nicardipine, or verapamil) are usually well tolerated. Adenosine is also a consideration for the treatment of vasospasm. Removal of the guide wire from the affected vessel may also be necessary, in refractory cases. A meticulous search for occult dissection also needs to be performed.

No-Reflow

As seen during coronary intervention, "no-reflow" may occur during infrapopliteal intervention, particularly when treating acute limb ischemia. As in the coronary circulation, the cause of no-reflow is often multifactorial, with distal embolization, vasospasm, and skeletal muscle edema as recognized contributors. Occult dissection and thrombosis certainly need to be considered when faced with this issue. A methodic approach to looking for, and treating, the above-mentioned causative mechanisms is required when faced with no-reflow during infrapopliteal intervention.

Thrombosis

Thrombosis that occurs during infrapopliteal intervention may be promptly resolved with catheter-based, mechanical, rheolytic thrombectomy, using the 0.014″ XMI AngioJet catheter. When arterial thrombosis occurs, the operator must be certain the appropriate doses of anticoagulation and antiplatelet therapy have been administered. Occult arterial dissection needs to be ruled out by meticulous angiography. If thrombus persists after catheter-based mechanical thrombectomy, and other causes for thrombosis have been ruled out, thrombolytic therapy should be considered if there are no contraindications.

Perforation

Arterial perforation most commonly occurs when treating long, total occlusions, or when using rotational atherectomy. The majority of perforations that occur during infrapopliteal intervention may be treated with prolonged balloon inflations. Rarely, reversal of anticoagulation and or platelet administration is necessary. For limb-threatening perforations that may not be controlled with prolonged balloon inflations, deployment of a coronary, covered stent would be an option (e.g., JoStent). This would be an exceedingly rare occurrence.

Flow-Limiting Dissection

The initial approach to managing a flow-limiting dissection that occurs during infrapopliteal intervention would be prolonged balloon inflation. If this approach fails, then bail-out stenting would be indicated. As above, 0.014″-based coronary stent systems would be used for this application. If the anatomic location is of concern for a possible crush point (e.g., proximal anterior-tibial artery), then a self-expanding coronary stent (e.g., Radius) would be preferred.

LONG-TERM FOLLOW-UP EVALUATION

One of the limitations in the historic performance of distal-limb endovascular techniques is the lack of close follow-up evaluation and noninvasive vascular surveillance. Our surgical colleagues are keenly aware of the need for bypass-graft surveillance (25). It has been the authors' experience that when continued surveillance is completed post-endovascular intervention, the limb-salvage rates are also improved. Importantly, neither clinical symptoms nor standard ABI measurements are as sensitive as duplex scanning for the detection of recurrent disease or restenosis. A peak systolic velocity greater than 200 cm per second, or a flow velocity of less than 45 cm per second distal to the lesion, is quite indicative of a stenosis of 50% or greater. As infrapopliteal intervention is becoming more common place, post-procedure testing should include an ABI evaluation prior to discharge, then duplex scanning at 3-, 6-, and 12-month intervals. A strict duplex-surveillance program should most certainly lead to higher secondary patency rates than clinical follow-up evaluation, alone.

An often overlooked rule that may not be over emphasized is repeat intervention must be completed, if there is evidence of recurrent vascular compromise prior to complete wound healing. Infrapopliteal intervention performed by experienced operators will rarely preclude the performance of a subsequent bypass graft, or alter previously planned surgery.

CONCLUSIONS

The endovascular treatment of infrapopliteal disease continues to improve and allows for successful limb salvage, in the majority of patients. The ability of percutaneous procedures to be repeated is often overlooked, and as discussed, it does *not* appear that long-term patency with endovascular techniques need match surgical results. Maintaining functional limb viability, with the lowest procedural and long-term mortality rates, should be the objective in the care of these patients. When chosen appropriately, both surgical bypass and endovascular therapy may benefit many patients. However, performing procedures that may lead to difficulty in healing or to prolonged hospitalization are not acceptable outcomes.

Treatment should not be entered into lightly or without a clear plan. A team approach, with a close working relationship between the interventionalist and surgeon, allows clear treatment goals and expected treatment outcomes to be determined. Whatever technique is used, the result should create straight-line, distal flow to the foot, preferably leading to distal pulsation. The patient should be followed closely for wound healing, and with noninvasive vascular surveillance to identify restenosis. Regular evaluation should also be continued for associated cardiovascular and cerebrovascular disease.

REFERENCES

1. London NJM, Srinavass R, Naylor AR, et al. Changing arteriosclerotic disease patterns and management strategies in lower-limb threatening ischemia. *Eur J Vasc Surg.* 1994;8:148–155.
2. Houghton AD, Taylor PR, Thurlow S, et al. Success rates for rehabilitation of vascular amputees: implications for preoperative assessment and amputation level. *Br J Surg.* 1992;79:753–755 .
3. Cheshire NJW, Wolfe JHN, Noone MA, et al. The economics of femorocrural reconstruction for critical limb ischemia with and without autologous vein. *J Vasc Surg.* 1992;15:167–175.
4. Veith FJ, Gupta SK, Ascer E, et al. Six-year prospective multicenter randomized comparison of autologous saphenous vein and expanded polytetrafluoroethylene grafts in infrainguinal arterial reconstructions. *J Vasc Surg.* 1986;3:104–114.
5. Harris PI, How TV, Jones DR. Prospectively randomized clinical trial to compare in situ and reversed saphenous vein grafts for femoropopliteal bypass. *Br J Surg.* 1987;74:252–255.
6. The Iloprost Bypass International Study Group. Effects of perioperative iloprost on patency of femorodistal bypass grafts. *Eur J Vasc Endovasc Surg.* 1996;12:363–371.
7. Schwartz ME, Harrington EB, Schanzer H. Wound complications after in situ bypass. *J Vasc Surg.* 1988;7:802–807.
8. Monteverde-Grether C, Valezy Tello de Meneses M, Nava Lopez G, et al. Percutaneous transluminal ultrasonic angioplasty: preliminary clinical report of ultrasound plaque ablation in totally occluded peripheral arteries. *Arch Invest Med Mexico.* 1991;22:171–179.
9. Brown KT, Moore ED, Getrajdman GI, et al. Infrapopliteal angioplasty: long term follow-up. *J Vasc Interv Radiol.* 1993;4:139–144.
10. Varty K, Bolia A, Naylor AR, et al. Infrapopliteal percutaneous transluminal angioplasty: a safe and successful procedure. *Eur J Vasc Endovasc Surg.* 1995;9:341–345.
11. Fraser SCA, Al-Kutoubi MA, Wolfe JNA. Percutaneous transluminal angioplasty of infrapopliteal vessels: the evidence. *Radiology.* 1996;200:33–36.
12. Ahn SS, Eton D, Moore WS. Endovascular surgery for peripheral arterial occlusive disease. *Ann Surg.* 1992;216:3–16.
13. Ansel G, George BS, Kander NH, et al. Successful limb salvage with superficial femoral artery Wall Stenting [abstr]. *Circulation.* 1997;96 (suppl 8):755.
14. Varty K, Bolosa A, Naylor AR, et al. Infrapopliteal percutaneous angioplasty: a safe and successful procedure. *Eur J Vasc Endovasc Surg.* 1995;9:341–345.
15. Angiomax Peripheral Procedure Registry of Vascular Events (APPROVE). Study. The Medicines Company. Protocol No TMC BIV 03 03 S1; US IND No. 35,756.
16. Iyer SS, Dorros G, Zaitown R, et al. Retrograde recanalization of an occluded posterior tibial artery by using a posterior tibial cutdown: two case reports. *Cathet Cardiovasc Diagn.* 1990;20:251–253.
17. Botti CF, Ansel GM, Silver MJ, et al. Percutaneous retrograde tibial access in limb salvage. *J Endovasc Ther.* 2003;10:614–618.
18. Bull PG, Mendel H, Hold M, et al. Distal popliteal and tibioperoneal transluminal angioplasty: long-term follow-up. *J Vasc Interv Radiol.* 1992;3:45–53.

19. Wagner HJ, Starch EE, McDermott JC. Infrapopliteal percutaneous transluminal revascularization: results of a prospective study on 148 patients. *J Interv Radiol.* 1993;8:81–90.

20. Matsi PJ, Manninen HI, Suhonen MT, et al. Chronic critical lower-limb ischemia: prospective trial of angioplasty with 1–36 months follow-up. *Radiology.* 1993;188:381–387.

21. Ansel GM, Botti C, Silver MJ. Cutting balloon angioplasty of the popliteal and infra-popliteal vessels for symptomatic leg ischemia. *Cath Cardiovasc Interv.* 2004;61(1):1–4.

22. Dorros G, Hull P, Prince C. Successful limb salvage after recanalization of an occluded infrapopliteal artery utilizing a balloon expandable (Palmer-Schatz) stent. *Cathet Cardiovasc Diagn.* 1993;28:83–88.

23. George BS, Ansel GM, Noethen AA, et al. Efficacy of rotational atherectomy in the treatment of patients with lower extremity (infra-femoral) ischemia. *Am J Cardiol* 1997;80(7A), 125.

24. LACI 2 Investigators. Laser Angioplasty for Critical Leg Ischemia. Report from Circulatory System Devices Advisory Panel of the US Food and Drug Administration (FDA). October 2, 2002. Washington, DC.

25. Green RM, McNamara J, Ouriel K, et al. Comparison of infrainguinal graft surveillance techniques. *J Vasc Surg.* 1990;11:207–215.

CHAPTER 15

Interventional Techniques in Venous Disease

Michael Wholey and Darren Postoak

W ith the rise in the peripheral vascular disease in the general population, there has also been an increased awareness of disorders of the peripheral venous circulation. Venous disorders affect both upper and lower extremities as well as the neck, chest, abdomen, and pelvis. The spectrum of venous disease is broad, including thrombosis caused by coagulopathies, occlusive disease from extrinsic compression, and venous insufficiency arising from malfunctioning valves. Deep venous thrombosis (DVT) receives the greatest attention because of the frequency of this event and the potentially life-threatening complication of embolization to the pulmonary venous circulation.

The objective of this chapter is to provide a description of the essentials of venous anatomy and venous pathology, and to summarize the interventional options in the treatment of venous disease.

ANATOMY

The venous circulation parallels much of the arterial system (Fig. 15-1).

In the infrainguinal region, the multitude of superficial veins of the lower extremity terminate in two saphenous veins: the small saphenous vein, which drains into the popliteal vein, and the greater saphenous vein, which drains into the common femoral vein. The deep veins closely parallel the arterial system and converge on the common femoral vein in the groin. Once in the

femoral veins, blood flows into the external and common iliac veins, toward the inferior vena cava and right atrium of the heart.

Similarly, venous blood from the upper extremities is returned from the superficial fascia by the cephalic and basilic veins that travel along the lateral and medial surfaces of the arm, respectively, and empty into the axillary and brachial veins, respectively. The deep veins travel along side their arterial counterparts, forming the brachial vein in the arm, which continues as the axillary and subclavian vein. Each subclavian vein unites the internal jugular vein, returning blood from the head and neck and forming the right and left innominate veins. The left innominate vein crosses the midline to join the right innominate vein and form the superior vena cava, which in turn drains into the right atrium.

Venous drainage from the pelvic viscera flows into the internal iliac vein and thereafter to the common iliac vein. Venous drainage from the abdominal viscera drains to the inferior vena cava. The azygous-hemiazygous system of veins forms an important link between the superior and inferior vena cavae, which serves an important function in patients with superior or inferior vena-caval obstruction. Located along the left side of the thoracic vertebral bodies, and receiving blood from the left chest wall and lung, the hemiazygous and accessory hemiazygous veins drain into the azygous vein, at the levels of the ninth and seventh thoracic vertebrae, respectively. In two-thirds of cases, the hemiazygous communicates directly with the left renal vein. The azygous vein is located along the right side of the

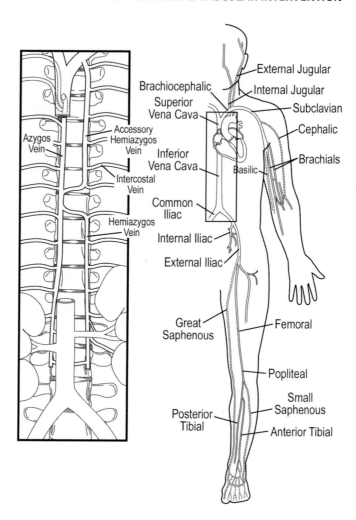

FIGURE 15-1 ● **Anatomy of the venous circulation.** Superficial veins in upper and lower extremity shown in dashed lines.

thoracic vertebral bodies, and has a similar source of drainage. Proximally, the azygous empties into the superior vena cava at the level of the fourth thoracic vertebra. Distally, the azygous vein is connected with the inferior vena cava, at the level of the renal veins.

PATHOLOGY OF VENOUS OCCLUSIVE DISEASE

The dominant etiologies underlying venous occlusive disease include: hypercoagulopathies, extrinsic compression from neoplasms and other masses, and iatrogenic causes (i.e., indwelling catheters, pacemaker leads). The relative importance of these etiologies varies, depending on the venous location, as summarized in Table 15-1.

In the lower extremities, venous thrombosis caused by a variety of hypercoagulopathies (both genetic and acquired) is the most common etiology. When extrinsic compression is responsible, it typically occurs at the level of the pelvis or abdomen, and occasionally at the level of the common femoral vein, such as when using manual compression following transfemoral cardiac catheterization. Compression of the left common iliac vein by the right common iliac artery, referred to as May-Thurner syndrome, is an uncommon cause of venous compression and lower extremity venous thrombosis.

Upper extremity venous occlusion in young, athletic males is typically seen at the level of the subclavian vein. At the thoracic inlet, the subclavian vein lies anterior to the first rib, medial to the scalenus anterior muscle and posterior to the clavicle, and is susceptible to compression during arm movements that involve shoulder abduction and external rotation (Paget-Von Schroetter syndrome). There is a high incidence of

> [!NOTE]
> ## TABLE 15-1

Etiologies of Venous Occlusive Disease Based on Venous Location

Venous Location	Etiology
Lower Extremity	Hypercoagulable states
	Extrinsic compression
	• Pelvic tumor
	• Abdominal tumor
	• May-Thurner syndrome—compression of left common iliac vein by right common iliac artery
	• manual compression post catheterization
Upper Extremity	Indwelling catheter (e.g., PICC line, central venous catheters)
	Extrinsic compression
	• Paget-Von Schroetter syndrome—compression of subclavian vein at the thoracic inlet prompted by shoulder abduction and external rotation
	Hypercoagulable states
Central	
SVC, Innominate	Indwelling central venous catheters
	Hemodialysis catheters
	Pacemaker/Defibrillation leads
	Extrinsic compression
	• Malignancy—Lung cancer
IVC	Extrinsic compression
	• Aneurysm
	• Abdominal neoplasm
	Extension of tumor (e.g., typically renal)
	Thrombus (e.g., on IVC filter)
Hemodialysis grafts	Venous anastomosis stenosis caused by intimal hyperplasia

PICC, peripherally inserted central catheter

associated anatomic abnormalities in this population. Among older patients, indwelling catheters and pacemaker wires are the most common causes of subclavian vein occlusive disease.

Central venous occlusive disease, involving the superior vena cava (SVC) and innominate veins, is most commonly related to the placement of central venous access catheters, hemodialysis catheters, and pacemaker or defibrillator wires (1,2). Extrinsic compression of the SVC most commonly results from lung malignancy. Inferior vena caval obstruction may be the result of extrinsic compression from abdominal tumors (e.g., aneurysms, benign or malignant neoplasms), extension of a tumor (typically renal), or thrombus formation (e.g., on a vena caval filter).

Patients on chronic hemodialysis represent a unique subset of patients that are susceptible to central venous obstructive disease (3). This is most commonly related to the use of percutaneous hemodialysis catheters, but may also be related to flow dynamics associated with their shunts. The impact of central venous stenosis for these patients is extremely serious, since it compromises the grafts and fistulas in the upper extremity. At the level of the arterial-venous fistulas (i.e., applies to both native Bresche-Cimino and PTFE grafts), in the upper extremity of patients on hemodialysis, venous obstruction also occurs at the site of the venous anastomosis and is caused by intimal hyperplasia. The cause of such hyperplasia is complex, but fluid dynamics with high pressures along the venous system seems to be major factor.

VENOUS OCCLUSIVE DISEASE—CLINICAL MANIFESTATIONS

The clinical manifestation of venous occlusive disease is dependent on the location and acuity of the occlusion, and the adequacy with which collaterals bypass the obstruction.

During the acute stage of thrombotic venous occlusion of extremity veins, the most common symptom is edema and swelling of the affected extremity. Under rare circumstance (i.e., typically involving the lower extremity), a near complete thrombotic-venous occlusion may manifest as a painful venous congestion of the extremity (i.e., phlegmasia cerulea dolens). Without aggressive treatment, this may progress to frank tissue loss (i.e., gangrene). In patients with significant peripheral arterial disease of the lower extremity, the increased venous pressure from venous obstruction may compromise arterial inflow and result in a pale, cool, ischemic leg (i.e., phlegmasia alba dolens). In the long term, deep venous thrombosis of the lower extremity may manifest as lower extremity edema resulting from incompetence of the valves of the deep veins.

For hemodialysis patients with stenoses that form at the venous anastomotic sites, or in the central veins, the most common complaint will be of lengthened dialysis times and eventually, thrombosed non-functioning grafts.

In patients with near occlusion of the superior vena cava who are without adequate collateralization, a constellation of symptoms referred to as the superior vena cava syndrome are typically manifest and include: a headache that is exacerbated by changes in position, facial, and bilateral upper extremity edema. Other symptoms occasionally include dyspnea, dysphagia, and cognitive dysfunction. The headache and cognitive symptoms result from cerebral venous hypertension and are caused by impairment of venous return.

Venous thrombosis in the deep veins of the extremity or central veins represents a potential source of embolization to the pulmonary circulation. In clinical practice, deep venous thrombosis of the pelvic and lower extremity veins (above the popliteal trifurcation) are responsible for more than 90% of all pulmonary emboli, and more commonly affect the lower pulmonary arteries. Depending upon the patient's condition, clot burden, and frequency of embolization, patients may be asymptomatic or have dyspnea stemming from hypoxia and elevated pulmonary pressures. Rarely, patients may experience right-sided heart failure, with hemodynamic collapse, and cardiopulmonary arrest.

DIAGNOSIS

In addition to the clinical history and examination findings outlined above, a variety of imaging studies, including angiography, are relevant in developing the proper strategy for treatment.

Noninvasive Techniques

Doppler ultrasound has proved very effective in diagnosing lower extremity venous disease and has become the screening modality of choice (5). With duplex imaging, the diagnosis of DVT is inferred from a variety of observations: (a) direct visualization of echogenic material in the vein, and incomplete collapse of the vein wall, in response to compression with the transducer, (b) abnormal Doppler flow waveform with evidence of decreased or absent Doppler flow, loss of respiratory variation, and loss of augmentation in flow with distal compression maneuvers, and (c) incomplete or absent color filling of the vein.

Venous enhanced subtracted peak arterial (VESPA) magnetic resonance (MR) venography has been shown to be comparable with conventional venography, for the diagnosis of femoral and iliac deep venous thrombosis (DVT) (6). In a small series by Laissy et al, the differences in sensitivity and specificity between MR venography and color Doppler sonography were not statistically significant (4). However, they found MR venography to be 95% sensitive and 99% specific in detecting the extension of deep venous thrombosis, compared with the 46% sensitivity and 100% specificity of color Doppler sonography (differences in sensitivity, $P < .01$) (7).

Duplex ultrasound, CT, and MR imaging are all useful in diagnosing upper extremity and central venous occlusive disease. Chronic venous thrombosis has been diagnosed by Doppler sonography by the presence of collateral veins, spread of thrombus to other major veins, and loss of normal vascular landmarks with poor visualization of the actual thrombus (8).

CT contrast studies and MRA are beneficial in detecting central stenosis in addition to the pathologic processes (i.e. extrinsic masses) that may have caused the central stenoses (9). CT angiography has the additional value of diagnosing acute pulmonary emboli with excellent sensitivity and specificity.

However, in the author's opinion, venograms remain the gold standard for the diagnosis of venous occlusive disease. This is based on the ability of venography to provide accurate delineation of the location, severity, and length of stenoses, occlusions, or thrombus in the venous circulation. These features are important in planning treatment. Occasionally, other findings such as arteriovenous fistulas or other causes for the symptomatology, will be detected.

Venogram Technique

By injecting contrast medium through peripheral intravenous access catheters in a superficial vein (i.e., typically in the arm), a rudimentary venogram of the central veins may be achieved. Views of the proximal portion of the extremity are obtained first and central images are then taken. When performed from the arm, contrast often pools in the axillary veins. Improved visualization of the central venous structures is accomplished by raising the arm to aid the drainage of contrast from the axillary veins. Alternatively, a small diameter angiographic catheter may be placed in the subclavian vein (i.e., through deep venous access) to provide improved central venous imaging.

Venograms of the lower extremities are rarely performed today, as a result of improved ultrasound imaging. If performed, a superficial vein on the dorsum of the foot should be used to gain venous access and contrast injected. For effective venography, one should use digital subtraction angiography (DSA) and large-sized image intensifiers.

One of the major limitations of ultrasound is its inability to visualize the iliac veins. For venography of this location, a 5-Fr to 6-Fr sheath is placed in the common femoral vein. Direct injection of contrast medium through this sheath, or through a pigtail catheter placed just inside the sheath, allows visualization of the iliac veins.

For examination of the inferior vena cava, a pigtail catheter (e.g., Omniflush catheter) is introduced through a common femoral venous sheath and positioned in the common iliac vein. Because of the large size and capacitance of the inferior vena cava, optimal visualization is achieved by using an automated injector that delivers contrast agent at a rate of 15 mL to 20 mL per second, for a total of 40 mL.

For pulmonary angiograms, the diagnostic catheter must be placed in the main pulmonary artery most commonly using common femoral or internal jugular venous access. A 6-Fr to 7-Fr angled-pigtail catheter is used, such as a Grollman catheter. With the catheter in place, pulmonary artery pressures are recorded and angiography is performed in anteroposterior (AP) and lateral views for each lung field. Usual injection rates are 15 mL to 20 mL per second, for a total of 30 mL. If pulmonary artery pressures are high, the rate is reduced, or the right and left pulmonary arteries are selectively engaged. During pulmonary angiography, it is important to be aware of the presence of any heart block (i.e., especially left bundle branch block), since the catheter may induce right bundle branch block and thus produce complete heart block.

INTERVENTIONAL TECHNIQUES FOR VENOUS DISEASE

Central Stenosis with Superior Vena Cava and Brachiocephalic Disease

Intervention for central venous disease is generally reserved for patients who require hemodialysis, or who have symptoms consistent with superior vena cava syndrome. The greater reluctance in treating central venous stenoses is because of the poor long-term results achieved with intervention of these vessels. For example, in a series of 29 patients who underwent angioplasty and occasional adjunctive stenting, the mean symptom-free period in follow-up evaluation was only 6.5 months (range, 4 to 36 months) (4). Recurrent edema led to additional angioplasty in 20 (63%) cases (4).

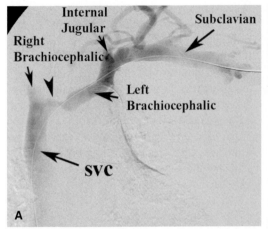

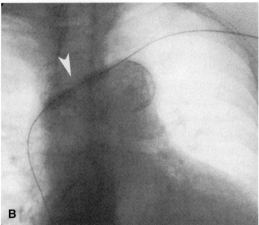

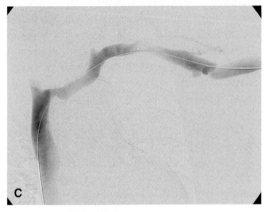

FIGURE 15-2 ● **Endovascular treatment of central vein stenosis in a hemodialysis patient. A:** Venogram showing high-grade stenosis at the junction of the superior vena cava (SVC) and left brachiocephalic vein. **B:** Lesion crossed with a 0.035″ wire and angioplasty performed using 12 mm diameter balloon (*arrowhead indicates site of stenosis*). **C:** Final venogram showing mild, residual stenosis at the lesion site.

For stenoses with a significant gradient located in the axillary, subclavian, or brachiocephalic veins, the first course of treatment is angioplasty. The authors generally see an improvement in gradients and elect to bring these patients back for re-angioplasty if symptoms recur, or if imaging studies suggest the return of severe disease. The choice of balloon catheters generally will be conservative, initially, and progress to the normal vessel segment diameter thereafter (Figs. 15-2[A–C] and 15-3 [A–C]).

The authors have not used cutting balloons for central lesions because of the inability to obtain the larger sizes in the US; these may help reduce the poor patency results seen with smaller sizes. The use of stents is reserved for those lesions that have a flow-limiting dissection, and self-expanding stents are generally preferred because external compression may be an issue in these locations.

In the management of superior vena cava syndrome caused by a high-grade stricture, the strategy will depend upon the underlying pathology. For benign strictures, one may use angioplasty alone, and for malignant strictures, angioplasty with self-expandable stents. Stents do not interfere with subsequent anti-tumor treatments and provide prompt relief of symptoms within 24 to 72 hours.

For complete occlusions of the subclavian, brachiocephalic, and superior vena cava, several treatment options exist (Fig. 15-4). The preferred method is to gain venous access from above (i.e., the internal jugular vein). The occlusion is crossed with a 0.035″ stiff glidewire (e.g., Terumo) supported by a diagnostic catheter (e.g., multipurpose, glide catheter). The authors have tried other systems to cross occlusions, including the Front Runner, but have not had success with these devices. Once across the occlusion, the glidewire is snared from below, through a

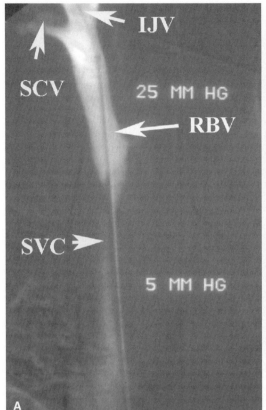

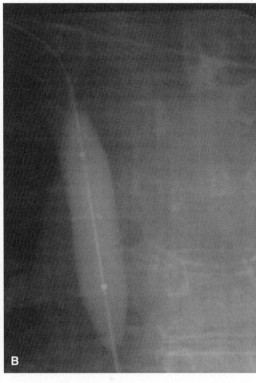

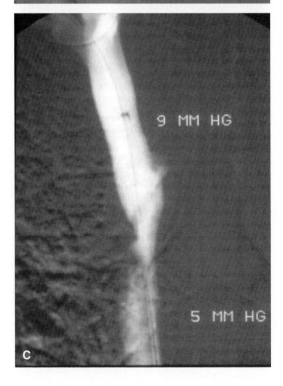

FIGURE 15-3 ● **Endovascular treatment of superior vena cava (svc) stenosis. A:** Catheter introduced from common femoral vein and positioned in right brachiocephalic vein. Venogram shows stenosis in SVC, and pressure measurements above and below the SVC confirmed the presence of a pressure gradient of 20 mmHg across the lesion. SCV, subclavian vein; IJV, right internal jugular vein; RBV, right brachiocephalic vein. **B:** Angioplasty of stenosis using 14 mm diameter balloon. **C:** Final venogram demonstrating moderate, residual stenosis. Repeat pressure measurement demonstrated residual 5 mmHg pressure gradient.

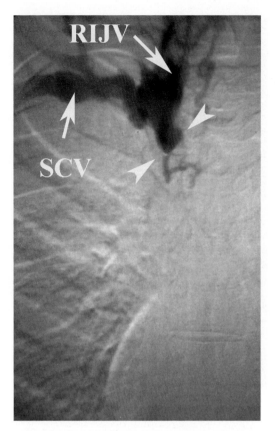

FIGURE 15-4 ● Right brachiocephalic vein and superior vena cava occlusion, in a patient with bronchogenic carcinoma, and symptoms consistent with superior vena cava syndrome. SCV, right subclavian vein; RIJV, right internal jugular vein; arrowheads indicate site of occlusion.

catheter introduced from the common femoral vein. Angioplasty and stenting are then performed through a guide or sheath, introduced through the common femoral vein. Other operators prefer to use common femoral venous access alone, and both cross the occlusion and introduce interventional equipment in a retrograde fashion. As in other central venous interventions, self-expanding stents are preferred in the SVC.

If there is angiographic evidence of significant clot burden associated with a central venous stenosis, an infusion catheter is introduced and thrombolytic therapy begun. Urokinase is our preferred thrombolytic agent, and is run at a medium dose of 120,000 units per hour, through the infusion catheter, in addition to heparin at 800 units to 1000 units per hour, through a periph-

eral IV. Thrombolysis is typically administered for 12 hours or less. This duration is sufficient to reduce the clot burden (Fig. 15-5[A–D]).

It is important to make sure that the patient is an appropriate candidate for lysis, as the incidence of serious complications, such as intracranial hemorrhage (ICH), with venous thrombolysis is 1 to 2%. Mechanical thrombectomy catheters may be helpful in reducing the lysis time, but may be only minimally helpful in large veins, such as the brachiocephalic and superior vena cava.

Hemodialysis Shunt Management

The management of stenosis or occlusions of hemodialysis shunts represents an important component of the multidisciplinary management of patients on chronic hemodialysis. Before embarking on such interventions, it is important to determine the following pieces of information.

1. *The types of shunts:*
   a. *Native fistulas* such as Brescia-Cimino fistulas are surgically made communications between the patient's artery and superficial vein, at the level of the wrist (using radial artery) or elbow (using branch of brachial artery).
   b. *Prosthetic grafts* composed of ePTFE in a straight or loop configuration connect the native artery (radial or branch of the brachial) to the cephalic or basilic vein in the arm. Prosthetic grafts are more likely to have issues with thrombosis and infection, and lower patency rates compared with native fistulas.

Both types of grafts are susceptible to failure from intimal hyperplasia at the venous anastomosis site, producing significant stenosis (Fig. 15-6[A–B]). This phenomenon may be complicated by thrombus formation and graft occlusion. Stenosis may also occur along the length of the main draining vein from the fistula. In both locations, the stenosis is amenable to treatment with angioplasty. Strictures rarely occur at the arterial anastomosis site, and are more difficult to treat, often requiring surgical intervention.

2. *Age of thrombotic occlusion.*
   Over time, the thrombus becomes fibrotic and more resistant to both pharmacologic and

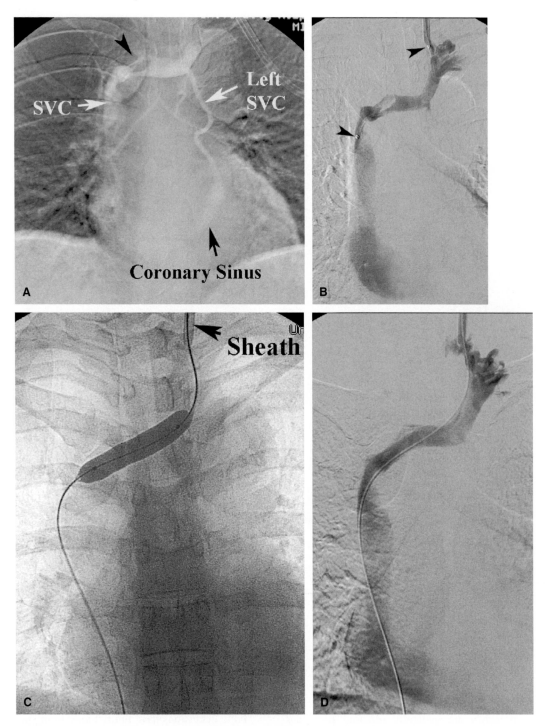

FIGURE 15-5 ● **Central vein thrombosis in a patient with a long-standing central venous catheter.**
A: Venogram showing large filling defect (*arrowhead*) in the left brachiocephalic vein. An incidental, persistent, left superior vena cava (SVC) that drains into the coronary sinus is labeled. **B:** A 5-Fr infusion catheter was positioned across the lesion and urokinase at 120,000 units per hour was administered, for 12 hours. Arrowheads indicate the active infusion length of the catheter. **C:** Subsequent angiography demonstrated a residual stenosis that was treated with a 14 mm diameter balloon catheter. **D:** Final venogram following angioplasty demonstrating improved flow and resolution of thrombus.

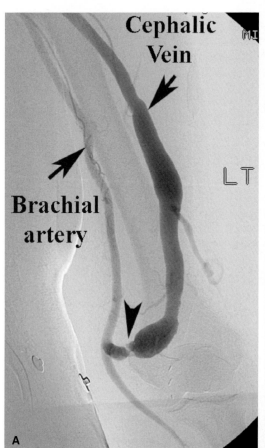
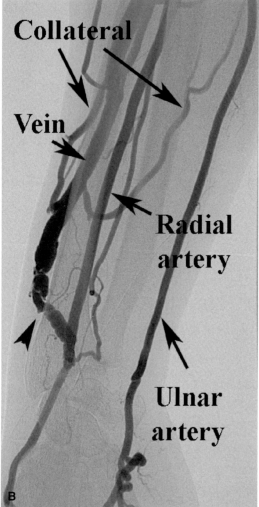

FIGURE 15-6 ● **Stenosis of native arteriovenous fistulas for hemodialysis. A:** Angiogram demonstrating native fistula from the cephalic vein to the brachial artery. There is a focal stricture at the venous anastomosis site (*arrowhead*). **B:** Native fistula linking the radial artery and a superficial vein along the lateral aspect of the forearm. There is stenosis at the venous anastomosis site (*arrowhead*). Collateral branches off the main draining vein, from the fistula, divert blood away from this vein and may interfere with its maturation.

particularly mechanical therapies. The endovascular procedure is most likely to be successful if the thrombotic occlusion is less than 2 to 3 days old, whereas surgical approaches are generally required for older occlusions.

3. *Temporal relation of occlusion to surgery.*

Early graft failure (i.e., within 2 to 3 weeks) following surgical implantation most likely reflects a surgical issue, and predicts a poor outcome with endovascular therapy.

4. *Size of the outflow vessels.*

If the outflow vein, such as the cephalic or basilic, is 4 mm or less, in diameter, then percutaneous attempts for the treatment of thrombotic occlusions have limited long-term success.

Endovascular Management of Hemodialysis Access Graft Stenosis

Stenoses at the venous anastomosis and venous outflow are easily treated with angioplasty, with minimal complications, regardless of the type of shunt employed. Access is obtained in an antegrade fashion, into the arterial limb of the graft, and a 6 Fr sheath is placed. Following venography and assessment of the venous stenosis, the stenosis is crossed with a wire and subsequently with the angioplasty balloon (i.e., starting with a 6 mm diameter balloon). A final balloon diameter 10 to 20% greater than the diameter of the adjacent vein is targeted. Should a dissection develop, low-pressure angioplasty for several minutes usually treats the problem.

A more common difficulty is recurrent stenosis that does not respond to angioplasty. The authors have tried leaving an accessory wire across the lesion at the time of angioplasty, to produce a 'cutting balloon effect', but this has not been particularly helpful. When larger cutting balloons finally become available in the US, one may employ them for these recalcitrant lesions. Stenting of venous anastomotic strictures is avoided, owing to the record of poor outcomes with stents in this location.

Endovascular Management of
Thrombotic Occlusion of Hemodialysis
Access Grafts

Occluded Native Fistulas
The authors have stopped trying to declot native fistulas. There have been several reports discussing successful thrombolysis of these native fistulas, but in the authors' opinion, the declot procedure is long, with poor success rates, and high rates of recurrent clotting. These patients should be referred for surgical revision of the fistula.

Occluded Prosthetic Grafts
There are several methods to declot prosthetic grafts. It is beyond the scope of this chapter to fully describe all of the strategies. The options that the authors employ include the following:

1. *'Lyse and wait' technique*
   This technique has proven fairly successful and simple. Antegrade access through the arterial inflow of the graft (i.e., pointing toward the venous anastomosis) is obtained with a 22-gauge angiocatheter, and a small aliquot of thrombolytics (e.g., urokinase 250,000 IU, tPA 2 mg to 5 mg) is administered while com-

pressing the arterial anastomosis to prevent reflux into the artery (Fig. 15-7[A-C]).

After 20 to 30 minutes, the patient is placed on the angiographic table, and an angiogram is performed through the angiocatheter to confirm lysis of the clot. In the presence of a venous anastomotic lesion, the angiocatheter is then exchanged for a sheath that allows angioplasty of the stenosis. Thereafter, the arterial plug that predictably forms at the site of the arterial anastomosis is dislodged. This requires a second, retrograde puncture into the venous segment of the graft. A Fogarty embolectomy balloon or regular, non-compliant angioplasty balloon, may be used to dislodge the plug.

2. *Mechanical thrombectomy*
   Mechanical thrombectomy, with an array of hydrodynamic aspiration (e.g., Angiojet,) and rotational fragmentation devices (e.g., Trerotola device,), has been used to remove clot from hemodialysis grafts. In a similar strategy to that described above, antegrade access is obtained on the arterial side of the graft, and thrombectomy of the venous limb is performed, followed by angioplasty of the venous anastomosis. A second retrograde puncture of the venous limb of the graft is then performed, to allow thrombectomy of the arterial limb. Care is taken not to activate these devices in the native artery or vein, unless thrombus is present at these sites. In such circumstances, the hydrodynamic aspiration devices may be less traumatic to the endoluminal surface of the vessel. Finally, if there is an arterial anastomosis stricture, an angioplasty is generally performed with a 5 mm balloon.

MANAGEMENT OF LOWER EXTREMITY DEEP VENOUS THROMBOSIS

Endovascular therapy for lower extremity deep venous thrombosis (DVT) is usually confined to patients with iliofemoral thrombosis. The following is a brief synopsis of our interventional strategy:

1. The extent of the venous occlusion is delineated, prior to the procedure, with non-invasive techniques. In the catheterization

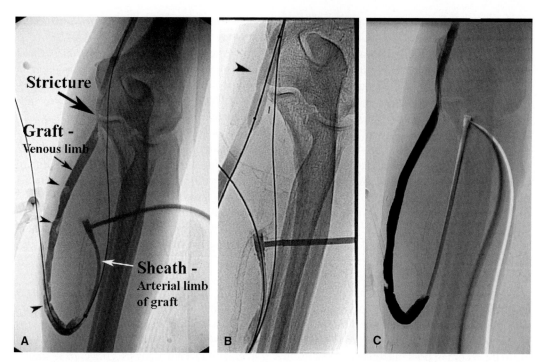

FIGURE 15-7 ● **Management of hemodialysis prosthetic graft thrombosis and stenoses. A:** A 6 Fr sheath was placed into the arterial limb of the graft, in the direction of the venous limb (i.e., antegrade). Angiography demonstrates PTFE graft, in loop configuration, linking the brachial artery and basilic vein. Thrombus is indicated by multiple filling defects (*arrowheads*). The stricture at the venous anastomosis site is labeled. Urokinase was infused (120,000 units) and allowed to dissolve the clot over the next 20 to 30 minutes (i.e., 'lyse and wait' technique). **B:** Following lysis, the venous stricture was treated through the same sheath, using a 7.0 mm diameter × 4.0 cm long balloon (*arrowhead*) inflated to high pressures. Access in the venous limb of the graft was then obtained, and angioplasty of an arterial stricture and angioplasty of the arterial plug was performed, using a 4.0 mm diameter × 4.0 cm long balloon. **C:** Final angiogram through the arterial limb of the graft showing near-complete resolution of thrombus and moderate residual stenosis at the venous anastomosis site.

suite, a venogram is performed. The patient is placed prone on the table, and using ultrasound guidance and a 4 Fr to 5 Fr micropuncture needle, the popliteal vein is accessed, and a 5 Fr sheath is placed. Attempting to perform this procedure from the contralateral common-femoral vein, passing retrograde across the venous valves, is usually very difficult and not recommended.

2. Injection of contrast through the popliteal vein sheath reveals the extent of the thrombus (Fig. 15-8[A–D]). The thrombotic occlusion is crossed with a wire, and an infusion catheter is then positioned to span the length of the thrombus. If the infusion catheter is of insufficient length an infusion wire may be passed through the infusion catheter, to extend the treatment length receiving thrombolytic therapy. The preferred thrombolytic agent is urokinase, administered at 120,000 units per hour, and given in conjunction with heparin at 800 to 1000 units per hour. Occasionally, one may use a hydrodynamic aspiration device (e.g., Angiojet) to reduce some of the clot burden, in an effort to shorten the duration of thrombolysis and the total dose of thrombolytic agent used. However, owing to the chronic nature of venous clot, these devices generally do not work well for this indication.

3. The patient returns to the catheterization suite the following day, having received a minimum of 12 hours of thrombolysis. At that point, a decision is made regarding whether or not further thrombolysis is required, or whether adjunctive angioplasty and stenting (using self-expanding stents) are required to treat a culprit lesion (e.g., left common iliac

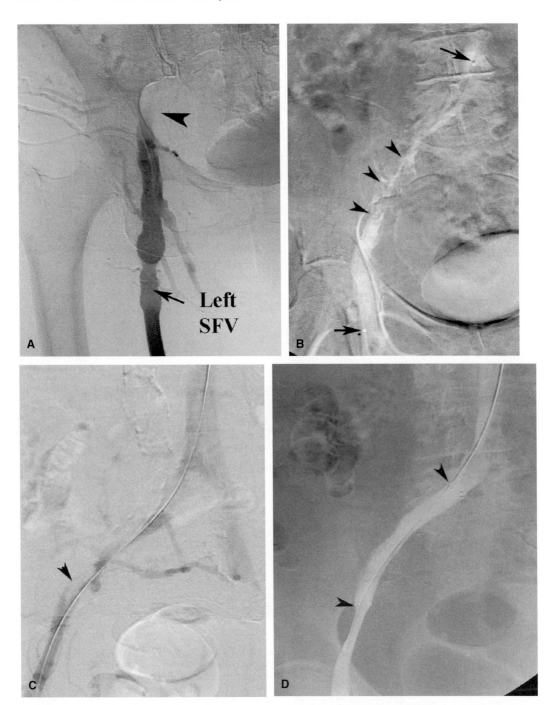

FIGURE 15-8 ● **Invasive management of ileofemoral vein thrombus in an 87 year-old male with a 2-week history of a swollen, painful, dusky appearing left lower extremity. A:** The patient was placed prone on the table and popliteal venous access was obtained using a micropuncture kit and ultrasound guidance. Venogram shows patent left superficial femoral vein, and occlusion (*arrowhead*) of the left external and common iliac veins. (Note that images are reversed because of prone position). **B:** A 5 Fr infusion catheter with an infusion length of 20 cm (*delineated by arrows*) was placed across the thrombotic occlusion (*arrowheads*). Urokinase at 120,000 units/hr was administered through the infusion catheter lumen, and heparin at 800 units per hour was administered through the popliteal venous sheath, for 12 hours. **C:** Follow-up venogram after thrombolysis demonstrating persistent thrombus in the left external iliac vein (*arrowhead*). **D:** Venogram following deployment of a self-expanding stent (i.e., 12 mm diameter × 80 mm length) at the site of residual thrombus.

vein stenosis in patients with May-Thurner syndrome).

PULMONARY ARTERY EMBOLI

Invasive management of pulmonary embolism is indicated, based on the clinical presentation of the patient. The current indications include:

- arterial hypotension (i.e., systolic blood pressure lower than 90 mmHg or rapid decrease of more than 40 mmHg)
- systemic hypoperfusion and hypoxemia
- right ventricular failure or pulmonary hypertension
- need for cardiopulmonary resuscitation
- arterial-oxygen alveolar gradient greater than 50 torr
- contraindication to anticoagulation

In these circumstances, the patient is taken to the catheterization laboratory for pulmonary angiography, to assess the treatment options. Venous access is obtained from the common femoral, or internal jugular vein, and a 7 Fr sheath is placed. An angled pigtail catheter, such as a 7 Fr Monty or Grollman catheter is advanced into the main pulmonary artery and then selectively, into the right and left pulmonary arteries. If pulmonary angiography reveals a large thrombus burden, and the patient is in critical condition, the typical strategy is to attempt to reduce the clot burden rapidly, with a mechanical thrombectomy device, and subsequently administer a bolus, followed by an infusion of a thrombolytic agent, for 12 to 24 hours.

Aspiration thrombectomy devices have an advantage over rotational fragmentation thrombectomy devices in that they do not disperse emboli particles to the distal pulmonary circulation. Some care with these devices is warranted, however. Asystole from adenosine release has been observed during use of the Angiojet

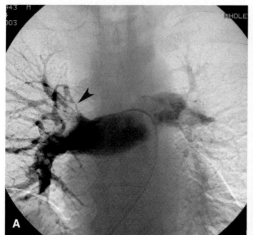

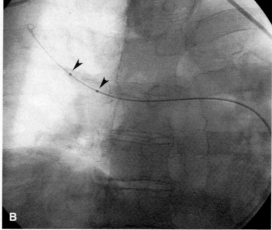

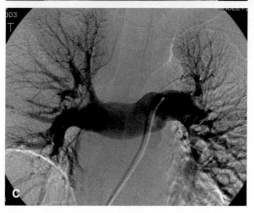

FIGURE 15-9 ● **Invasive management of symptomatic pulmonary embolus in 65-year-old male with underlying carcinoma. A:** PA pulmonary angiogram of right lung demonstrating multiple defects. Large filling defect in ascending branch of right pulmonary artery is indicated by arrowhead. **B:** Attempts to break up the clot in the right upper and middle lobe branches with a 8.0 mm diameter × 4.0 cm length balloon (*arrowheads*) were unsuccessful. An infusion catheter with a 20 cm infusion length was placed across the thrombus, in the right pulmonary artery, and urokinase at 120,000 units per hour was administered, overnight. **C:** Final pulmonary angiogram showing marked improvement in filling of right upper and mid-lung fields, with some residual defects in the right upper lobe arteries.

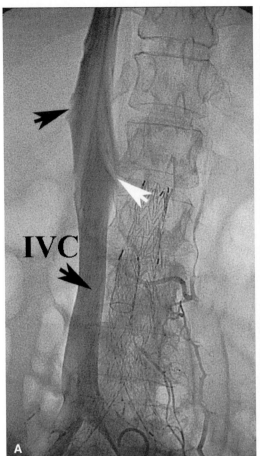
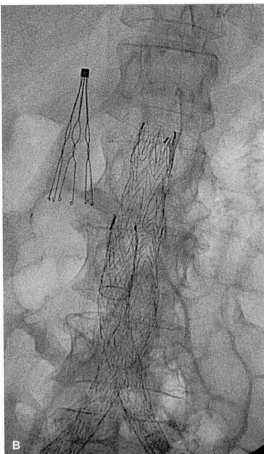

FIGURE 15-10 ● **Placement of inferior vena cava filter. A:** Venogram of inferior vena cava, performed with pigtail introduced from internal jugular vein, and positioned in the left common iliac vein. The position of the left (*white arrow*) and right (*black arrow*) renal veins is inferred from the negative contrast effect of non-contrast-filled renal blood entering the contrast-filled inferior vena cava (IVC). **B:** Deployed Greenfield® filter, with the apex of the filter positioned opposite the renal venous inflow.

rheolytic thrombectomy device, for this indication, and there have been cases of pulmonary artery perforation with both kinds of thrombectomy devices. The experience with angioplasty, alone, for the treatment of pulmonary emboli has been disappointing. If the patient is more stable, thrombolytic therapy alone may be attempted. (Fig. 15-9[A–C]).

When there is a perceived risk that a recurrent pulmonary embolic event might be fatal, or that the risk of a recurrent event is very high (e.g., free floating ileocaval thrombus), it is justified to place a filter in the inferior vena cava during the same procedure. A venogram of the inferior vena cava is performed to identify the location of the lowest renal vein (i.e., usually the

left) and confirm the absence of IVC thrombus at this location. The filter is delivered through a sheath, from the internal jugular or common femoral vein, and deployed such that its body lies between the renal vein and IVC bifurcation (Fig. 15-10[A,B]). Currently there are nine IVC filters available for use. Of these, three are retrievable and may be safely removed 2 to 3 weeks later, if needed.

REFERENCES

1. Sticherling C, Chough SP, Baker RL, et al. Prevalence of central venous occlusion in patients with chronic defibrillator leads. *Am Heart J.* 2001;141(5):813–816.
2. Gonsalves CF, Eschelman DJ, Sullivan KL, et al. Incidence of central vein stenosis and occlusion following

upper extremity PICC and port placement. *Cardiovasc Intervent Radiol.* 2003;26(2):123–127.

3. Criado E, Marston WA, Jaques PF, et al. Proximal venous outflow obstruction in patients with upper extremity arteriovenous dialysis access. *Ann Vasc Surg.* 1994;8(6):530–535.

4. Sprouse LR II, Lesar CJ, Meier GH III, et al. Percutaneous treatment of symptomatic central venous stenosis angioplasty. *Vasc Surg.* 2004;39(3):578–582.

5. Donnelly R, Hinwood D, London NJ. ABC of arterial and venous disease. Non-invasive methods of arterial and venous assessment. *Br Med J.* 2000;320(7236):698–701.

6. Fraser DG, Moody AR, Davidson IR, et al. Deep venous thrombosis: diagnosis by using venous enhanced subtracted peak arterial MR venography versus conventional venography. *Radiology.* 2003;226(3):812–820.

7. Laissy JP, Cinqualbre A, Loshkajian A, et al. Assessment of deep venous thrombosis in the lower limbs and pelvis: MR venography versus duplex Doppler sonography. *Am J Roentgenol.* 1996;167(4):971–975.

8. Weissleder R, Elizondo G, Stark DD. Sonographic diagnosis of subclavian and internal jugular vein thrombosis. *J Ultrasound Med.* 1987;6(10):577–587.

9. Finn JP, Zisk JH, Edelman RR, et al. Central venous occlusion: *MR Angiography Radiology.* 1993;187(1):245–251.

CHAPTER 16

Management of Extra-Aortic Arterial Aneurysms

Albert W. Chan and Christopher J. White

An aneurysm has been traditionally defined as a localized dilation of an arterial segment by more than 50% of the reference diameter (1). Although more than 95% of the arterial aneurysms are located in the aorta, they may develop in any artery of the body. A true aneurysm is one that involves dilation of all three layers (i.e., adventitia, media, and intima) of the arterial wall, characterized pathologically by extensive atrophy of the media. In contrast, a false aneurysm, or pseudoaneurysm, is the result of the disruption of at least one of the three layers of the vessel wall, and blood is contained within the adventitia or by the surrounding tissue. While pseudoaneurysms are mainly caused by trauma, a myriad of etiologies are related to the formation of true aneurysms (Table 16-1).

With the refinement of endovascular technologies, many aneurysms may be managed by an endovascular approach, rather than by surgery. Endovascular therapy has the advantage of lowering morbidity (e.g., perioperative myocardial infarction, infection, prolonged recovery) by obviating the need for general anesthesia, avoiding blood loss, and by reducing in-hospital recuperation time, when compared to surgical treatment. This chapter reviews the contemporary endovascular management of the aneurysms in the extra-aortic vessels.

INDICATIONS FOR REPAIR

In general, the indications for aneurysm repair include: (1) symptom(s) caused by the aneurysm (e.g., thromboembolism, compression on surrounding tissues and organs); (2) prevention of impending rupture; (3) evidence of aneurysm expansion detected by serial imaging studies.

It is important to realize that angiography only provides a lumenogram of an artery, and the actual size of the aneurysm may be underestimated in the presence of a layered, intramural thrombus. Imaging modalities such as ultrasound, computed tomography (CT), or magnetic resonance imaging (MRI), should be performed in order to identify the vessel wall and to provide the actual measurement of the size of an aneurysm.

STRATEGIES OF ENDOVASCULAR TREATMENT OF ANEURYSMS

Many factors should be taken into consideration when determining the appropriate management strategy for an aneurysm. These include the patient's clinical presentation, comorbidities, the location, size, and morphology (saccular or fusiform) of the aneurysm, and the anatomy of the vascular bed involved. The treatment aim is to exclude the aneurysmal sac, while maintaining the long-term patency of the parent vessel.

Endovascular strategies for aneurysm repair may be classified into two categories, namely *stent graft* placement (Table 16-2, Figs. 16-1 and 16-2) and *embolization* (Table 16-3).

Stent grafts exclude the aneurysm and maintain long-term patency of the main vessel. Both self-expanding and balloon-expandable stent grafts are available. For a fusiform aneurysm, the presence of a proximal and distal neck is

TABLE 16-1

Etiology of Aneurysms

Atherosclerosis/Degenerative

Trauma

Vasculitis

Infection

Fibromuscular Dysplasia

Chronic Dissection

Connective Tissue Disorders

TABLE 16-3

Embolization Coils and Delivery Catheters That May Be Used for Transcatheter Embolization of an Aneurysm in the Catheterization Laboratory

Coils	Delivery Catheters
Flipper® detachable embolization coil*	Tapered angiographic catheters
Hilal® embolization microcoil*	Tracker® coaxial infusion catheter
Tornado® embolization microcoil*	MicroFerret® infusion catheter
Microplex®Ψ	Heishima® Microcatheter
Hydrocoil®Ψ	
GDC® detachable coilΦ	

*Cook Inc, Bloomington, IN.
ΨMicroVention, Aliso Viejo, CA.
ΦBoston Scientific Inc, Natick, MA.
GDC: Guglielmi Detachable Coil.

---

necessary for successful endovascular repair. The choice of stent graft largely depends on the location of the aneurysm, and the size of the parent vessel. For a large vessel subject to compression or flexion, a self-expanding Wallgraft (Figure 16-2[A]) or Viabahn may be used, with a large delivery sheath (larger than 9 Fr) (Table 16-2).

The Wallgraft endoprosthesis is composed of a stainless steel, monofilament wire, covered by polyethylene (PET) graft material. The Viabahn endoprosthesis is made up of polytetrafluoroethylene (PTFE) lining, with an external nitinol skeleton extending along its entire length. Since a self-expanding stent graft may resist deformation, it would best suit aneurysms located in vascular regions that are subject to compression or flexion, such as those in the common carotid artery, proximal internal carotid artery,

axillary artery, femoral artery, and popliteal artery (Figs. 16-3 and 16-4). The size of a self-expanding stent graft should be 0.5 mm to 1.0 mm larger than the estimated reference diameter of the target vessel, in order to minimize shortening of the stent graft, and to ensure

---

TABLE 16-2

Various Intraluminal Stent Grafts Available for the Treatment of Extra-aortic Aneurysm*

Type	Delivery System	Guidewire	Diameter	Length
Wallgraft[1]	9 Fr to 12 Fr sheath	0.035″	6.0 mm to 14.0 mm	20 mm to 70 mm
Viabahn[2]	8 Fr to 14 Fr sheath	0.035″ for 5 mm to 8 mm stents 0.025″ for 9 mm to 13 mm stents	5.0 mm to 13.0 mm	2.5 cm to 15 cm
Jostent[3]	6 Fr guide	0.014″	3.0 mm to 5.0 mm	12 mm to 26 mm
ICAST[4]	7 Fr	0.035″	5.0 mm to 12 mm	39 mm and 59 mm

*Not FDA-approved for use in peripheral artery in the United States.
[1]Boston Scientific/Meditech, Natick, MA.
[2]W.L. Gore, Flagstaff, AZ.
[3]Abbott Vascular Devices, Redwood City, CA.
[4]Atrium, Hudson, NH.

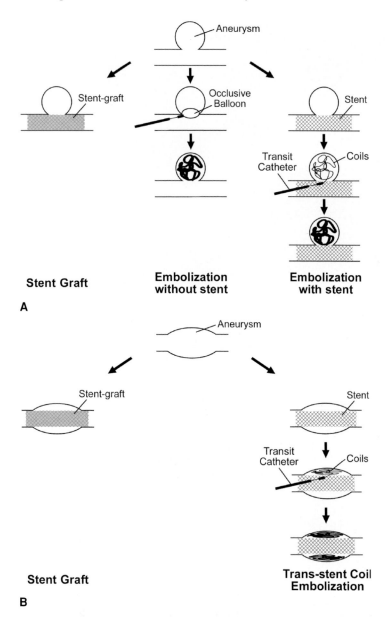

FIGURE 16-1 ● Schematic diagrams depicting the strategies of endovascular repair of **(a)** a saccular aneurysm, and **(b)** a fusiform aneurysm. In **(a)**, the aneurysm may be isolated by a stent graft within the parent artery, treated with embolization coil(s) alone, or bare metal stent placement and embolization within the parent vessel. In **(b)**, the aneurysm may be treated with a stent graft or a bare metal stent combined with embolization coil(s) within the perigraft space to induce thrombosis.

adequate apposition of the stent with the vessel wall.

For vessels with smaller diameters (up to 5.0 mm), a balloon-expandable, covered-stent (e.g., Jostent) may be used with the advantage of precise stent placement, and immediate exclusion of the aneurysm (Figures 16-2[B] and 16-5).

The Jostent is constructed by sandwiching an ultrathin layer of PTFE graft material between two stents that are welded at the ends. Recently, premounted Jostents have become available. The diameter of these stents is chosen to match the reference diameter of the target vessel. Occasionally, operators may find it useful to perform

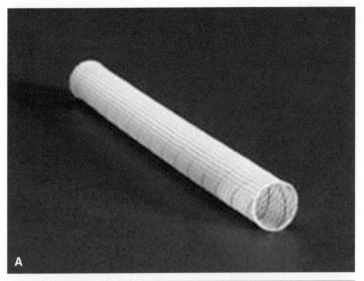

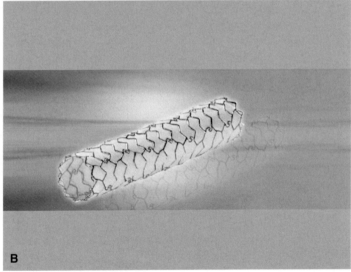

FIGURE 16-2 ● **A:** Wall-graft™; **B:** Jostent™ covered stent.

intravascular ultrasonography, to determine the reference vessel diameter. High-pressure inflation (12 atmospheres to 18 atmospheres) should be used to ensure full expansion and apposition of the stent. For aneurysms in larger vessels (i.e., 75 mm) that are not subject to compression or flexion, the ICAST covered balloon-expandable stent offers an important low-profile alternative to self-expanding covered stents.

Before discussing embolization strategies for the treatment of aneurysms, it is worth providing a brief outline of the coils that have been developed for vascular occlusion. Most coils are composed of stainless steel or platinum, with at-

tached Dacron strands to enhance thrombogenicity. The coils are delivered from within a hollow, linear, metal tube (i.e., called the loading canula/cartridge) and when released, assume a variety of shapes: straight, curved, helical, or tapered helical (e.g., tornado). Coils are also defined by the diameter of the metal coil (e.g., 0.018″ – 0.052″), the diameter assumed by the unconstrained coil (e.g., 2 mm to 10 mm), and the linear length of the coil when constrained in its linear form by the loading canula (e.g., 2 cm to 10 cm).

In general, delivery of the coil is achieved by putting the metal loading canula into the

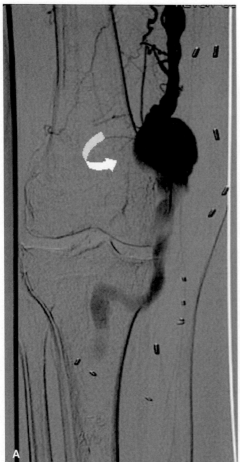

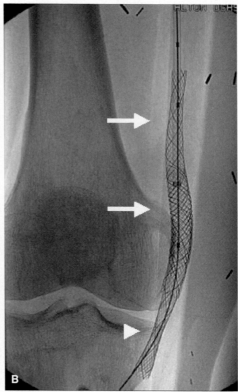

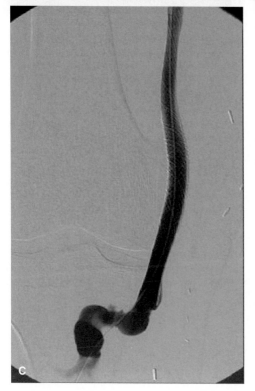

FIGURE 16-3 ● **Endovascular treatment of popliteal artery aneurysm.** This patient had a history of coronary artery bypass surgery, ischemic cardiomyopathy, and infrarenal abdominal aortic aneurysm repair with an endovascular graft. Endovascular exclusion of the popliteal artery aneurysm (*curved arrow*) was performed because of multiple embolic events to the foot **(A).** Antegrade arterial access with a 12 F sheath was established in the right common femoral artery. Over a stiff-angled glidewire, two 10 mm diameter × 70 mm long Wallgraft stents (*arrows*) were placed sequentially across the popliteal artery aneurysm. Postdilation with 10 mm diameter × 40 mm long balloon catheter was performed. A residual leak was demonstrated on repeat angiography and this necessitated placement of a 12 mm diameter × 50 mm long Wallgraft (*arrow-head*) placed distally followed by postdilation with a 12 mm diameter × 40 mm long balloon catheter **(B).** Final angiogram revealed adequate exclusion of the aneurysm **(C).** Aspirin, clopidogrel, and warfarin were provided after the procedure.

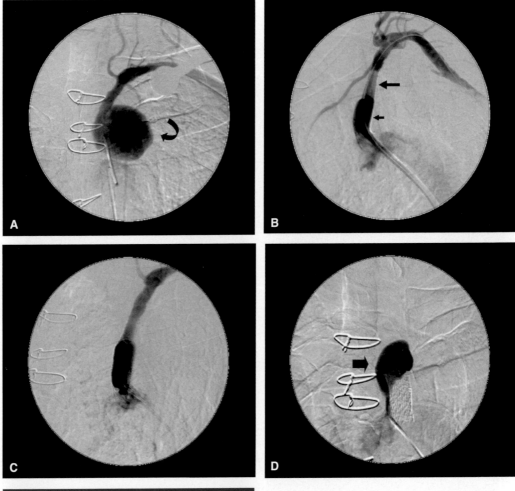

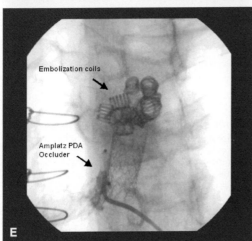

Embolization coils

Amplatz PDA
Occluder

FIGURE 16-4 ● **Endovascular repair of left subclavian artery pseudoaneurysm.** This 79-year-old man complained of left upper extremity numbness following coronary bypass surgery (involving the use of a left internal mammary artery conduit). He had a history of hypertension and surgical repair of an abdominal aortic aneurysm 20 years ago. A large pseudoaneurysm (*curved arrow*) was demonstrated in the proximal left subclavian artery **(A).** Via a 12 Fr sheath inserted through the right common femoral artery, an 11 mm diameter × 50 mm long Viabahn endoprosthesis (*large arrow*) was advanced over a 0.018″ Roadrunner wire and was deployed across the aneurysm. Postdilation was performed with a 12 mm diameter × 40 mm long balloon catheter. A 12 mm diameter × 26 mm long Intrastent®(*small arrow*) was deployed within the inflow of the covered stent in a bid to seal off the residual leak **(B).** A year later, repeat angiography revealed a patent subclavian artery and persistence of a large perigraft aneurysmal sac (**C & D,** *block arrow*). Via a 4 Fr multipurpose catheter, a total of three Flipper® detachable embolization coils (0.035″ × 5 cm × 8 mm, two 0.035″ × 12 cm × 8 mm), two Hilal® embolization coils (0.038″ × 8 cm × 5 mm), and eight embolization coils (0.038″ × 8 cm × 5 mm) were deployed. An Amplatz PDA® occluder (8 mm × 6 mm) was deployed via a 7 Fr Shuttle sheath in order to seal to entrance of the aneurysm **(E).**

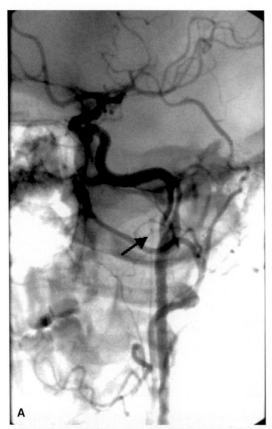

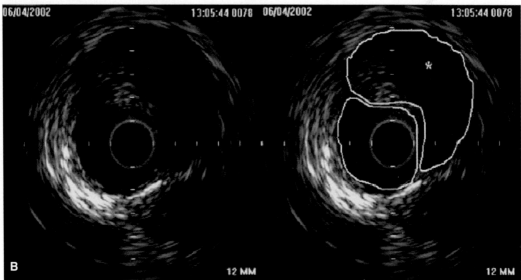

FIGURE 16-5 ● **Endovascular treatment of internal carotid artery aneurysm.** This 41-year-old woman complained of left-sided tinnitus and right-sided hemiparesthesia. **A:** Angiogram revealed an aneurysm in the distal left internal carotid artery associated with dissection. FMD was evident in the vertebral artery as well as the renal arteries. A 0.014″ BMW wire was placed across the aneurysmal segment (*arrow*). **B:** Intracarotid ultrasound across the lesion demonstrated simultaneous filling of both chambers with agitated saline contrast. ("*" denotes the false lumen) (*continued*)

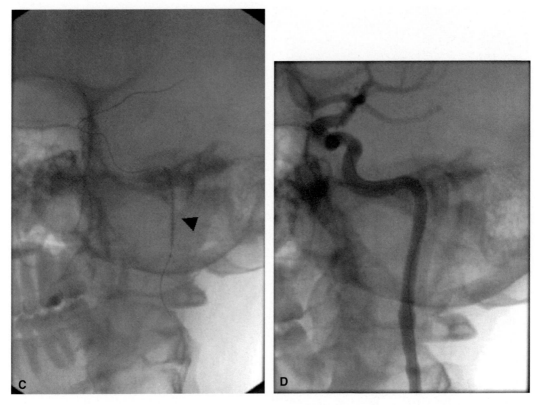

FIGURE 16-5 ● (*Continued*) **C:** The Jostent (*arrowhead*) was placed across the distal part of the aneurysm over a Synchro® Neuro guidewire. **D:** Sequential placement of two Jostent covered stents resulting in complete coverage of the aneurysm and dissection. Symptoms were resolved postprocedure, and the patient was started on daily aspirin and clopidogrel. Ultrasound revealed a patent vessel at 1 year. (Reprint from: Chan et al. Endovascular repair of carotid artery aneurysm with Jostent™ covered stent: initial experience and one-year result. *Cathet Cardiovasc Intervent.* 2004;63(1):15–20. with permission from Wiley-Liss)

hub of the delivery catheter whose tip has been positioned at the desired location for coil delivery. The coil is then extruded from the loading canula into the delivery catheter by pushing a wire guide into the proximal end of the loading canula. Continued advancement of the wire results in extrusion of the coil from the distal end of the delivery catheter.

For each coil, the manufacturer provides the recommended minimum and maximum internal diameter of the delivery catheter. Strict adherence to these recommendations is advised. A variety of delivery catheters are available (Table 16-3). The use of polyurethane catheters is discouraged because of the risk of the coil becoming lodged in the catheter. For each coil, the manufacturer will also recommend the appropriate diameter of the wire guide. This will vary from 0.018″ to 0.035″. While certain guide wires are available for use with specific delivery catheters (e.g., Tracker), the stiff end of any appropriately sized wire may be used. Attention to coil sizing during treatment of aneurysms is important. If a coil is too small, there is an increased risk of embolization. Alternatively, using too large a coil will result in the coil remaining elongated, and decrease the likelihood of occlusion of the aneurysmal sac. In addition, the proximal end of the coil may protrude through the neck of the aneurysm, or the interstices of a stent, and provide a nidus for thrombus formation.

Saccular aneurysms may be effectively treated using coil embolization, with or without stent placement, in the main vessel. When embolization coils are used, placing a stent within the parent vessel may prevent coil herniation and hence promote thrombogenesis within

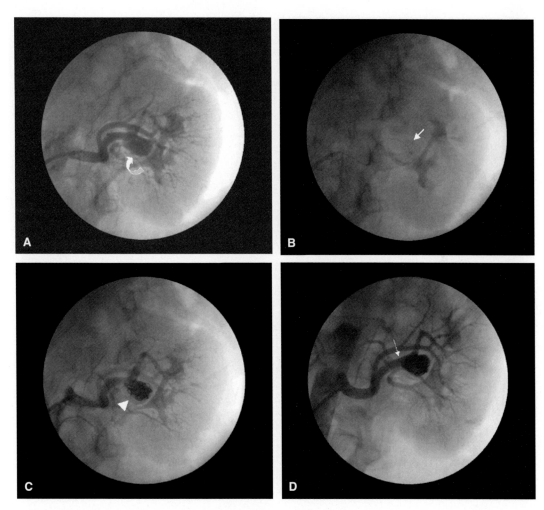

FIGURE 16-6 ● **Endovascular repair of left renal artery aneurysm and right renal artery stenosis. A:** A 67 year-old woman with a long-standing history of refractory hypertension was referred for back pain and investigation revealed a large left renal artery saccular aneurysm (*curved arrow*) associated with bilateral fibromuscular dysplasia. **B:** Through a 6 Fr Hockey Stick Pinnacle sheath and over a Choice PT wire, a 4 Fr Transit catheter (*white arrow*) was advanced into the aneurysmal sac. Unfractionated heparin was given for anticoagulation. **C:** Four Hydrocoils (i.e., 20 mm × 20 mm, 14 mm × 20 mm, 14 mm × 15 mm, 12 mm × 20 mm) and 2 Microplex detachable coils (i.e., 18 mm × 43 mm, 12 mm × 27 mm) were inserted into the aneurysm (*arrow-head*). **D:** A 5 mm diameter × 31 mm long Magic Wallstent (*white arrow*) was placed within the dysplastic main renal artery and covered the entry of the aneurysm. (*continued*)

the aneurysm (Figs. 16-1[A] and 16-1[B]). For a narrow neck, saccular aneurysm, an occlusion balloon catheter (e.g., Fogarty balloon catheter) may be first advanced into the aneurysm over a directionally controlled guidewire (Figure 16-1[A]). With the balloon inflated, the catheter is then pulled back snugly to the neck, to prevent coil embolization. Alternatively, coil embolization may be performed via a microcatheter (e.g., Transit catheter) within the aneurysm (Figs. 16-1[A] and 16-6).

For fusiform aneurysms, a bare metal, self-expanding stent may be deployed across the lesion (Figure 16-1[B]). A Transit catheter may then be placed within the aneurysm, through the stent struts, over a 0.014″ guidewire. The guidewire is then removed, and coils may be deployed into the aneurysmal cavity by pushing with the stiff end of a 0.018″ wire through the Transit catheter. The number of coils needed is determined by the size of the cavity. Attention needs to be paid to avoid disengaging the

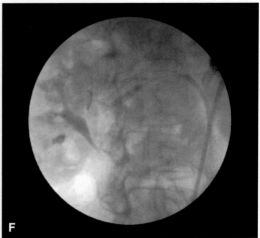

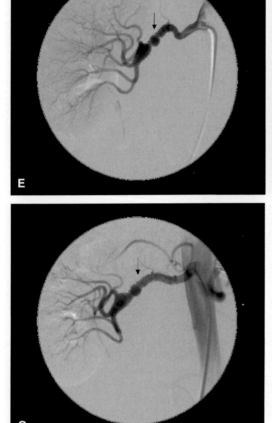

FIGURE 16-6 ● (*Continued*) **E:** Fusiform aneurysms within right renal artery fibromuscular dysplasia. **F:** Balloon angioplasty with balloon catheter that matched the reference diameter of the vessel. **G:** Typical post-angioplasty appearance of FMD does not appear differently from that before angioplasty.

Transit catheter out of the aneurysm while deploying the coils. The diameter of the coil should be about 1 mm larger than that of the target vessel.

Endoleaks (Table 16-4) occur as a result of failure of a graft to seal an aneurysm completely, the presence of collateral flow, or tears in the fabrics, leading to incomplete, spontaneous thrombosis after stent graft implantation.

Persistence of an endoleak may result in continuous aneurysmal expansion and rupture. Patients should be followed up with ultrasound, CT angiography, or invasive angiography, to detect the presence of any endoleak after endovascular repair of an aneurysm. Coil embolization may be considered for treatment of endoleaks (Fig. 16-4).

TABLE 16-4

Classification of Endoleaks

Types	Description
I	Inadequate seal at the proximal or distal neck
II	Retrograde filling of the aneurysmal sac through a side branch
III	Leak as a result of stent migration or arterial remodeling
IV	Contrast blush through the stent graft as a result of graft porosity

SPECIFIC CONSIDERATIONS

Extracranial Carotid Artery

Aneurysms located in the common carotid artery are usually caused by atherosclerosis, trauma, or post-infectious changes, while those in the carotid bulb are most commonly seen after surgical endarterectomy. Carotid aneurysms related to fibromuscular dysplasia (FMD) are usually located in the distal internal carotid artery. The presence of carotid FMD should prompt a search for FMD in other arterial territories, particularly within the vertebral, renal, and intracranial arteries (2). Spontaneous dissections are frequently associated with FMD (Fig. 16-5).

Extracranial carotid aneurysms may be asymptomatic, and may only be detectable by palpation underneath the angle of the jaw, on physical examination. Occasionally, the lesions may be associated with cervical pain, transient ischemic attacks (TIAs), or stroke resulting from embolization. Patients may provide a history of invasive tests or cervical manipulation (e.g., insertion of internal jugular venous catheter). Though ultrasonography, CT angiography, or magnetic resonance angiography (MRA) usually is the initial imaging modality, contrast angiography is often required both for confirmation of the diagnosis and guidance of management. Knowledge of the intracranial vascular anatomy, and any associated cerebrovascular obstructive disease or dissection, is necessary in order to select appropriate management strategy.

The natural history of an untreated carotid aneurysm is not known. In the past, surgical repair was recommended because cerebral ischemia was common, and most patients remained asymptomatic after surgery (3–5). Endovascular repair has become a more attractive approach because it eliminates general anesthesia and the potential complications related to surgery (e.g., cranial nerve palsy or stroke). Percutaneous treatment is the therapy of choice for patients with suitable lesions.

The technique of carotid angiography and choice of guide catheters has been described in Chapter 6. During angiography, it is critical to identify the location of the neck of the aneurysm, in order to ensure complete coverage. For aneurysms located in the common carotid artery or at the carotid bifurcation, coil embolization or stent graft placement have been performed successfully for both aneurysms (i.e., saccular or fusiform) and pseudoaneurysms (6–9). The balloon-expandable covered stent, Jostent, has been used for treatment of distal internal carotid artery aneurysms (Fig. 16-5) (10). All patients should undergo ultrasound and Doppler study prior to discharge, and again in 1 month, 6 months, 1 year, and annually thereafter.

Vertebral Artery

Extracranial vertebral artery aneurysms are exceedingly rare, and the majority of them are related to trauma. FMD of the vertebral artery could result in a spontaneous dissection and pseudoaneurysm formation. Symptoms may range from cervical or occipital pain, to vertebrobasilar insufficiency (e.g., nausea, vertigo, diplopia, hemiplegia, hemiparesis). Coil embolization or stent graft placement may be considered for symptomatic patients. A stent graft is contraindicated if a major side branch (e.g., posterior inferior cerebellar artery) is involved in the aneurysm.

Renal Artery

Renal artery aneurysms (RAA) are reported in 0.1 to 1.0% of all patients undergoing renal angiography (11,12). Bilateral RAA may occur in about 15% of these patients (11,13). They are usually discovered as an incidental finding during imaging studies, but occasionally they may present with rupture (13). RAA may result in secondary hypertension, by causing ischemia stemming from compression of the artery, altering antegrade blood flow, or causing renal infarction arising from embolization of mural thrombus. Pregnancy poses a particular risk for rupture (14). The indications for RAA repair include: the presence of symptoms, demonstration of progressive enlargement, expectation of pregnancy, intractable hypertension, and renal infarction (15). Whether or not the size of the aneurysm should be a factor in determining treatment remains debatable. In the surgical literature, a minimum size of 2 cm in the diameter of an aneurysm has been required by some centers for surgical repair

(15–19), while others reported that rupture may still occur even when the aneurysm was smaller than 2 cm (20).

Surgical ligation and renal artery reconstruction have been the standard treatment for RAA, but percutaneous treatment has become available in the past several years. Aneurysms in the main renal artery may be treated with coil embolization or implantation of a stent graft (21). Those located in the distal renal arteries may be treated with coil embolization, using microembolization coils (Table 16-3), resulting in small, segmental, renal infarction and elimination of the aneurysm. This may be achieved by advancing a Transit catheter to the target renal artery over a 0.014″ floppy coronary guidewire, and one or more microembolization coils may be used to fill up the artery that feeds the aneurysm.

FMD in the renal artery is usually associated with fusiform aneurysms (22). These typically appear as a "string of beads," representing a series of stenoses with intervening areas of dilation, and are typically located proximal to the first branch of the main renal artery (Fig. 16-6[E]). Duplex ultrasound, CT angiography, and MRI are the noninvasive modalities that may be used to detect this pathology (Fig. 16-7). Blood pressure usually responds to angioplasty, alone, in FMD (23), and placement of a bare metal stent is indicated only for failed angioplasty. Long-term patency of a balloon-expandable covered stent has been reported in the treatment of FMD-related RAA (24).

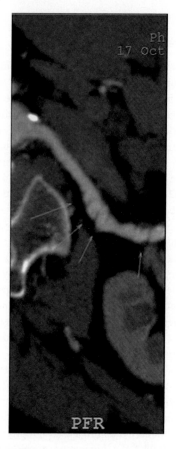

FIGURE 16-7 ● Computed tomography angiogram of FMD (arrows) within a renal artery.

Iliofemoral Artery

The prevalence of an iliac artery aneurysm (IAA) ranges from 0.01 to 0.03% of the United States population, many of which are in continuity with infrarenal aortic aneurysms (25–27). Most IAAs are caused by atherosclerosis. These aneurysms may be detected incidentally, during physical examination, or during investigation for obstructive arterial disease in the extremities. They may also be diagnosed as a result of complaints related to ureteral obstruction, hydronephrosis, or rupture (28,29). IAAs appear more likely to be under diagnosed, relative to abdominal aortic aneurysms, but the mortality rate (i.e., 50%) associated with IAA rupture is comparable to that of aortic aneurysm rupture (27,29). Therefore, early recognition and prompt treatment of IAAs, to prevent rupture, are important.

A longitudinal study reported by the Veterans Administration Medical Center suggested that the expansion rate of IAA of less than 3.0 cm in diameter was about 0.11 +/− 0.02 cm per year; this became significantly greater when the size of IAA was 3.0 cm to 5.0 cm (i.e., 0.26 +/− 0.10 cm per year) (30). In addition, all patients suffering from IAA rupture in that series had a diameter of more than 4.0 cm. Hence, in addition to symptoms and evidence of aneurysm enlargement, an aneurysm larger than 3.0 cm is an indication for repair (25,26,29–31). The success rate for endovascular therapy of anatomically suitable IAA is nearly 100% (32–35). The primary patency rates of the stent grafts are 88 to 92%, at 3 years (33,34). There is no evidence of aneurysm

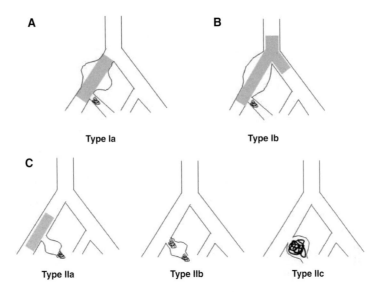

FIGURE 16-8 ● **Various endovascular treatment options for solitary common and internal iliac artery aneurysms. A:** Type 1a: common iliac artery aneurysm with a proximal neck; coil embolization of the internal iliac artery is needed to avoid retrograde feeding of the aneurismal sac via pelvic collaterals into the internal iliac artery. **B:** Type 1b: common iliac artery aneurysm without a proximal neck; this necessitates stent graft placement in the aortic bifurcation. **C:** Internal iliac artery aneurysm may be treated with distal coil embolization combined with either proximal stent graft coverage (type 2a) or coil embolization (type 2b). Coil embolization alone may be used for those without a proximal neck (type 2c). Illustrations adapted from reference (32).

expansion after successful exclusion. Successful placement of a stent graft relies on the presence of a suitable, proximal, and distal anchor zone. For isolated IAA repair, Wallgraft placement has been successful (36,37). When the proximal neck is absent, or an infrarenal aortic aneurysm coexists, an aortic bifurcated stent graft (e.g., AneuRx; Vanguard; Excluder) with an iliac extender cuff is required (38–40).

Fahrni et al described five morphologies of iliac aneurysms that may be treated successfully with a stent graft, combined with coil embolization of the internal iliac artery (Fig. 16-8) (32). When a stent graft is required for treating a common, or external iliac artery aneurysm, coil embolization of the internal iliac artery is important, to prevent retrograde filling of the aneurysmal sac and late rupture.

Isolated femoral artery aneurysms are mostly of the fusiform type and are related to degenerative changes secondary to atherosclerosis. Saccular aneurysms at this location are typically pseu-

doaneurysms related to iatrogenic trauma (e.g., after catheterization).

Popliteal Artery

Popliteal artery aneurysms are the most common, extra-aortic, arterial aneurysm, and account for 70% of all extra-aortic aneurysms (41). They have been documented in one of every eight to 15 patients with abdominal aortic aneurysms, with a male predominance (i.e., greater than 95%) (41,42). Under-reporting, owing to the absence of symptoms, implies that this disease is more prevalent than the reported numbers. Pooling the results from 29 published reports that included a total of 1673 patients with popliteal aneurysms, Dawson and coworkers reported that ischemic events during follow-up evaluation occurred at a mean rate of 36% (43).

Symptoms are manifested as "blue toes" or "trash-foot", and mortality or amputation rates with these conditions may be as high as 20%

(44). Repair of the popliteal artery aneurysm has been recommended not only for the symptomatic patients, but also for asymptomatic patients with aneurysm sizes greater than 2.0 cm (45). Conservative follow-up evaluation of an aneurysm of up to 2.0 cm appears to be safe (41,46). Thrombolysis may be used for acute or recent thrombotic occlusion (47,48). Failed thrombolysis may indicate poor runoff, and may predict poor, long-term outcome, with revascularization (49). Several centers have suggested that placement of a self-expanding stent graft is reasonable, with primary and secondary patency rates, at 18 months, of between 47 to 74% and 67 to 92%, respectively (Fig. 16-3) (50,51). These results are comparable to the surgical results (i.e., 2-year graft patency rate is about 75 to 80%) (43,52). Adequate outflow (i.e., at least two vessels runoff) is beneficial in maintaining long-term patency of the stent graft (53).

Axillo-Subclavian Artery

Aneurysms in the axillo-subclavian artery are extremely rare, and the majority of these are, in fact, pseudoaneurysms secondary to trauma (Fig. 16-4). As a result, the experience with endovascular repair of these aneurysms is in case report form only. Overall, these reports suggest that endovascular repair is feasible, and may be an alternative to surgical treatment. An aneurysm associated with thoracic-outlet syndrome probably should be treated surgically, rather than with stents (54).

REFERENCES

1. Johnston KW, Rutherford RB, Tilson MD, et al. Suggested standards for reporting on arterial aneurysms. Subcommittee on Reporting Standards for Arterial Aneurysms, Ad Hoc Committee on Reporting Standards, Society for Vascular Surgery and North American Chapter, International Society for Cardiovascular Surgery. *J Vasc Surg.* 1991;13:452–458.
2. Cloft HJ, Kallmes DF, Kallmes MH, et al. Prevalence of cerebral aneurysms in patients with fibromuscular dysplasia: a reassessment. *J Neurosurg.* 1998;88:436–440.
3. Moreau P, Albat B, Thevenet A. Surgical treatment of extracranial internal carotid artery aneurysm. *Ann Vasc Surg.* 1994;8:409–416.
4. Pulli R, Gatti M, Credi G, et al. Extracranial carotid artery aneurysms. *J Cardiovasc Surg (Torino).* 1997;38:339–346.
5. Sahlman A, Salo J, Kostiainen S, et al. Extracranial carotid artery aneurysms. *Vasa.* 1991;20:369–373.
6. Assali AR, Sdringola S, Moustapha A, et al. Endovascular repair of traumatic pseudoaneurysm by uncovered self-expandable stenting with or without transstent coiling of the aneurysm cavity. *Catheter Cardiovasc Interv.* 2001;53:253–258.
7. Bush RL, Lin PH, Dodson TF, et al. Endoluminal stent placement and coil embolization for the management of carotid artery pseudoaneurysms. *J Endovasc Ther.* 2001;8:53–61.
8. Redekop G, Marotta T, Weill A. Treatment of traumatic aneurysms and arteriovenous fistulas of the skull base by using endovascular stents. *J Neurosurg.* 2001;95:412–419.
9. Mukherjee D, Roffi M, Yadav JS. Endovascular treatment of carotid artery aneurysms with stent grafts. *J Invasive Cardiol.* 2002;14:269–272.
10. Chan AW, Yadav J, Kreiger D, et al. Endovascular repair of carotid artery aneurysm with Jostent™ covered stent: initial experience and one-year result. *Catheter Cardiovasc Interv.* 2004;63(1):15–20.
11. Tham G, Ekelund L, Herrlin K, et al. Renal artery aneurysms. Natural history and prognosis. *Ann Surg.* 1983;197:348–352.
12. Stanley JC, Rhodes EL, Gewertz BL, et al. Renal artery aneurysms. Significance of macroaneurysms exclusive of dissections and fibrodysplastic mural dilations. *Arch Surg.* 1975;110:1327–1333.
13. Henke PK, Cardneau JD, Welling TH III, et al. Renal artery aneurysms: a 35-year clinical experience with 252 aneurysms in 168 patients. *Ann Surg.* 2001;234:454–462.
14. Cohen JR, Shamash FS. Ruptured renal artery aneurysms during pregnancy. *J Vasc Surg.* 1987;6:51–59.
15. Martin RS III, Meacham PW, Ditesheim JA, et al. Renal artery aneurysm: selective treatment for hypertension and prevention of rupture. *J Vasc Surg.* 1989;9:26–34.
16. Dzsinich C, Gloviczki P, McKusick MA, et al. Surgical management of renal artery aneurysm. *Cardiovasc Surg.* 1993;1:243–247.
17. Soussou ID, Starr DS, Lawrie GM, et al. Renal artery aneurysm. Long-term relief of renovascular hypertension by in situ operative correction. *Arch Surg.* 1979;114:1410–1415.
18. Hageman JH, Smith RF, Szilagyi E, et al. Aneurysms of the renal artery: problems of prognosis and surgical management. *Surgery.* 1978;84:563–572.
19. Bastounis E, Pikoulis E, Georgopoulos S, et al. Surgery for renal artery aneurysms: a combined series of two large centers. *Eur Urol.* 1998;33:22–27.
20. Reiher L, Grabitz K, Sandmann W. Reconstruction for renal artery aneurysm and its effect on hypertension. *Eur J Vasc Endovasc Surg.* 2000;20:454–456.
21. Schneidereit NP, Lee S, Morris DC. Endovascular repair of a ruptured renal artery aneurysm. *J Endovasc Ther.* 2003;10:71–74.
22. Alimi Y, Mercier C, Pellissier JF, et al. Fibromuscular disease of the renal artery: a new histopathologic classification. *Ann Vasc Surg.* 1992;6:220–224.
23. Sos TA, Pickering TG, Sniderman K, et al. Percutaneous transluminal renal angioplasty in renovascular hypertension due to atheroma or fibromuscular dysplasia. *N Engl J Med.* 1983;309:274–279.
24. Bisschops RH, Popma JJ, Meyerovitz MF. Treatment of fibromuscular dysplasia and renal artery aneurysm with

use of a stent-graft. *J Vasc Interv Radiol.* 2001;12:757–760.

25. Lawrence PF, Lorenzo-Rivero S, Lyon JL. The incidence of iliac, femoral, and popliteal artery aneurysms in hospitalized patients. *J Vasc Surg.* 1995;22:409–415; discussion 415–416.

26. Brunkwall J, Hauksson H, Bengtsson H, et al. Solitary aneurysms of the iliac arterial system: an estimate of their frequency of occurrence. *J Vasc Surg.* 1989;10:381–384.

27. Vammen S, Lindholt J, Henneberg EW, Fasting H. A comparative study of iliac and abdominal aortic aneurysms. *Int Angiol.* 2000;19:152–157.

28. Unno N, Kaneko H, Uchiyama T, et al. The fate of small aneurysms of the internal iliac artery following proximal ligation in abdominal aortic aneurysm repair. *Surg Today.* 2000;30:791–794.

29. Minato N, Itoh T, Natsuaki M, et al. Isolated iliac artery aneurysm and its management. *Cardiovasc Surg.* 1994;2:489–494.

30. Santilli SM, Wernsing SE, Lee ES. Expansion rates and outcomes for iliac artery aneurysms. *J Vasc Surg.* 2000;31:114–121.

31. Kasirajan V, Hertzer NR, Beven EG, et al. Management of isolated common iliac artery aneurysms. *Cardiovasc Surg.* 1998;6:171–177.

32. Fahrni M, Lachat MM, Wildermuth S, et al. Endovascular therapeutic options for isolated iliac aneurysms with a working classification. *Cardiovasc Intervent Radiol.* 2003;26(5):443–447.

33. Henry M, Amor M, Henry I, et al. Percutaneous endovascular treatment of peripheral aneurysms. *J Cardiovasc Surg (Torino).* 2000;41:871–883.

34. Scheinert D, Schroder M, Steinkamp H, et al. Treatment of iliac artery aneurysms by percutaneous implantation of stent grafts. *Circulation.* 2000;102:III253–III258.

35. Henry M, Amor M, Cragg A, et al. Occlusive and aneurysmal peripheral arterial disease: assessment of a stent-graft system. *Radiology.* 1996;201:717–724.

36. Curti T, Stella A, Rossi C, et al. Endovascular repair as first-choice treatment for anastomotic and true iliac aneurysms. *J Endovasc Ther.* 2001;8:139–143.

37. Kumins NH, Owens EL, Oglevie SB, et al. Early experience using the Wallgraft in the management of distal microembolism from common iliac artery pathology. *Ann Vasc Surg.* 2002;16:181–186.

38. Zarins CK, White RA, Moll FL, et al. The AneuRx stent graft: four-year results and worldwide experience 2000. *J Vasc Surg.* 2001;33:S135–S145.

39. Zarins CK, White RA, Schwarten D, et al. AneuRx stent graft versus open surgical repair of abdominal aortic aneurysms: multicenter prospective clinical trial. *J Vasc Surg.* 1999;29:292–305; discussion 306–308.

40. Kibbe MR, Matsumura JS. The Gore Excluder US multicenter trial: analysis of adverse events at 2 years. *Semin Vasc Surg.* 2003;16:144–150.

41. Duffy ST, Colgan MP, Sultan S, et al. Popliteal aneurysms: a 10-year experience. *Eur J Vasc Endovasc Surg.* 1998;16:218–222.

42. Diwan A, Sarkar R, Stanley JC, et al. Incidence of femoral and popliteal artery aneurysms in patients with abdominal aortic aneurysms. *J Vasc Surg.* 2000;31:863–869.

43. Dawson I, Sie RB, van Bockel JH. Atherosclerotic popliteal aneurysm. *Br J Surg.* 1997;84:293–299.

44. Wingo JP, Nix ML, Greenfield LJ, et al. The blue toe syndrome: hemodynamics and therapeutic correlates of outcome. *J Vasc Surg.* 1986;3:475–480.

45. Szilagyi DE, Schwartz RL, Reddy DJ. Popliteal arterial aneurysms. Their natural history and management. *Arch Surg.* 1981;116:724–728.

46. Galland RB, Magee TR. Management of popliteal aneurysm. *Br J Surg.* 2002;89:1382–1385.

47. Dorigo W, Pulli R, Turini F, et al. Acute leg ischaemia from thrombosed popliteal artery aneurysms: role of preoperative thrombolysis. *Eur J Vasc Endovasc Surg.* 2002;23:251–254.

48. Varga ZA, Locke-Edmunds JC, Baird RN. A multicenter study of popliteal aneurysms. Joint Vascular Research Group. *J Vasc Surg.* 1994;20:171–177.

49. Marty B, Wicky S, Ris HB, et al. Success of thrombolysis as a predictor of outcome in acute thrombosis of popliteal aneurysms. *J Vasc Surg.* 2002;35:487–493.

50. Tielliu IF, Verhoeven EL, Prins TR, et al. Treatment of popliteal artery aneurysms with the Hemobahn stent-graft. *J Endovasc Ther.* 2003;10:111–116.

51. Gerasimidis T, Sfyroeras G, Papazoglou K, et al. Endovascular treatment of popliteal artery aneurysms. *Eur J Vasc Endovasc Surg.* 2003;26:506–511.

52. Sarcina A, Bellosta R, Luzzani L, et al. Surgical treatment of popliteal artery aneurysm. A 20 year experience. *J Cardiovasc Surg.* 1997;38:347–354.

53. Lagana D, Mangini M, Marras M, et al. Percutaneous treatment of femoral-popliteal aneurysms with covered stents. *Radiol Med.* 2002;104:322–331.

54. Phipp LH, Scott DJ, Kessel D, et al. Subclavian stents and stent-grafts: cause for concern? *J Endovasc Surg.* 1999;6:223–226.

CHAPTER 17

Percutaneous Transcatheter Closure of Patent Foramen Ovale and Atrial Septal Defects

Ivan P. Casserly and E. Murat Tuzcu

Mills and King are credited with performing the first nonoperative atrial septal defect (ASD) closure in a human subject using a double-umbrella device (1). Although this procedure took place in 1976, a further decade elapsed before the clam-shell device sparked a broader interest in the concept of non-operative ASD closure. Although the technical deficiencies of this device (i.e., metal arm fractures, high rates of residual shunting) resulted in its subsequent withdrawal from use, it formed the basis for further generations of similar devices and other novel devices that have been successfully implanted in thousands of patients.

Coincident with these developments, the concept of persistent patent foramen ovale (PFO) in adults, as a risk factor for cryptogenic stroke, gained momentum (2,3), and is now corroborated by impressive epidemiologic data (4). Paradoxic embolism of venous thrombus into the arterial circulation across the PFO is the presumed pathogenic mechanism of stroke in these patients. Percutaneous closure of these defects is a logical therapeutic strategy, and many devices originally designed for ASD closure were used for PFO closure. In addition, specific PFO closure devices were developed.

Cardiac interventionists have embraced the techniques of nonoperative ASD/PFO closure. These procedures fall under the umbrella of non-coronary cardiac intervention. For most cases, the technical requirements of the procedures are reasonably straight forward. The greater challenge is to appropriately select patients who are suitable candidates for percutaneous PFO/ASD closure. This requires an understanding of the embryology of these defects, and the anatomy of the PFO or ASD that one plans to close percutaneously. Additionally, it is imperative to incorporate echocardiographic guidance in the pre-procedural assessment, performance of the procedure, and post-procedural surveillance of these patients. For most interventionists, this will require establishing a strong partnership with their echocardiographic colleagues. Nevertheless, the interventionist needs to become familiar with the interpretation of these studies, and have a fundamental understanding of the features that relate significantly to a successful procedural outcome.

THE ATRIAL SEPTUM— EMBRYOLOGY AND ANATOMY

In utero, the common atrial chamber is divided into right and left atria by the atrial septum (Fig. 17-1) (5). This is a composite structure, derived from the septum primum and septum secundum. Initially, the sickle-shaped septum primum grows into the common atrium from the dorsal wall, and fuses with the endocardial cushions.

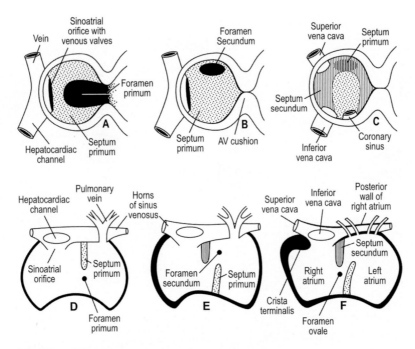

FIGURE 17-1 ● Embryologic development of the atrial septum as viewed from the right atrium **(A–C),** and in cross-section **(D–F).** See text for details. Reproduced with permission from Fitzgerald MJT. Thoracic organs. In: Fitzgerald MJT, ed. *Human Embryology.* Baltimore, MD: Harper & Row; 1976:83–105.

During this process, a defect forms in the rostral portion of the septum primum, termed the foramen secundum. Subsequently, the sickle-shaped septum secundum grows into the atrium on the right side of the septum primum. The septum secundum covers the foramen secundum in the septum primum, but stops short of forming a complete interatrial membrane. The defect found between its free margin and the dorsal wall of the atrium is termed the foramen ovale, and the septum primum forms the floor of this foramen.

Prior to birth, blood from the inferior vena cava is directed across the foramen ovale, which functions as a valve-like channel, allowing only right-to-left flow. Following birth, loss of umbilical blood flow (i.e., from the placenta), and increased pulmonary blood flow results in decreased right atrial and increased left atrial pressures, respectively. The effect is to oppose the septum primum to the septum secundum, and result in fusion of the two components, eliminating the communicating channel between the two chambers. In approximately 25% of individuals, this fusion is incomplete, leaving a persistent,

crescent-shaped, valve-like channel, termed the foramen ovale (Fig. 17-2).

A further anomaly of the atrial septum important to our discussion is the atrial septal aneurysm (ASA). Classically, this anomaly will appear as a thin, redundant, billowing membrane in the area of the fossa ovalis that is hypermobile (Fig. 17-3).

It represents an abnormality in the septum primum portion of the septum, and its incidence as assessed by transesophageal echocardiography (TEE) is about 2%. An associated PFO is found in a very high percentage (more than 50%) of patients with an ASA. Despite the classic description, ASAs have a very heterogenous phenotype, which has resulted in a remarkable inconsistency in the definitions used to categorize the presence or absence of an ASA. These definitions focus on two fundamental attributes of the aneurysm: (1) mobility—this is defined as either the entire excursion of the septum into both the left and right atrium, or the maximal excursion of the septum into either the right or left atria from the midline. Various authors have used an entire excursion distance of 10 mm, 11 mm, or

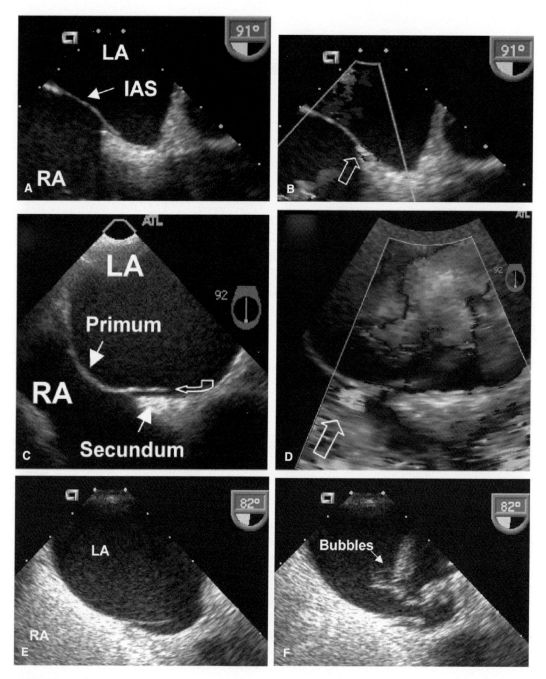

FIGURE 17-2 ● TEE images of a short PFO **(A)** and tunnel-type PFO **(C).** Color Doppler of these PFOs demonstrates a small amount of left-to-right shunting *(open arrows in **B** and **D**.)* **E–F.** Right-to-left shunting of bubbles across a PFO is demonstrated. PFO, patent foramen ovale; RA, right atrium; LA, left atrium; IAS, interatrial septum.

15 mm, or a maximal excursion distance into either atrium of 10 mm, to define the presence of an ASA; (2) diameter of the base of the aneurysm—most authors have used a base diameter of 15 mm as one of the criteria to diagnose an ASA.

ASDs represent a through-and-through communication between both atria, at the level of the septum (6), and they account for 6 to 11% of all congenital cardiac anomalies (7). Thus, an ASD is anatomically very distinct from a PFO, which

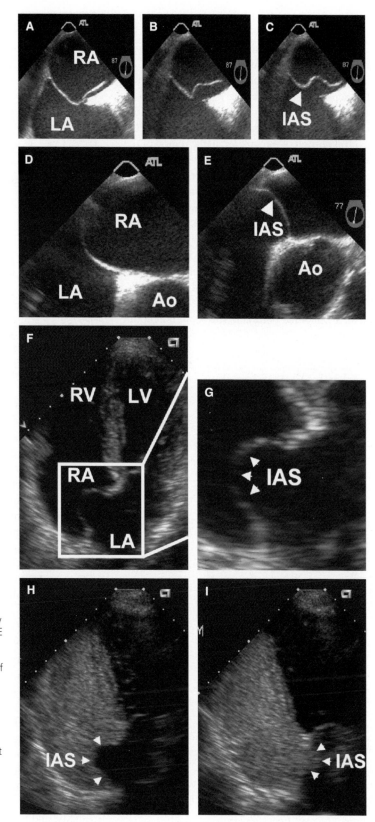

FIGURE 17-3 ● **Anatomic variations of atrial septal aneurysm. A–C.** TEE image demonstrating focal hypermobility of the interatrial septum. **D–E.** TEE image demonstrating hypermobility of the entire septum. **F–I.** Classic appearance of an atrial septal aneurysm by TTE. The redundant septum primum typically bows into the right atrium. Venous injection of bubbles clearly delineates the aneurysmal septum **(H).** The septum may also bow into the left atrium depending on the instantaneous pressures in both atria **(I).** LA, left atrium; RA, right atrium; IAS, interatrial septum; Ao, aorta.

functions as a valve-like channel rather than a true defect. Approximately two-thirds of all ASDs are of the secundum type. This defect type is thought to represent abnormal development, abnormal resorption, or ectopic cellular death of the septum primum, in the region of the fossa ovalis that the septum secundum does not adequately cover. They are therefore found in the central portion of the septum, in the region of the fossa ovalis (Fig. 17-4).

Apart from this classic description, there are many important anatomic variants to be appreciated that, cumulatively, are present in the majority of patients: (8) ASDs are multiple or fenestrated (i.e., also termed 'cribriform') in about 8 to 20% of cases (Fig. 17-5); deficiency of the superior-anterior and inferior-posterior rim of the defect occurs in about 40% and 10% of cases, respectively, and the defect may occur in an aneurysmal portion of the septum in about 8% of cases.

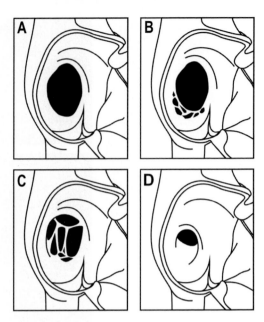

FIGURE 17-5 ● Anatomic variation of atrial secundum defects. **A.** defect occupies entire fossa ovalis. **B.** Large defect with fenestrations in inferior section. **C.** Entire defect is fenestrated. **D.** Small defect in superior portion of fossa ovalis.

The locations of the remaining types of ASD are illustrated (Fig. 17-4). Since these defect types are not amenable to percutaneous closure, they will not be discussed further, but an awareness of their existence is important, as patients with these defects will occasionally be referred to interventionists for consideration for closure.

An understanding of the spatial orientation of the atrial septum, and the spatial relationship of various structures to the septum, are fundamental to performing transcatheter closure of PFOs and ASDs. In the adult, the atrial septum is oriented as follows: the superior and inferior portions of the septum are directed anteriorly and posteriorly, respectively, and right and left portions of the septum are directed posteriorly and anteriorly, respectively. The septum forms the posteromedial wall of the right atrium, and the anterolateral wall of the left atrium. From the right atrial side, the most prominent anatomic landmark is the fossa ovalis, which is a shallow, translucent depression facing the opening of the inferior vena cava (Fig. 17-6). In relation to the fossa, the inferior and superior vena cavae lie inferolaterally and superolaterally, the aorta lies superomedially, the tricuspid valve lies inferomedially, and the coronary sinus lies inferiorly.

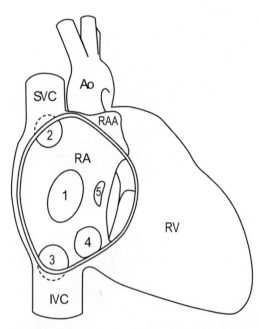

FIGURE 17-4 ● View of the atrial septum from the right atrial side demonstrating the typical location of the various types of ASD. 1. secundum, 2. sinus venosus—superior vena caval type, 3. sinus venosus—inferior vena caval type, 4. coronary sinus, 5. primum. RAA, right atrial appendage: Ao, aorta: SVC, superior vena cava: IVC, inferior vena cava: RV, right ventricle. Reproduced with permission from Valdes-Cruz LM, Caryre RO. Atrial septal defects. In: Valdes-Cruz LM, Caryre RO, eds. *Echocardiographic Diagnosis of Congenital Heart Disease.* Philadelphia: Lippincott-Raven; 1999:187–213.

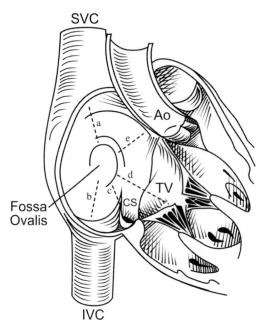

SVC

Ao

a

e

d

c

b

TV

CS

Fossa
Ovalis

IVC

FIGURE 17-6 ● View of the atrial septum from the right atrial side demonstrating the relationship of the fossa ovalis with the surrounding structures. Reproduced with permission from Harper RW, Mottram PM, McGaw DJ. Closure of secundum atrial septal defects with the Amplatzer septal occluder device: techniques and problems. *Catheter Cardiovasc Interv* 2002;57(4):508–524.

THE DEVICES

Devices that are currently approved or available under human device exemption (HDE) for the percutaneous closure of PFOs or ASDs are described in Table 17-1, and shown in Fig. 17-7 and Fig. 17-8.

In most centers, investigators choose to use one or two devices, and become proficient in their use. This is an appropriate strategy, particularly in the early stages of development of a percutaneous PFO/ASD closure program. It is not possible to describe all of the details of the devices available. However, it is important to understand some of the basic concepts of device design for PFO/ASD occluders.

Current devices are all double-disc devices, essentially, containing right and left atrial discs, which oppose the atrial septum, and a central connecting waist element that rests in the PFO or ASD. The discs are composed of a metal frame that supports a fabric promoting occlusion of the defect. Various metals and metal alloys and fabrics have been used, and the

ratio of the two components varies between devices.

The ideal characteristics of a PFO/ASD occluder device are listed in Table 17-2.

Many of these characteristics are interrelated, and are dependent on the multiple constituent elements of the device, the delivery system, and the deployment mechanism. Achieving an effective seal is dependent on adequate and rapid endothelialization of the device. It is still uncertain which fabric, metal constituent, or device design is superior in this respect. Generally, it has been thought that reduced metal-to-fabric ratios would favorably impact reendothelialization and defect closure, but this has not been borne out in clinical practice. The principle safety issues with these devices relates to stability of the device, the likelihood of device thrombosis, metal fatigue leading to fracture, and device impingement on adjacent structures.

• Stability of the Device Across the Defect

Device stability is generally produced by the passive counter tension between both atrial discs. The integrity of this mechanism is what prevents device embolization (i.e., assuming appropriate deployment of the device) and is critical to the design of any device. Additional locking mechanisms have been added to some devices (e.g., HELEX), but it remains unclear if this significantly reduces the incidence of device embolization.

• Likelihood of Device Thrombosis

The prevailing wisdom is that minimizing the metal content in devices and metal exposure in the left atrium, together with a reduction in device profile should reduce the risk of thrombosis. However, this has not been borne out in clinical studies, where the risk of thrombosis with the relatively bulky Amplatzer device with a high metal-to-fabric ratio is no higher than devices with lower profiles and low metal-to-fabric ratios (e.g. CardioSEAL). Clearly, the fabric element is also an important consideration in device thrombosis.

• Fatigue in the Metal Components Leading to Fracture

Metal fatigue is a concern with all occluder devices with metal components. This has led to a switch away from stainless steel formulations

TABLE 17-1

Descriptive Summary of PFO/ASD Closure Devices That Are Currently Available for Use or Under Active Investigation

	CardioSEAL®[1]	STARFlex®[2]	Amplatzer PFO Occluder	Amplatzer ASD Occluder	HELEX Septal Occluder	PFO-Star[7]	Sideris Buttoned Occluder[8]
Manufacturer	Nitinol Medical Technologies Inc	Nitinol Medical Technologies Inc	AGA Medical Corporation	AGA Medical Corporation	WL Gore and Associates Inc	Applied Biometrics Inc	Custom Medical Devices
Design							
Metal frame support	MP35n	MP35n	Nitinol	Nitinol	Nitinol	Nitinol	Teflon-coated stainless steel
Occlusive material	Polyester	Polyester	Polyester	Polyester	PTFE	Ivalon	Polyurethane foam
Description	Two square-shaped polyester umbrellas each supported by 4 metal alloy arms (MP35n) connected to central hinge point. Each metal arm has 3 spring coils for flexibility	Same as CardioSEAL with following modifications: nitinol microsprings sutured to the tip of each metal arm and attached in alternating fashion between opposing arms of umbrellas	Self-expandable double-disc device made from nitinol wire mesh. Thin connecting waist of fixed size between discs. Polyester patches sewn within discs and waist using polyester thread	Same as Amplatzer PFO occluder except: • diameter of the waist varies between devices • left atrial disc is larger than right atrial disc	An expanded PTFE patch with hydrophilic coating supported by single length of nitinol super-elastic wire.[6] When deployed the occluder takes on a double-disc shape	Two square-shaped Ivalon sails connected by either 3 mm or 5 mm center posts. Sails supported by 4 or 6 nitinol wires with titanium end caps. Ivalon is attached to the outer surface of the left sail	Consists of left atrial occluder (square-shaped polyurethane foam supported by X-shaped wire skeleton) and right atrial counteroccluder (rhomboid-shaped polyurethane foam covering single strand of wire skeleton) joined by a central button/counter button mechanism
Use							
PFO	Yes	Yes	Yes	No	Yes	Yes	Yes
ASD	Yes	Yes	No	Yes	Yes	No	Yes
Centering	Noncentering	Self-centering	Noncentering	Centering	Noncentering	Noncentering	Noncentering
Fixation	Passive counter tension	Passive counter tension	Passive counter fixation	Passive counter fixation	Passive and active with locking mechanism	Passive Counter fixation	Sutured counter button

Delivery Sheath	11 Fr	10 Fr	8–9 Fr	6–12 Fr	9 Fr	9–10 Fr	8–11 Fr
Device Size (mm)	17,23,28,33,40	23,28,33,38[3]	18,25,35[4]	4 to 20 mm—in 1 mm increments, 22 to 38 mm in 2 mm increments	15,20,25,30,35	18,22,26,30,35	25 to 60 mm in 5 mm increments
Approval Status							
United States	Investigational	Investigational	Investigational	Approved 2001	Investigational	Investigational	Investigational
Europe	Approved 1997	Approved 1998	Approved 1998	Approved 1998	Investigational	Investigational	Investigational
Characteristics							
Profile	++	++	+++	++++	+	++	++
Metal surface area	++	++	++++	++++	+	++	++
Retrievable and repositionable after right atrial disc deployed	No	No	Yes	Yes	Yes	Yes	No
Clinical experience	++++	++	++	+++	+	+	++++
Additional features		• Allows closure of larger defects (up to 25 mm stretch diameter) than CardioSEAL • Lower profile than CardioSEAL	Very user friendly device	Very user friendly device	• Deployment technique is currently more demanding than most devices • Has additional safety cord which minimizes risk of device embolization	Deployment technique similar to CardioSEAL and Amplatzer device	Complex implantation technique Increased risk of device embolization

[1] Evolved from Bard Clamshell Septal Umbrella.
[2] Evolved from CardioSEAL device.
[3] 6 arm device.
[4] Sized according to right atrial disc size.
[5] Sized according to device waist diameter.
[6] PTFE, polytetrafluoroethylene.
[7] Data relate to third-generation device.
[8] Data relate to fourth-generation device.

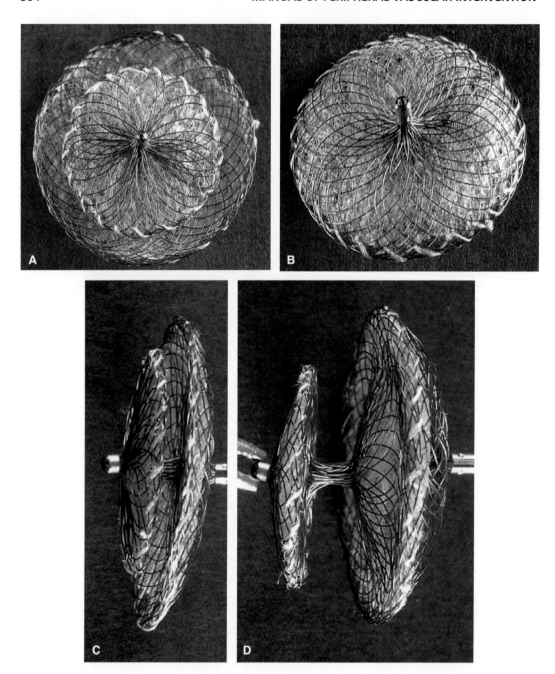

FIGURE 17-7 ● Photographs of the Amplatzer PFO **(A–D)** and ASD **(E–H)** occluder devices as viewed from the left atrial side (A,E), right atrial side (B,F), in cross-section (C,G), and in cross-section with traction on the right and left atrial components to demonstrate the waist section of each device (D,H).

toward the use of nitinol and other metal alloys in many devices, and the incorporation of specific design modifications, such as the addition of spring coils in the metal arms of the CardioSEAL and STARFlex devices.

- The Impingement of the Device on Adjacent Structures

In addition to the size of the device, this characteristic is impacted particularly by the profile

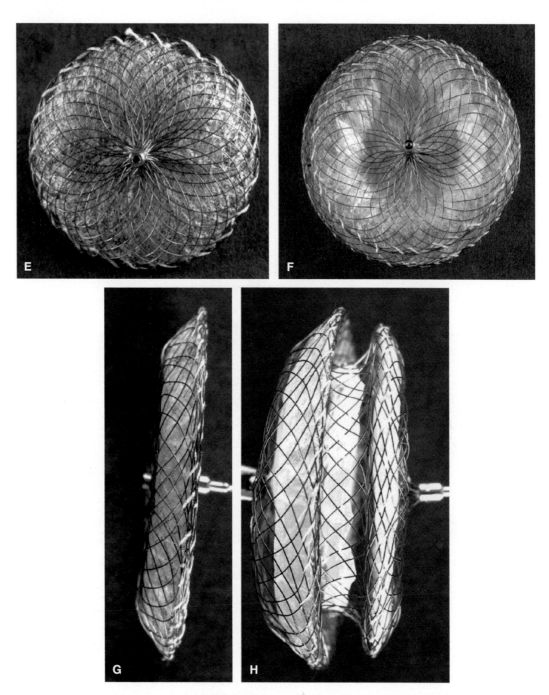

FIGURE 17-7 ● *(Continued).*

of the device, the smoothness of the transition between the device and septal tissue, and the ability of the device to conform to the curvature of the septum. Devices such as the CardioSEAL, STARFlex, PFO-Star, and HELEX, have an advantage over the Amplatzer device, in this regard.

The feasibility of ASD/PFO closure with a given device is dependent on a number of factors.

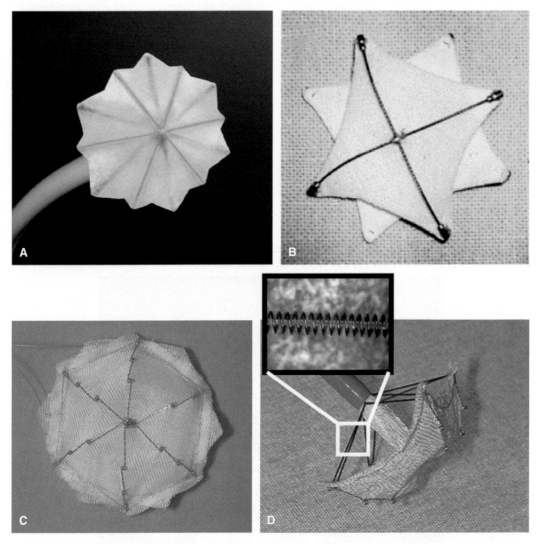

FIGURE 17-8 ● **A–B.** Enface view of third-generation **(A)** and first-generation **(B)** PFO-Star device. **C–D.** Enface view of 38 mm STARFlex device and partially deployed STARFlex device demonstrating nitinol microsprings (magnified in inset image) that are attached between opposing arms of the umbrellas and serve to center the device across the defect. **E–F.** HELEX occluder in both linear **(E)** and helical configurations **(F)**. **G–H.** CardioSEAL device in side profile **(G)** and en-face (H) views.

From a practical standpoint, the more generations of a device that have been developed, the more user-friendly the device and the associated equipment are likely to be. The deployment mechanism of the Amplatzer, CardioSEAL, STARFlex, and PFO-Star devices are all similar and straight forward, compared with more complex implantation techniques with the HELEX and Buttoned Occluder. Finally, the ability to reposition the device following deployment of the right atrial disc device is an important consideration. The nitinol

metal frame of the Amplatzer and HELEX devices confers the property of deformability, allowing easy retrieval and repositioning of the device, which is not true for the CardioSEAL and STARFlex devices. The latter devices may not be reused if retrieved following deployment of the right atrial disc.

Most of the devices developed have been designated for dual use in PFO and ASD closure, although specific design modifications have been made in the case of the Amplatzer PFO occluder

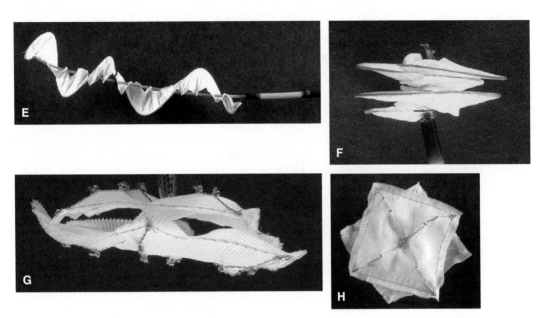

FIGURE 17-8 ● *(Continued)*

and PFO-Star devices. These modifications center largely on the waist region of the device that is purposefully narrow, in the case of PFO-specific occluders. The Amplatzer device also makes the right atrial disc larger than the left atrial disc, for its PFO occluder. The majority of the devices are "non-centering," meaning that there is no mechanism to ensure that the device sits in the center of the defect. This is not an issue when closing PFOs, since the defect is generally small, but it does impact the closure of large ASDs, where self-centering devices (e.g., STARFlex, Amplatzer ASD occluder, buttoned COD) may allow the closure of larger defects than their noncentering counterparts (i.e., CardioSEAL, buttoned devices).

TABLE 17-2

List of Ideal Characteristics of a PFO/ASD Closure Device

Characteristic
Primary
Effectively close defect
Safe
Technically feasible
Secondary
Conform to septal curvature without distortion
Low profile
Low radial stiffness
Smooth transitions between implant and septal tissue
User-friendly
Have minimal metal surface area in frame (debatable)

PATIENT SELECTION

PFO Closure

Prevention of Paradoxic Embolism

The dominant indication for percutaneous PFO closure is the prevention of recurrent cerebral embolic events, in patients who present with cryptogenic stroke or transient ischemic attack (TIA) (Table 17-3). The prevailing hypothesis is that a significant percentage of cryptogenic strokes (i.e., up to 35%) are caused by paradoxical embolism of deep venous thrombus, across the PFO, into the systemic cerebral circulation. Only in rare instances where paradoxical embolism is visualized may we be certain of the stroke/TIA mechanism (9). In the remaining patients, pre-procedural evaluation is required to determine the likelihood that the clinical stroke, or TIA, occurred on the basis of paradoxical

TABLE 17-3

Indications for Percutaneous PFO Closure

Indication
Prevention of paradoxical embolism
Cryptogenic stroke and PFO
Prevention of neurologic complications in deep sea divers
Hypoxia secondary to right-to-left shunting
Platypnea-Orthodeoxia
Refractory hypoxia (e.g. post RV infarction, acute pulmonary embolism)
Migraine (with aura)

PFO, patent foramen ovale; RV, right ventricle.

TABLE 17-4

Features in Clinical History, PFO Anatomy, and Ancillary Investigations That Argue in Favor of Paradoxical Embolism as the Cause of Cryptogenic Stroke

Clinical
    Young age <40 years
    DVT temporally related to event
    No history of atrial arrhythmias
    No structural heart disease
    Absence of atherosclerotic risk factors
    No history of atherosclerosis in any vascular territory
PFO Anatomy
    Large PFO
    Large right-to-left shunt at rest/minimal provocation
    Associated atrial septal aneurysm
Ancillary Laboratory/Imaging Studies
    Multiple strokes in multiple cerebral territories
    Normal carotid ultrasound
    Negative hypercoagulability panel

DVT, deep venous thrombosis; PFO, patent foramen ovale.

embolism, and hence that closure of the PFO is likely to reduce the risk of recurrent events. This requires a synthesis of the clinical history of the patient, together with appropriate laboratory and imaging studies (Table 17-4).

Clinical

In younger patients, the presence of a PFO is a much stronger predictor of cryptogenic stroke than in older patients. A close, temporal relationship between lower or pelvic deep venous thrombosis and the cerebrovascular event strongly suggests paradoxical embolism. Important negative clinical characteristics supporting the mechanism of paradoxical embolism include: (1) the absence of atherosclerotic risk factors or proven atherosclerosis in any vascular territory, which lessens the likelihood that aortic atheroma or carotid/vertebral atheroma contributed to the event; and (2) the absence of structural heart disease (i.e., either valvular or myocardial) or a history of atrial fibrillation/flutter, which lessens the likelihood that embolism of left atrial or ventricular thrombus could occur.

PFO Anatomy

The anatomic attributes of the PFO, itself, are important in decision-making. A small number of studies have suggested that larger PFOs and those with larger right-to-left shunts that are provoked at rest, or minimal provocation, are more likely

to be associated with cryptogenic stoke, and by inference with recurrent stroke (10). The association of an atrial septal aneurysm with the PFO is a well established risk factor for cryptogenic stroke and probably warrants a more aggressive approach to PFO closure (4).

Imaging and Laboratory Studies

The routine imaging and laboratory studies performed prior to percutaneous PFO closure are listed in Table 17-5.

Many significant, hypercoagulable abnormalities will require oral anticoagulant therapy in the setting of a cryptogenic stroke, which reduces the indication for PFO closure. Brain imaging with computed tomography (CT) or magnetic resonance imaging (MRI) is useful to document not only the presence of the presenting stroke, but also determine if other 'silent strokes' have occurred in the past. The presence of multiple strokes in multiple cerebral territories argues in favor of an embolic etiology, and an aggressive approach to PFO closure.

Baseline Screen Recommended in Patients with Cryptogenic Stroke and PFO to Exclude Causes Other Than Paradoxical Embolism

Investigation
Hypercoagulability panel
Prothrombin time
Activated Partial Thromboplastin Time
Free Protein S
Total Protein S
Antithrombin III
Protein C
Factor V Leiden resistance
Cardiolipin antibody—IgA, IgM, IgG
Transesophageal ECHO
Rule out
— left atrial/left ventricular thrombus
— aortic atheroma
Carotid ultrasound
24-hour Holter monitor
— rule out paroxysmal atrial fibrillation/atrial flutter

It is clear that the decision regarding the likelihood that the cerebrovascular event occurred on the basis of paradoxical embolization requires careful consideration. An honest assessment of this likelihood is shared with the patient, together with the information on the therapeutic options. Currently, PFO closure by surgical means is difficult to justify, unless the patient is undergoing open-heart surgery for another primary indication. There are no randomized trials comparing medical therapy versus percutaneous closure for the prevention of recurrent events following cryptogenic stroke, in patients with PFO. In the absence of such data, the authors advocate a conservative approach, with the following indications for percutaneous PFO closure: (1) patients who have recurrent events while on antiplatelet or anticoagulant therapy, (2) patients who are intolerant of anticoagulant or antiplatelet therapy, (3) patients who express a strong preference for percutaneous closure, despite education regarding the absence of randomized data, and (4) patients who, on the basis of their PFO anatomy and physiology, or the presence of multiple prior strokes, are deemed at high risk for recurrent events.

Prevention of Neurologic Injury in Deep-Sea Divers

With ascent during both diving and altitude activities, the decrease in ambient pressure is associated with dissolved inert gas (i.e., usually nitrogen) coming out of solution from tissues and forming venous bubbles (11). Paradoxic embolization of these venous bubbles into the arterial circulation, across a PFO toward small subcortical cerebral vessels, resulting in cerebral infarcts, is thought to contribute in part to the neurologic complications of decompression sickness (DCS-Type II) and to asymptomatic cerebral infarcts in divers. The epidemiologic data supporting this hypothesis are somewhat inconsistent, although most would agree that the presence of a PFO increases the risk of Type II DCS two- or threefold, and increases the incidence of cerebral lesions in divers twofold. This has caused some organizations to advocate screening for PFO among divers, and closure of the PFO, in the primary and secondary prevention of Type II DCS and cerebral lesions. The effectiveness of these strategies has not been tested, and no clear guidelines with regard to the appropriateness of PFO closure in this group exist.

Hypoxia Syndromes: Platypnea-Orthodeoxia Syndrome (POS) and Persistent Hypoxia from Right-to-Left Shunts

Platypnea-orthodeoxia is a rare syndrome typically seen in elderly patients that is characterized by dyspnea and arterial oxygen desaturation induced or accentuated by the upright position. A subset of these cases is caused by accentuation of right-to-left shunting across the atrial septum. Associated conditions that are believed to contribute to the phenomenon are usually present including: prior pneumonectomy or lobectomy (i.e., right greater than left), recurrent pulmonary emboli, chronic lung disease, thoracic aortic aneurysm or ectasia, thoracic kyphoscoliosis, loculated pericardial effusion, and hypovolemia (12–15). Typically, these patients will have normal right atrial and pulmonary artery pressures suggesting that the mechanism of the right-to-left shunting is the result of preferential blood flow, streaming from the superior vena cava or more commonly, the inferior vena cava, toward the left atrium. Several cases series of percutaneous PFO closure for patients with POS have been described with a variety of closure devices (Amplatzer, CardioSEAL, Buttoned). The results have been encouraging, with improvement in symptoms and arterial oxygen saturation rates (i.e., to greater than 95%) in the upright posture, in most patients (12,15). Based on these data, it is reasonable to attempt percutaneous PFO closure in symptomatic patients with POS.

A distinct clinical entity from POS is persistent hypoxia, from right-to-left shunting associated with elevated right atrial or pulmonary artery pressures. This is typically encountered as an acute event in the setting of right ventricular infarction, acute pulmonary embolism, or acute tricuspid regurgitation (e.g., immediately post-cardiac transplantation). Since many of these events are associated with gradual resolution of elevated right atrial and pulmonary pressures, it is wise to adopt a conservative approach and avoid percutaneous PFO closure unless the hypoxia is severe.

Migraine

Recent epidemiologic and observational data suggest a possible link between the presence of a PFO and migraine with aura. In two separate studies involving young patients with cryptogenic stroke, the presence of a PFO was associated with an odds ratio for migraine of 1.75 and 4.8 respectively (16,17). A retrospective, observational study of patients who underwent PFO or ASD closure, reported either complete or partial resolution in 18 of 21 (86%) patients with migraine (18). While these data are provocative, more robust, randomized trial data are required before PFO closure should be recommended for patients with migraine with aura. It may be offered as a last resort for patients with incapacitating symptoms unresponsive to medical therapy.

Atrial Septal Defect Closure

There is considerably less controversy over the indications for percutaneous atrial septal defect (ASD) closure (19). Where there is a clinical indication to close a secundum-type defect, the only barrier to percutaneous closure is the technical feasibility of the procedure. Referral for surgery is reserved for those patients in whom percutaneous closure is not possible.

In adult patients, the presence of a significant left-to-right shunt (i.e., Qp/Qs greater than 1.5), together with evidence of right-sided volume overload, is generally considered grounds for ASD closure. In the absence of right-sided volume overload, the significance of the shunt should be questioned and a conservative approach may be warranted. Additionally, the presence of right-sided volume overload that is out of proportion to the ASD size should alert the operator to the possibility of anomalous pulmonary-venous drainage.

Patients with secundum ASDs and pulmonary hypertension represent an important and challenging subset. Vogel reported an incidence of pulmonary hypertension (i.e., mean pulmonary artery pressure of more than 30 mmHg) of about 9% in patients with secundum ASDs (20). While pulmonary hypertension was an exclusion factor in many of the ASD device registries, it is not a contraindication to ASD closure. The more critical determinant of feasibility is the pulmonary vascular resistance (PVR). Significant increases in the PVR will result in right-to-left shunting across the ASD, and closure of the ASD in this circumstance may result in elevation in pulmonary pressures and a worsening in clinical status. There is no widely accepted measurement in patients with ASDs and pulmonary hypertension that may be used to decide whether ASD closure will be safe or not. In a large multicenter study, the presence of a PVR greater than 7 Wood units, or the presence of a right-to-left shunt at the atrial level with a peripheral arterial saturation of less than 94%, were used as exclusion criteria (21). Other authors have suggested alternative thresholds of PVR of 10 to 12 Wood units and a resting oxygen saturation of less than 90% (19). These patients require careful assessment of all variables by an experienced interventionist, and a physician with an expertise in pulmonary hypertension, before proceeding with percutaneous closure.

Only secundum-type ASDs are recommended for percutaneous closure. As described above, these defects occupy a typical central location, and are easily identified by transesophageal echocardiography (TEE) or intracardiac echocardiography (ICE). Defects following prior ASD operative repair, or following valvular surgery (i.e., typically mitral valve) where an atrial septal opening was not adequately repaired, have also been successfully closed percutaneously.

The anatomy of the secundum or postoperative defect is also critical. Defects larger than 40 mm in maximal diameter are not amenable to percutaneous closure. It is important to be aware of which devices are available at your institution, since ASDs larger than 30 mm may only be closed with the Amplatzer septal-occluder device (see below) and this may limit one's ability to offer percutaneous closure for such defects. For defects smaller than 25 mm, this is not an issue, as all devices come in sizes capable of closing these defects. The distance of the margin between the defect and adjacent structures (i.e., aortic root, superior and inferior vena cava, coronary sinus, mitral valve, right upper pulmonary vein) is also a critical factor. Generally, it is advised that a 5 mm margin with these structures is required. In the case of a deficient aortic rim, the ability to splay the right and left atrial components over the aortic root may allow defect closure with a lesser margin. Similarly, a lesser margin to the coronary sinus may be tolerated, as the large size of the coronary sinus ostium will generally allow overlap of the device without compromise of venous flow. It is not advisable to close a defect with two or more deficient rims, as this may result in device instability, and either immediate or delayed device embolization (22).

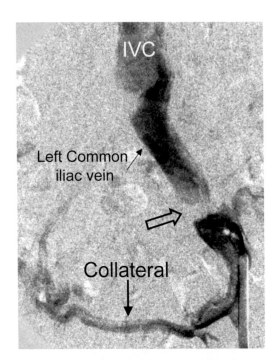

FIGURE 17-9 ● Left femoral venous angiogram from a patient undergoing percutaneous PFO closure demonstrating a filling defect in the left common iliac vein *(arrow)* (presumably thrombus) with collateral formation toward the contralateral iliac veins.

INTERVENTIONAL TECHNIQUE

Pre-procedure Care and Venous Access

Prior to the procedure, our practice is to administer aspirin, 325 mg daily, and clopidogrel, 75 mg daily (i.e., following a loading dose of 300 mg), for a minimum of 3 days. Just prior to the procedure, 1 gm of intravenous cefazolin is routinely administered (or 1 gm of vancomycin, intravenously, in penicillin-allergic patients). At the authors' institution, all procedures in adults are performed under conscious sedation.

When ICE is planned, access in the left femoral vein is obtained, and a long (i.e., 35 cm) 11-Fr sheath is inserted with its tip in the distal,

inferior vena cava to facilitate passage of the ICE catheter, distal to the pelvic veins. Venous access is obtained in the right femoral vein for device delivery, and the sheath size inserted will depend on the device to be used, and the predicted defect size. Caution is warranted during the insertion of venous sheaths, particularly in patients with a history of deep venous thrombosis. The authors have encountered two cases of previously unrecognized iliac vein thrombosis that did not allow venous access on that side (Fig. 17-9).

Following insertion of the venous sheaths, a bolus of intravenous heparin is administered in a dose of 70 mg/kg of body weight, to achieve an activated clotting time (ACT) of approximately 300 seconds.

Imaging Guidance—TEE and ICE

Most operators use adjunctive echocardiographic imaging to guide percutaneous PFO and ASD closure procedures. ICE has significant advantages over TEE: (1) it requires no added sedation, whereas TEE requires heavy sedation at a minimum, and in some cases, general anesthesia;

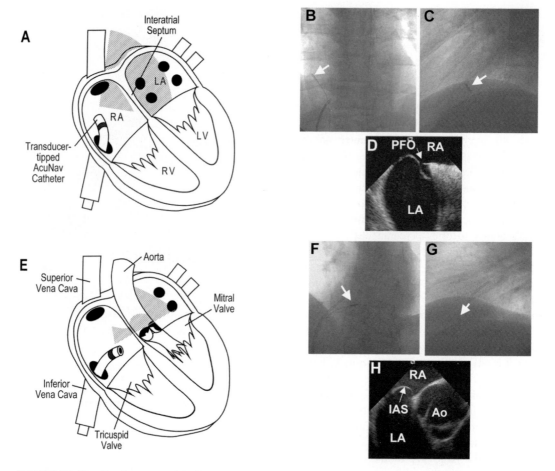

FIGURE 17-10 ● Illustration of the longitudinal (A–D) and cross-sectional (E–H) views of the atrial septum generated using intracardiac echocardiography (ICE). Arrows point to the position of the catheter tip of the ICE probe in PA (B,F) and lateral (C,G) fluoroscopic views. RA, right atrium; LA, left atrium; RV, right ventricle; LV, left ventricle; PFO, patent foramen ovale; Ao, aorta; IAS, interatrial septum.

(2) ICE provides superior visualization of the inferoposterior portion of the septum, compared to TEE; and (3) ICE gives the interventionist more autonomy during the procedure, which results in greater procedural insight for the operator, and more efficient use of time.

While it is not possible to describe ICE comprehensively in this chapter, the basic fundamentals are outlined, since the interventionist is responsible for the generation and interpretation of ICE images (Fig. 17-10).

ICE is currently performed using a 10-Fr Acunav diagnostic ultrasound catheter transducer that is interfaced with the Sequioa, Aspen, or Cypress ultrasound imaging platforms. The catheter has a directionally controlled tip that may be moved in four directions (anterior, posterior, right, and left), with an excursion of 160° in each direction. Within the catheter tip, there is a multifrequency 5.0 MHz to 10 MHz, 64-element vector, phased-array transducer that provides high-resolution 2D and Doppler imaging (including color Doppler). The scan plane is along the axis of the catheter, and by varying the frequency of the transducer, the depth of tissue penetration may vary from 2 cm to 12 cm.

During PFO/ASD closure procedures, two ICE views are particularly helpful (Fig. 17-10): (1) longitudinal view of the septum—this view is generated by advancing the ICE probe to the level of the mid-atrium, rotating the entire catheter clockwise, and moving the tip to the right (i.e., lateral retroflexion) and slightly anterior; and

(2) short-axis view of the septum—this view is generated by rotation of the entire catheter clockwise followed by rotation of the catheter tip to the right and arteriorly. In this position the catheter tip is very near or through the tricuspid valve. In most cases, these two views will allow an adequate assessment of the septal defect at baseline, and an assessment of the device position following deployment. Either of these two views will also function as a working view to monitor the various steps of the procedure. There is a locking mechanism that stabilizes the catheter tip position for this purpose.

Assessment of Qp/Qs and Pulmonary Angiography

Prior to ASD closure, our practice is to perform a comprehensive assessment of oxygen saturations from the innominate vein, SVC, IVC, right atria and ventricle, and pulmonary artery, using a Goodale-Lubin catheter. It is important to ensure that the patient is not on supplemental oxygen, for these measurements. This allows an assessment of the Qp/Qs, and confirms the location of the step-up in oxygen saturation, at the level of the atrial septum. Anomalous pulmonary venous drainage to the innominate vein, SVC (most commonly), or IVC will often be detected with careful adherence to this practice.

Some operators also perform a pulmonary, or left atrial angiogram, prior to ASD closure. Pulmonary angiography may be performed with an NIH catheter or angiographic Berman catheter, placed directly in the pulmonary artery, or with a similar catheter in the IVC or right atrium. The main purpose of pulmonary angiography is to exclude the presence of anomalous pulmonary venous drainage, which will be manifest by early filling of the right atrium, relative to the left atrium during the delayed levo-phase. The PA or left anterior oblique (LAO) cranial view also clearly documents the presence of the left-to-right shunt across the ASD (Fig. 17-11).

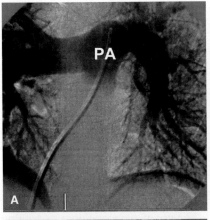

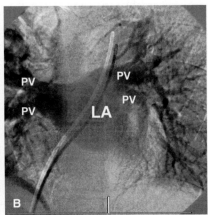

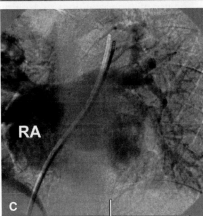

FIGURE 17-11 ● Pulmonary angiogram (LAO cranial view) from a patient with an atrial septal defect demonstrating initial filling of the pulmonary arteries (A), followed by filling of the pulmonary veins and left atrium, and subsequent filling of the right atrium due to left-to-right shunting across the defect. PA, pulmonary artery; PV, pulmonary vein; LA, left atrium; RA, right atrium.

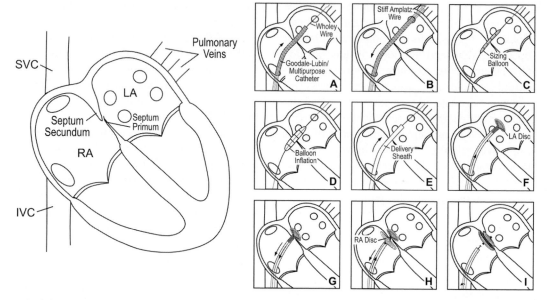

FIGURE 17-12 ● **Schematic of the technique used to perform percutaneous PFO or ASD closure.** Device depicted is an Amplatzer PFO occluder. See text for complete details. RA, right atrium; LA, left atrium. SVC, superior vena cava; IVC, inferior vena cava.

Left atrial angiography is performed with the angiographic catheter at the right upper pulmonary vein/left atrial junction. This will not exclude anomalous pulmonary venous drainage, but will give good definition of the left-to-right shunt, across the ASD (LAO cranial view).

Delivering the Stiff Support Wire into the Pulmonary Vein

A 5 Fr Multipurpose or Goodale-Lubin catheter is advanced into the right atrium over an 0.035″ wire. The catheter is then directed to the left and posteriorly (with clockwise rotation), and advanced across the PFO or ASD (Fig. 17-12[A]). This is where the use of biplane angiography is useful, with the lateral camera allowing easy determination of the posterior orientation. The catheter is then manipulated into the left upper pulmonary vein (Fig. 17-11[B]). Since the pulmonary veins are located posteriorly in the left atrium, direct cannulation is usually achieved by further clockwise rotation and advancement of the catheter. When this is not possible, a soft-tipped Wholey wire is used to find the ostium of the pulmonary vein, using the catheter to direct the wire. This minimizes the risk of trauma or

arrhythmias from manipulation in the left atrium. When the catheter tip is in the left upper pulmonary vein, it will extend beyond the left margin of the cardiac silhouette. If any doubt exists regarding the catheter position, one may directly inject contrast to visualize the pulmonary vein. The Wholey wire is then exchanged for a stiff Amplatz wire whose tip (in a J shape) is positioned 3 to 5 cm into the pulmonary vein, to ensure stability, and the catheter is then withdrawn.

Sizing Balloons and Defect Stretch Diameters

The use of sizing balloons to determine the size of the PFO defect, prior to closure, is controversial. During our initial experience, the authors performed balloon sizing prior to all PFO closures. This experience demonstrated that the stretch diameter of the PFO may vary markedly, and reinforced the concept of varying lengths of the PFO tunnel in different patients (Fig. 17-13). However, the findings rarely altered the decision regarding device size, and the authors have largely abandoned this step prior to PFO closure.

In contrast, it is mandatory to measure the defect size prior to ASD closure, as the stretch

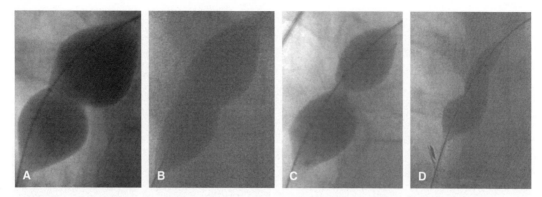

FIGURE 17-13 ● **Fluoroscopic images (PA) obtained after balloon inflation across various PFOs.** Note the variability in size and shape of the stretch diameter of the defect, and the cylindric tunnel appearance of the PFO in image D. PA, posteroanterior; PFO, patent foramen ovale.

diameter of the defect is critical in deciding device size. There are two basic methods used to assess the defect size. The first is a 'static' balloon measurement technique, using a highly compliant balloon that is inflated across the defect (e.g., Amplatzer, NuMED PTS) (Table 17-6) until an indentation is visualized. The waist is then measured fluoroscopically, using calibration markers on the balloon shaft or by ICE/TEE (Fig. 17-14).

Alternatively, a less compliant balloon (e.g., Meditech) is inflated in the left atrium, to a diameter about 5 mm greater than the estimated ASD

diameter. The balloon is then withdrawn onto the atrial septum; while the operator maintains continuous traction on the balloon, an assistant slowly deflates the balloon until it pops through the defect. The volume of contrast medium in the balloon, at this point, is carefully recorded and the balloon deflated. Outside of the body, the balloon is reinflated with the same volume of contrast, and a sizing plate is used to determine the stretch diameter of the defect.

The static technique does not perform as well in sizing large ASDs, owing to the tendency of

TABLE 17-6

Description of Balloons Used to Perform Static Technique for Assessment of Stretch Diameter of PFO/ASD

Amplatzer Balloon	Max Defect Size (mm)	Max Inflated Balloon Diameter (mm)	Balloon Length (cm)	Usable Length (cm)	Guidewire (inch)	Shaft Size (Fr)	Max Balloon Inflation Volume (cc)
24	≤22	30–31	4.5	70	0.035	7.0	30
34	≤40	42–43	5.5	70	0.035	7.0	90

NuMed PTS®	Balloon Length (cm)	Usable Length (cm)	Guidewire (inch)	Shaft Size (Fr)	Rated burst pressure (atm)
20	3.0	80	0.035	8	1.5
25	3.0	80	0.035	8	1.5
30	3.0	80	0.035	8	1.0
40	3.0 and 5.0	80	0.035	8	0.5

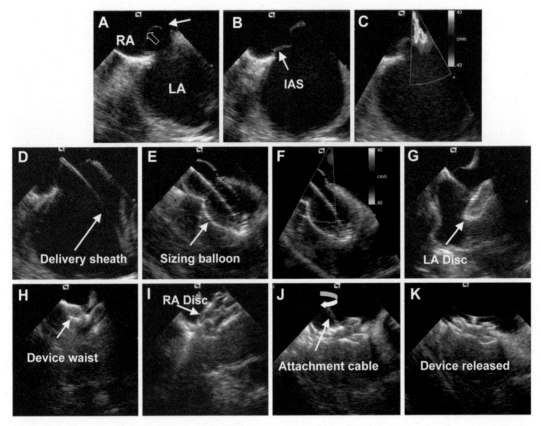

FIGURE 17-14 ● Sequential intracardiac echocardiographic images obtained from a patient undergoing closure of an atrial septal defect *(arrow in Figure A)* using an Amplatzer ASD occluder device. RA, right atrium; LA, left atrium; IAS, interatrial septum. Curved arrow: device is detached by performing counterclockwise rotation of the delivery cable. Open arrow: aneurysmal septum.

the balloon to 'melon-seed' (i.e., slip into right or left atrium) across the defect. There may also be a tendency to oversize the defect, using this technique. Despite these limitations, the static method is the most widely practiced because it is technically simple to perform.

From a technical standpoint, the sizing balloon is advanced directly over the stiff support wire, though the femoral venous access sheath (Fig. 17-12[C]). Using currently available sizing balloons, the sheath will need to be at least 8 Fr to accommodate the balloon. Some operators prepare the balloon outside the body by filling the balloon with contrast and deflating it again on multiple occasions. This is done as a precaution to remove air from the balloon in case the balloon ruptures during inflation, although this is rare. In practice, the inflation-deflation of the balloon prior to insertion makes

delivery of the balloon though the sheath more difficult (i.e., generally requires a 10-Fr sheath).

It is important to use dilute contrast (i.e., 25% contrast, 75% saline) in these balloons, which serves to facilitate balloon inflation and deflation. One must also exercise care to avoid trauma to the septum during balloon inflation. During balloon inflation in one ASD, the authors observed a clear expansion of the defect size, most likely due to fusion of the defect with fenestrations at the defect margin (Fig. 17-15). While this is generally not a problem, it did result in the use of a larger device size than would otherwise have been required. Frank tearing of the septum is also possible with the use of the sizing balloon, and is to be avoided. One should also ensure that the balloon is fully deflated prior to removal.

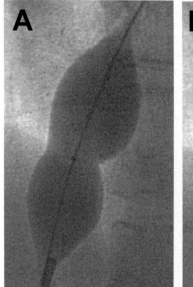
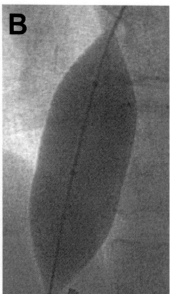

FIGURE 17-15 ●
Fluoroscopic image obtained
following sizing balloon inflation
across an atrial septal defect **(A)**.
Subsequent inflation of the balloon
across the defect resulted in
expansion of the defect **(B)**, likely
due to the presence of
fenestrations at the margin of the
defect.

The Delivery Sheath

Following removal of the sizing balloon, the femoral sheath is removed and the delivery sheath is inserted. Many devices come with a proprietary delivery sheath. However, a standard Mullins sheath may also be used. In either case, the sheath should be carefully flushed prior to insertion. Inserting a mandrel (i.e., wire introducer) into the valve of the sheath, and flushing from the side arm, helps to eliminate air that tends to lodge in the sheath between the side arm and the valve. To reduce the risk of arterial-air embolism, it is advisable to remove the dilator from the delivery sheath in the inferior vena cava, and flush the sheath in that location. Injection of about 5 to 10 mL of contrast medium to fill the delivery sheath will then allow the operator to confirm the absence of air bubbles in the sheath, using fluoroscopy. The sheath is then advanced such that its tip lies in the mid-left atrium (Figure 17-11[E]). This attention to detail is required to eliminate the risk of producing air emboli.

Device Size, Preparation, Delivery, and Deployment

Choosing the appropriate device size is an important consideration from a safety and economic standpoint. Extreme care is required in deciding the device size for ASD closure, since the risk of device embolization arising from undersizing, and mechanical complications as a result of over sizing, is so much greater in this setting compared to PFO closure. All of the available devices have recommendations for device size, based on measurement of the stretch diameter of atrial septal defects (i.e., the device size: stretch diameter ratio) (Table 17-7).

In general, the ratio is between 1.5 to 2.0:1, and is slightly less for self-centering devices, compared to non-centering devices. The Amplatzer device is the exception, with the device size chosen being about 2 mm larger than the stretch diameter of the defect. Most current devices will not allow closure of defects with stretch diameters of more than 25 mm. Again, the Amplatzer septal occluder is the exception, owing to its unique property of stenting the defect with the waist of the device, and may be used for defects with stretch diameters up to 40 mm.

The decision regarding device size for PFO closure is simpler than that for ASD closure. Some operators advocate a one-size-fits-all strategy, whereas others advocate using a slightly larger device for patients with an associated floppy or aneurysmal septum, with a long interatrial channel, or a larger stretch diameter PFO size. The typical stretch diameter of a PFO will be approximately 5 mm to 15 mm. For those devices with a device size: stretch diameter

TABLE 17-7

Suggested Device Size Recommended, Based on Stretch Balloon-Diameter Measurement of ASD for the Most Commonly Used Devices

Device	Device Size: Stretch Diameter Ratio	Maximum Stretch Diameter That May Be Safely Closed (mm)
Amplatzer septal occluder	1–2 mm larger than SD	40
CardioSEAL	1.5–2.2:1[59]	25
STARFlex	1.6:1[60]	25
HELEX	1.6:1 [61]	22
Buttoned	1.8–2:1[62]	30

SD: stretch diameter

ratio of between 1.5 to 2.0:1 (e.g., CardioSEAL, STARFlex, HELEX, PFO-Star), it is reasonable to use a 26-mm to 30-mm device for PFO closure, and to use some judgment in relation to the anatomy of the PFO. In the case of the Amplatzer device, our practice is to use the 25-mm device in most instances, and to use the 35-mm device where the anatomic features listed above are present, to a significant degree.

All devices have specific issues related to device preparation and delivery. Current designs require the device be attached to a delivery cable. Different attachment mechanisms exist, such as a screw-in mechanism in the case of the Amplatzer device, a pin-to-pin locking mechanism for the CardioSEAL and STARFlex devices, and attachment to a delivery forceps in the case of the PFO-Star device. Following attachment, the device is withdrawn into a short delivery catheter, for insertion into the delivery sheath. All of the devices require careful flushing and insertion into the delivery sheath under heparinized saline, to minimize the risk of air embolization.

The device is advanced through the delivery sheath and the left atrial component is deployed into the left atrium (Fig. 17-12[F]). Both the delivery cable and sheath are then withdrawn as a unit, until the left atrial component abuts the septum (Fig. 17-12[G]). Advancement of the delivery cable and withdrawal of the delivery sheath then results in deployment of the right atrial component (Fig. 17-12[H]).

At this point, it is imperative that the operator ensures that the device is in its proper position and is secure. Using echocardiography, this involves visualizing the atrial septum between both the right and left atrial components both superoanterior and inferoposterior to the defect. Because of the thicker septum secundum superoanterior to the defect, and the tendency for the right and left atrial components to splay over the aortic root, the task of ensuring proper device placement superoanterior to the defect is usually straightforward. Inferoposteriorly, this may be more difficult due to the generally thin septum primum and careful manipulation of the echo probe to ensure adequate imaging of this area is required. Usually, the issue of doubt is whether the right atrial component is truly on the right atrial side of the septum. This may be inferred if the right atrial component does not move in unison with the left atrial component. For operators who do not use echocardiography during the procedure, a right atrial or IVC injection of contrast is performed (i.e., 20-mL to 30-mL power injection) in the LAO projection, to confirm the position of the device (Fig. 17-16).

Using this technique, it is important to examine the position of the device during opacification of the right atrium, to confirm adequate placement. Additionally, under fluoroscopy alone, a 'pacman' sign is typically created by the splaying apart of the superior portions of the right and left atrial components of the device, by the thicker septum secundum located superiorly (Fig. 17-17) (23). Failure to observe this appearance should raise serious concern that the left and right

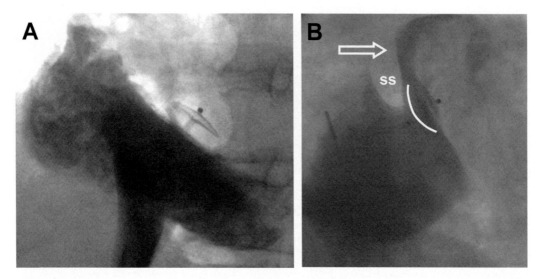

FIGURE 17-16 ● **A.** Inferior vena cavogram following placement of Amplatzer PFO occluder demonstrating normal placement of the device with the right and left atrial discs in the right and left atria respectively. **B.** Inferior vena cavogram following placement of Amplatzer PFO occluder demonstrating the right and left atrial discs in the left atrium, persistence of the PFO with prominent right-to-left shunting (open arrow), and clear evidence that the superior portion of the device does not straddle the thickened septum secundum. SS, septum secundum; solid curved black line, delineates the surface of the right atrial disc.

atrial components of the device are in one atrial chamber.

Having confirmed appropriate positioning of the device, the stability of the device is discerned by advancing and retracting the delivery cable that remains attached to the device (Fig. 17-18).

The attempt is to reproduce an exaggeration of the movement of the deployed device, and discern the risk of embolization. Once stabil-

ity has been confirmed, the device is released by removing the delivery catheter from the device, the mechanism of which will depend on the attachment mechanism. Following release, the device usually assumes a more superior orientation, owing to release of the inferior traction created by the attachment to the delivery catheter (Fig. 17-18[E]). This usually results in a better alignment of the device, in relation to the septum.

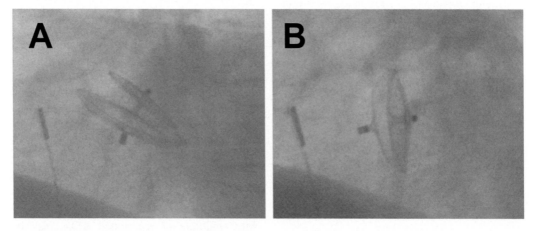

FIGURE 17-17 ● Lateral fluoroscopic image of an Amplatzer PFO occluder device demonstrating the normal 'PACMAN' sign appearance of the device when the superior portions of the right and left atrial discs straddle the septum secundum **(A).** When the superior portions of the right and left atrial discs fail to straddle the septum secundum, the appearance in image **B** is seen.

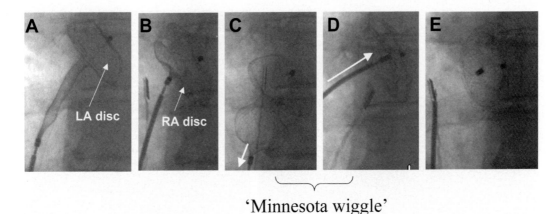

'Minnesota wiggle'

FIGURE 17-18 ● Sequential fluoroscopic images (PA) showing typical deployment of Amplatzer ASD occluder device. Pulling downward (C) and pushing forward (D) on the device following deployment of the right atrial disc is termed the 'Minnesota wiggle' and is used by some operators to assess device stability. Note the more superior orientation of the device following detachment (compare B with E). LA, left atrium; RA, right atrium; PA, posteroanterior.

Postprocedural Care

Following the procedure, all venous sheaths are required using manual pressure to achieve hemostasis, and specifically the use of protamine to reverse the anticoagulant effects of heparin is avoided. Patients are generally admitted for observation, overnight. Two further doses of cefazolin or vancomycin are administered intravenously at 8 and 16 hours following the procedure. A surface echocardiogram, and CXR (PA and lateral) is performed on the day of discharge, to confirm device placement, and assess the baseline degree of shunting across the device (if any).

Patients are discharged on aspirin, 325 mg daily, and clopidogrel, 75 mg daily, for a minimum treatment duration of 6 months. This is entirely empiric, and the medical regimen may need to be modified according to the clinical situation. Patients are advised to avoid physical-contact sports for a minimum of 1 month following the procedure, as individual cases of device embolization have been linked with such activity. In addition, all patients are advised to practice endocarditis prophylaxis, for a minimum of 6 months following device implantation.

Challenging Technical Subsets

Large ASDs with Deficient Rims

Large ASDs (i.e., greater than 30 mm) with deficient rims remain a challenging subset that often

requires some modification to the technique described above. An important concept in closing such defects is that the chances of success are maximized if one may maintain the device in a plane perpendicular to the defect (Fig. 17-19) (24).

Pulling the device across the defect, at an angle, increases the risk that the left atrial disc (i.e., usually the superior margin) will cross the defect and come to rest on the right atrial side. There are two fundamental approaches to this problem. The first is to alter the curve of the delivery sheath. This may be accomplished by withdrawing the sheath, and remolding it with the dilator in place to create a greater curve, or by using a different, preformed, delivery sheath (e.g. Hausdorf Sheath). The second approach is to alter the orientation of the device, with respect to the septum, by applying clockwise or counterclockwise rotation to the delivery sheath before deployment of the left atrial disc, and maintaining this position during pull back of the left atrial disc onto the septum. Guidance from ICE or TEE will allow the operator to determine which maneuver results in the optimal orientation of the device, with respect to the septum.

Multiple or Fenestrated ASDs

Most multiple or fenestrated ASDs may be treated with a single closure device. For umbrella-type devices (e.g., CardioSEAL), this is achieved because the right and left atrial

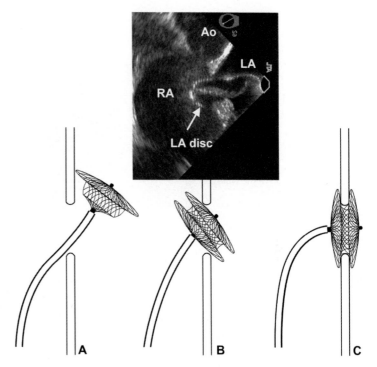

FIGURE 17-19 ● Illustration of the tendency of the left atrial component of ASD closure devices to come through the defect in the absence of a perpendicular orientation with the septum. TEE image (rotated to allow orientation with the schematic picture) demonstrates this phenomenon in a real case. Ao, aorta; RA, right atrium; LA, left atrium.

components of the device are generally large enough that they cover adjacent defects or fenestrations. The fenestrated Amplatzer device, a special fenestrated device that contains the waist of the Amplatzer PFO-occluder, but has the left and right atrial disc configuration of the Amplatzer ASD-occluder, is an alternative option. In the absence of this type of device, a PFO-occluder seems a better option in such cases, rather than using multiple, smaller, ASD-occluder devices. For multiple and fenestrated ASDs, it is ideal to try to position the waist of the device through the central area of the fossa, although this is not always possible. Most operators would also use a slightly larger device in such circumstances, to maximize the chance of closure of more peripheral defects.

For multiple, discrete defects that are widely separated (i.e., defined as more than 7 mm apart), two separate devices are often required. In this circumstance, venous access from both groins is obtained, and both defects are crossed with sizing balloons (Fig. 17-20[A]) and the stretch diameters measured.

With both balloons inflated, careful TEE or ICE examination with color flow should document the absence of any further left-to-right shunting across the septum. The smaller defect is generally closed first, followed by the second-larger defect (Fig. 17-20[B]). This approach appears to work well in cases where there is an adequate rim of tissue between the defects and in the absence of aneurysmal tissue. When these conditions do not apply, a suggested approach is to fuse both defects together, using a balloon atrial-septostomy technique, and then close the new larger defect with an appropriately sized device (25).

Device Entrapment by Right Atrial Structures

Problems created by right atrial structures, such as Chiari networks and redundant Eustachian valves, have been reported in the literature. The main problem posed by these structures is that they, rarely, entrap the right atrial component of the device during deployment, and result in incomplete opposition of the right atrial component of the device, with the right atrial surface of the septum (Fig. 17-21). One author has suggested the use of a directionally controlled radiofrequency ablation catheter (e.g. Stinger catheter) to help displace these structures (26), although exercising some care not to dislodge the device during these maneuvers is warranted.

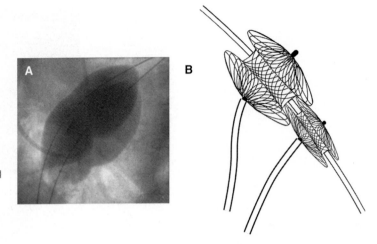

FIGURE 17-20 ● **A.** Fluoroscopic image following balloon inflation across two separate atrial septal defects. **B.** Schematic illustration of the typical placement of devices in such cases: the smaller defect is closed first followed by the larger defect such that the discs of the larger device straddle the smaller device.

Inferior Vena Caval Filters

A small percentage (less than 10%) of cryptogenic stroke patients referred for PFO closure will have had a documented deep venous thrombosis, and some will have received an IVC filter. The presence of an IVC filter is not a contraindication to percutaneous PFO closure. The authors have successfully closed PFOs using femoral venous access in several patients. The practice is to obtain femoral venous access with a short sheath, and perform an inferior vena cavogram, to confirm the absence of significant thrombus on the filter (Fig. 17-22).

Thereafter, a Wholey wire is carefully passed across the filter, and the short sheath exchanged for a long sheath (i.e., usually 35 or 55 cm, in length) within its tip, located between the IVC filter and the right atrium. The remainder of the procedure is identical to that described above. Of note, the ICE probe may also be carefully manipulated across an IVC filter using fluoroscopic guidance, or through a long sheath placed across the IVC filter.

Tunnel-Type PFOs

A number of operators have advocated a unique approach to closing PFOs in patients with long interatrial channels. The concern of these operators is that the oblique interatrial channel results in poor apposition of the left atrial component to the septum, because these devices were designed to close flat hole type defects. This issue is overcome by performing a transseptal puncture of the septum primum, thus creating a flat-hole defect,

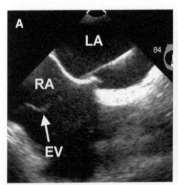
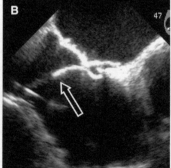
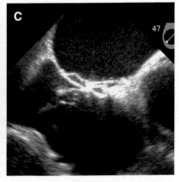

FIGURE 17-21 ● **A–C.** Series of TEE images demonstrating interference by a prominent Eustachian valve remnant **(A)** with deployment of the right atrial component of a CardioSEAL device (open arrow in **B**). Gentle manipulation of the device resulted in relief of this constraint and satisfactory device position **(C).** EV, Eustachian valve; RA, right atrium; LA, left atrium.

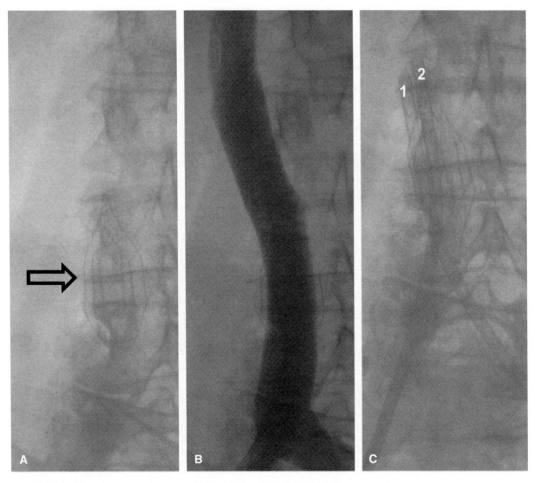

FIGURE 17-22 ● Illustration of steps taken prior to percutaneous PFO/ASD closure in patients with IVC filters (*open arrow in **A***). An IVC gram is performed to confirm the absence of overt thrombus **(B),** and sheaths are placed across the filter to allow for passage of the device and ICE probe (1,2 in C).

and facilitating a more appropriate device position across the septum (Fig. 17-23) (27,28).

CLINICAL OUTCOMES OF PERCUTANEOUS ASD/PFO CLOSURE

With rare exception, the technical feasibility of device placement for PFO closure is consistently 100%, in large case series. Based on intention to treat, the success rate of device placement for ASD closure is usually less (about 95%) because of extra challenges posed particularly by anatomically complex lesions, namely, large defects, deficient rims, multiple defects, and septal aneurysms (8,22,29,30).

Following successful device placement, the clinical outcome of the procedure is then determined by the balance between the success in treating the underlying condition (i.e. efficacy) and the risk of procedural and post-procedural complications.

Efficacy

The effectiveness outcome measures following PFO closure and ASD closure are distinct. Following PFO closure for treatment of paradoxical embolism, the primary outcome measure of interest is the incidence of recurrent TIA, stroke, or peripheral embolization. Currently, these data are derived from several registries, which have reported an incidence of recurrent TIA or stroke, at 1 year, of 0 to 4.9%. In the absence of randomized

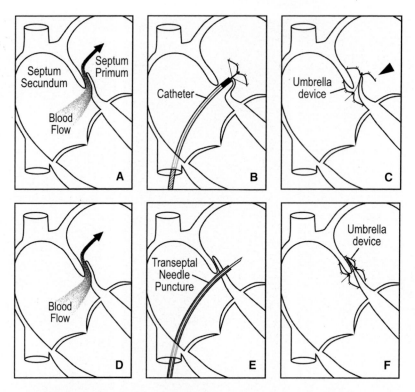

FIGURE 17-23 ● Illustration of the difficulty in placement of PFO closure devices in tunnel-type PFOs. The oblique orientation of the tunnel may result in failure of apposition of the device against the septum **(A–C)**. This is overcome by transseptal puncture, which creates a flat defect, facilitating adequate apposition of the device against the septum **(D–F)**. Reproduced with permission from Ruiz CE, Alboliras ET, Pophal SG. The puncture technique: a new method for transcatheter closure of patent foramen ovale. *Catheter Cardiovasc Interv* 2001;53(3):369–372. PFO, patent foramen ovale.

data, it is unclear whether this represents a superior, equivalent, or inferior outcome to medical therapy alone, but nonrandomized data suggest that it is superior (29).

The variability in outcome between studies is likely related to issues of patient selection, adequacy of follow-up evaluation, and variations in operator experience and type of device used. A useful, surrogate, end-point of efficacy is the elimination of right-to-left shunting. Immediately following device placement, complete closure is achieved in 40 to 80% of cases. In most studies, the rate of complete closure at 6 months approaches 95 to 100%. Most residual shunts are small, but in rare cases, placement of a second device for the treatment of significant residual shunts is required. Although individual studies have suggested that the presence of any residual right-to-left shunt is associated with an increased risk of recurrent events (30), this is not a

consistent finding. This inconsistency is concerning, as it calls into question the hypothesis that supports percutaneous PFO closure. However, it seems likely that relatively small sample sizes and numbers of outcomes, together with variability in the determination of right-to-left shunting, may explain much of this inconsistency.

For ASD closure procedures, the goal is to eliminate left-to-right shunting, which will relieve right-sided volume overload, and prevent future pulmonary vascular injury and atrial arrhythmias, and ultimately improve quality of life and the functional status of the patient. Percutaneous closure is associated with a complete closure rate of 95 to 100% at least 6 months from the time of device implantation (21,33–35). Most residual shunts are trivial or small, and do not warrant any further therapy. There are some data to suggest that residual shunts, following use of the CardioSEAL and STARFlex devices, may be more frequent than with the use of the ASO device, but it seems unlikely that this increased rate of largely minor shunts will translate into any clinical effect.

Relief of volume overload is reflected by a reduction in right atrial (RA) and right ventricular (RV) volume, and right ventricular end-diastolic diameter measurements (36–38). Studies that have examined the timing of these changes have been inconsistent, with one study demonstrating the bulk of these changes in the first 24 hours following closure (36), and another demonstrating the majority of change between 24 hours and 3 to 6 months following the procedure (37). The presence of minor residual shunts did not impact these changes in RA and RV dimensions. Compared with controls, the RV volume returned to normal but the RA area remained larger than normal at 24-month follow-up evaluation (37). Other notable alterations noted following percutaneous ASD closure include a decrease in the left atrial area, and an increase in left ventricular dimensions and function, presumably due to improved left ventricular filling (36).

The influence of percutaneous ASD closure, in patients with pulmonary hypertension, mirrors that seen with surgical closure. In a retrospective analysis of 29 patients with secundum-type ASD with pulmonary hypertension, who were undergoing percutaneous closure, the mean-peak systolic pulmonary pressure decreased from 64 ± 23 mmHg, at baseline, to 34 ± 11 mmHg at a mean follow-up evaluation of 21 months (39). Because of the limited, long-term follow-up monitoring in patients with percutaneous ASD closure, the influence on the long-term risk of atrial fibrillation and other atrial arrhythmias is unknown. It is reasonable to extrapolate from the older surgical literature and speculate that early percutaneous closure of ASDs, which halts and promotes the regression of pulmonary hypertension, will be associated with a reduced risk of subsequent atrial arrhythmias (40).

COMPLICATIONS

While the safety of percutaneous PFO and ASD closure has improved dramatically over the last decade, there remains a definite risk associated with these procedures. Although there is a lack of uniformity in the definition and reporting of complications following percutaneous PFO and ASD closure, a reasonable estimate of the risk of a major or minor complication associated with device implantation is about 0.5 to 1.5% and approximately 5 to 8%, respectively (31,41). Most of these complications apply to all devices and to both PFO and ASD closure. The low frequency of individual complications likely explains the variability in the reported frequencies between different studies.

Device Embolization

This is one of the feared complications of percutaneous PFO and particularly of ASD closure. It may occur during the procedure (i.e., just following detachment of the device from the delivery mechanism) or at any time following the procedure (i.e., in the first few weeks to months). Operator error certainly plays a role in device embolization; the use of an undersized device during ASD closure, and failure to ensure the appropriate placement of the right and left atrial components of the device on either side of the septum in all planes, are likely the key errors contributing to device embolization. It is intuitive that earlier generations of devices are also more susceptible to this risk as the inventors of the devices and operators discover the design flaws of a particular device. Additional factors include mechanical defects or operator error in the attachment mechanism, and anatomic features of the PFO or ASD, such as the presence of a septal aneurysm, a large ASD with deficient rims, or a PFO with a long interatrial channel. Embolization may occur leftward, into the left atrium, where it may lodge, or cross the mitral valve to the left ventricle. Further migration is generally constrained by the left ventricular outflow tract, although embolization to the descending thoracic and abdominal aorta has been reported (42). Alternatively, the device may dislodge into the right atrium, and travel toward the right ventricle or pulmonary artery, where it is typically constrained.

Retrieval may be performed percutaneously or surgically. It should be appreciated that retrieval of the Amplatzer devices is likely more difficult than the remaining devices because of the need to grasp the relatively small right atrial screw pin in order to allow retraction of the device into the retrieval sheath. If the device is mobile, as it is likely to be in the cardiac chambers, this is expected to be a very difficult task, and early surgical assistance should be sought. When percutaneous retrieval is attempted, it is prudent to place a large retrieval sheath (i.e., 14 Fr) close to the location of the device. Most operators use snare devices and, rarely, forceps devices to capture the errant device, but forceps should be used with caution, owing to the increased risk of perforation.

Thrombus Formation

Device thrombosis is an uncommon but feared complication of percutaneous PFO/ASD closure. Based on prospective TEE data with an older device (i.e., ASDOS), it is thought that a layer of thrombotic material manifest by a plane layer of echodense material (i.e., 2 to 8 mm in thickness) is normal for 1 to 2 months following device placement (43). Pathologic thrombus formation is diagnosed by the presence of a nonplane, partially mobile, spheric structure adherent to the surface of the device. Thrombus has been observed on both the right or left atrial components of the device, and both during the procedure and at widely varying periods following the procedure (44–46). Fortunately, most of these events have been asymptomatic, but the risk of neurologic sequelae for left-sided thrombus is probably high. A recent analysis of 1000 consecutive patients from a single center, who were undergoing percutaneous PFO/ASD closure, suggests that the risk of device thrombosis is increased with umbrella-type devices (i.e., 5 to 7%) compared with the Amplatzer-type devices (0%) (47).

Once diagnosed, management is generally with anticoagulation, initially intravenously with heparin, followed by prolonged oral anticoagulation with warfarin. Complete resolution of thrombus is usually observed over the course of 4 to 6 weeks. The use of thrombolytic agents, with or without glycoprotein IIb/IIIa inhibitors, in this setting is controversial, and should be reserved for exceptional circumstances (34). Preprocedural dual antiplatelet therapy, for 2 to 3 days, with aspirin and clopidogrel, together with aggressive intraprocedural anticoagulation (i.e., ACT longer than 300 seconds) may eliminate some of the risk of procedure-related thrombus. It also makes intuitive sense that a similarly aggressive dual antiplatelet regimen following device placement will provide better protection against left-sided arterial thrombus formation, compared to anticoagulant therapy.

Wire Fractures

Of the contemporary ASD/PFO devices, fracture of the metal arms of the device has been found most commonly with the CardioSEAL/STARFlex and PFO-Star devices. The frequency of wire fractures has continually decreased with subsequent generations of the devices due to the use of different metal alloys and design modifications. The concern with wire fracture is that friction lesions from rubbing of the fractured device may injure adjacent structures and potentially result in perforation. Additionally, wire fracture could theoretically predispose to embolization of metal fragments. Despite these theoretic risks, there is no clear evidence that metal arm fracture in contemporary devices is associated with adverse outcomes (48).

Cardiac/Aortic Perforation

Individual cases of cardiac perforation of the right or left atrium have been reported intraprocedurally, related to manipulation of the delivery sheath (32) or guidewire. Post-procedural cardiac perforation was initially observed with older devices, and was blamed on the rigid structure of these devices. However, perforation has also been recently observed with contemporary devices (49–51). In this circumstance, perforation is caused by repetitive injury between the right or left atrial components and the various surrounding structures, which may result in free-wall perforation with pericardial tamponade or fistula formation (e.g., aorto-right atrial). These events have occurred within 24 hours of the procedure and up to 3 months following the procedure, highlighting the need for vigilance in the care of these patients.

Air Embolization

Air embolism has been reported in individual cases in most case series, and typically occurs during insertion of the delivery sheath in the left atrium or following deployment of the left atrial component of the device. This is typically manifest by embolization to the right coronary artery, producing transient ST-segment elevation that is usually asymptomatic. Rarely, neurologic sequelae have been observed, which are generally reversible (32). This complication often occurs during the early experience of an operator, and is corrected by more careful attention to purging of air from the delivery sheath and from the device and delivery system.

Pericardial Effusion

Detection of a pericardial effusion in any patient, either early or late, following percutaneous PFO/ASD closure should always be regarded as evidence of perforation until proven otherwise. Individual cases of pericardial effusion have been reported in the absence of perforation, the etiology of which is obscure (41). In the absence of clinical evidence of tamponade, these cases may be managed medically with careful observation to document resolution of the effusion.

Arrhythmia

Supraventricular arrhythmias (i.e., atrial fibrillation, atrial flutter, and supraventricular tachycardia) account for the majority of rhythm disturbances encountered following ASD/PFO occlusion, and occur in about 2% of cases. These arrhythmias have been reported early (i.e., in hospital) and late (i.e., within several weeks) following device implantation and may be self-limited or may require medical or electric cardioversion to sinus rhythm. Heart block (i.e., complete and second degree) is rare, and reports are generally confined to the ASD closure literature. It has been observed immediately following device deployment and later during follow-up (22). In the latter instance, permanent pacemaker implantation is required. It should also be noted that there is a significant increase in the frequency of supraventricular ectopics in the first 24 hours following device placement that is generally regarded as a benign finding (52).

Nickel Sensitivity

Most current devices use a nitinol framework, which is composed of 45% titanium and 55% nickel. This has raised some concerns regarding the potential for ASD and PFO closure devices to produce allergic reactions in nickel-sensitive individuals. Blood samples taken from patients before and after implantation of the ASO demonstrate a significant increase in serum nickel concentrations within 24 hours (i.e., from 0.47 ng per mL, at baseline, to 1.27 ng per mL) of the proce-

dure, and peaks at 1 month (i.e., 1.5 ng per mL). Levels remain elevated at 3 months (i.e., 1.24 ng per mL), and return to normal by 12 months (i.e., 0.25 ng per mL) (53). Isolated cases of what clinically was interpreted as a systemic allergic reaction to a PFO/ASD closure device have been reported (54). It is unclear if these cases represent an allergic response to nickel, which typically has a dermatologic manifestation (e.g. urticaria, generalized nickel dermatitis, eczema). Despite these reports, the development of nickel sensitivity to any PFO/ASD device is unproven, and performance of skin testing for nickel allergy prior to device implantation is not required.

Infection

Fortunately, infection of PFO/ASD closure devices is very rare. Two separate cases of infection of a CardioSEAL and Amplatzer device with *Bacillus pumilis* and *Staphylococcus aureus* species, respectively, are reported in the literature (55,56). Although rare, these events highlight the importance of strict antiseptic technique in the catheterization laboratory during these procedures. Our practice is to institute the same standards as apply to pacemaker implantation. This will require some education of the support staff in laboratories that are more accustomed to performing coronary interventions alone. It is also appropriate to avoid the implantation of these devices in patients with evidence of infection or with febrile illnesses of uncertain etiology. Most laboratories use routine antibiotic prophylaxis, pre- and postprocedure, to minimize the risk of device infection.

Miscellaneous

Further rare complications have also been reported. For example, myocardial ischemia, caused by compression by a PFO-closure device of an anomalous circumflex artery arising from the right coronary sinus, and taking a typical retro-aortic course, has been observed (57). Ewert et al. have reported in a subset of elderly patients undergoing ASD closure that there was a marked increase in left atrial pressure, associated with a restrictive filling pattern across the mitral valve (i.e., increase in E/A ratio) (58). In these patients there was an increased risk of left ventricular failure stemming from loss of the decompressive impact of the ASD. These rare events highlight the need for vigilance in monitoring patients undergoing these relatively novel procedures.

CONCLUSION

Percutaneous closure of PFOs and secundum-type ASDs is now a reality. Developments in device technology, ancillary imaging, and procedural technique have all contributed in making these procedures both feasible and safe. While there are adequate data to support the efficacy of percutaneous ASD closure, compared to surgical therapy (21), the results of ongoing studies (CLOSURE, RESPECT, CARDIA), comparing the efficacy of percutaneous PFO closure versus current medical therapy, are eagerly awaited.

REFERENCES

1. Mills NL, King TD. Nonoperative closure of left-to-right shunts. *J Thorac Cardiovasc Surg*. 1976;72(3):371–378.
2. Webster MW, Chancellor AM, Smith HJ, et al. Patent foramen ovale in young stroke patients. *Lancet*. 1988;2(8601):11–12.
3. Lechat P, Mas JL, Lascault G, et al. Prevalence of patent foramen ovale in patients with stroke. *N Engl J Med*. 1988;318(18):1148–1152.
4. Overell JR, Bone I, Lees KR. Interatrial septal abnormalities and stroke: a meta-analysis of case-control studies. *Neurology*. 2000;55(8):1172–1179.
5. Fitzgerald MJT. Thoracic organs. In: Fitzgerald MJT, ed. *Human Embryology*. Baltimore, Md: Harper & Row, 1976: 83–105.
6. Ferreira Martins JD, Anderson RH. The anatomy of interatrial communications—what does the interventionist need to know? *Cardiol Young*. 2000;10(5):464–473.
7. Valdes-Cruz LM, Caryre RO. Atrial septal defects. In: Valdes-Cruz LM, Caryre RO, eds. *Echocardiographic Diagnosis of Congenital Heart Disease*. Philadelphia, Pa: Lippincott-Raven, 1999: 187–213.
8. Podnar T, Martanovic P, Gavora P, et al. Morphological variations of secundum-type atrial septal defects: feasibility for percutaneous closure using Amplatzer septal occluders. *Catheter Cardiovasc Interv*. 2001;53(3):386–391.
9. Kessel-Schaefer A, Lefkovits M, Zellweger MJ, et al. Migrating thrombus trapped in a patent foramen ovale. *Circulation*. 2001;103(14):1928.
10. Kerut EK, Norfleet WT, Plotnick GD, et al. Patent foramen ovale: a review of associated conditions and the impact of physiological size. *J Am Coll Cardiol*. 2001;38(3):613–623.
11. Saary MJ, Gray GW. A review of the relationship between patent foramen ovale and type II decompression sickness. *Aviat Space Environ Med*. 2001;72(12):1113–1120.
12. Rao PS, Palacios IF, Bach RG, et al. Platypnea-orthodeoxia: management by transcatheter buttoned device implantation. *Catheter Cardiovasc Interv*. 2001; 54(1):77–82.
13. Landzberg MJ, Sloss LJ, Faherty CE, et al. Orthodeoxia-platypnea due to intracardiac shunting—relief with transcatheter double umbrella closure. *Cathet Cardiovasc Diagn*. 1995;36(3):247–250.
14. Godart F, Rey C, Prat A, et al. Atrial right-to-left shunting causing severe hypoxaemia despite normal right-sided pressures. Report of 11 consecutive cases corrected by percutaneous closure. *Eur Heart J*. 2000;21(6):483–489.
15. Waight DJ, Cao QL, Hijazi ZM. Closure of patent foramen ovale in patients with orthodeoxia-platypnea using the Amplatzer devices. *Catheter Cardiovasc Interv*. 2000;50(2):195–198.
16. Milhaud D, Bogousslavsky J, van Melle G, et al. Ischemic stroke and active migraine. *Neurology*. 2001; 57(10):1805–1811.
17. Lamy C, Giannesini C, Zuber M, et al. Clinical and imaging findings in cryptogenic stroke patients with and without patent foramen ovale: the PFO-ASA Study. Atrial Septal Aneurysm. *Stroke*. 2002;33(3):706–711.
18. Wilmshurst PT, Nightingale S, Walsh KP, et al. Effect on migraine of closure of cardiac right-to-left shunts to prevent recurrence of decompression illness or stroke or for haemodynamic reasons. *Lancet*. 2000;356(9242):1648–1651.
19. Landzberg MJ. Closure of atrial septal defects in adult patients: justification of the "tipping point." *J Interv Cardiol*. 2001;14(2):267–269.
20. Vogel M, Berger F, Kramer A, et al. Incidence of secondary pulmonary hypertension in adults with atrial septal or sinus venosus defects. *Heart*. 1999;82(1):30–33.
21. Du ZD, Hijazi ZM, Kleinman CS, et al. Comparison between transcatheter and surgical closure of secundum atrial septal defect in children and adults: results of a multicenter nonrandomized trial. *J Am Coll Cardiol*. 2002;39(11):1836–1844.
22. Du ZD, Koenig P, Cao QL, et al. Comparison of transcatheter closure of secundum atrial septal defect using the Amplatzer septal occluder associated with deficient versus sufficient rims. *Am J Cardiol*. 2002;90(8):865–869.
23. Meier B. Pacman sign during device closure of the patent foramen ovale. *Catheter Cardiovasc Interv*. 2003;60(2):221–223.
24. Harper RW, Mottram PM, McGaw DJ. Closure of secundum atrial septal defects with the Amplatzer septal occluder device: techniques and problems. *Catheter Cardiovasc Interv*. 2002;57(4):508–524.
25. Carano N, Hagler DJ, Agnetti A, et al. Device closure of fenestrated atrial septal defects: use of a single Amplatz atrial septal occluder after balloon atrial septostomy to create a single defect. *Catheter Cardiovasc Interv*. 2001;52(2):203–207.
26. McMahon CJ, Pignatelli RH, Rutledge JM, et al. Steerable control of the eustachian valve during transcatheter closure of secundum atrial septal defects. *Catheter Cardiovasc Interv*. 2000;51(4):455–459.
27. McMahon CJ, El Said HG, Mullins CE. Use of the transseptal puncture in transcatheter closure of long tunnel-type patent foramen ovale. *Heart*. 2002;88(2):E3.
28. Ruiz CE, Alboliras ET, Pophal SG. The puncture technique: a new method for transcatheter closure of patent foramen ovale. *Catheter Cardiovasc Interv*. 2001;53(3):369–372.

29. Demkow M, Ruzyllo W, Konka M, et al. Transvenous closure of moderate and large secundum atrial septal defects in adults using the Amplatzer septal occluder. *Catheter Cardiovasc Interv* 2001;**52**(2):188–193.

30. Suarez De Lezo J, Medina A, Pan M, et al. Transcatheter occlusion of complex atrial septal defects. *Catheter Cardiovasc Interv* 2000;**51**(1):33–41.

31. Khairy P, O'Donnell CP, Landzberg MJ. Transcatheter closure versus medical therapy of patent foramen ovale and presumed paradoxical thromboemboli: a systematic review. *Ann Intern Med* 2003;**139**(9):753–760.

32. Windecker S, Wahl A, Chatterjee T, et al. Percutaneous closure of patent foramen ovale in patients with paradoxical embolism: long-term risk of recurrent thromboembolic events. *Circulation* 2000;**101**(8):893–898.

33. Butera G, De Rosa G, Chessa M, et al. Transcatheter closure of atrial septal defect in young children: results and follow-up. *J Am Coll Cardiol* 2003;**42**(2):241–245.

34. Fischer G, Stieh J, Uebing A, Hoffmann U, et al. Experience with transcatheter closure of secundum atrial septal defects using the Amplatzer septal occluder: a single centre study in 236 consecutive patients. *Heart* 2003;**89**(2):199–204.

35. Lee CH, Kwok OH, Fan K, et al. Transcatheter closure of atrial septal defect using Amplatzer septal occluder in Chinese adults. *Catheter Cardiovasc Interv* 2001;**53**(3):373–377.

36. Du ZD, Cao QL, Koenig P, et al. Speed of normalization of right ventricular volume overload after transcatheter closure of atrial septal defect in children and adults. *Am J Cardiol* 2001;**88**(12):1450–1453, A9.

37. Kort HW, Balzer DT, Johnson MC. Resolution of right heart enlargement after closure of secundum atrial septal defect with transcatheter technique. *J Am Coll Cardiol* 2001;**38**(5):1528–1532.

38. Veldtman GR, Razack V, Siu S, et al. Right ventricular function and function after percutaneous atrial septal defect device closure. *J Am Coll Cardiol* 2001;**37**(8):2018–2113.

39. de Lezo JS, Medina A, Romero M, et al. Effectiveness of percutaneous device occlusion for atrial septal defect in adult patients with pulmonary hypertension. *Am Heart J* 2002;**144**(5):877–880.

40. Gatzoulis MA, Freeman MA, Siu SC, et al. Atrial arrhythmia after surgical closure of atrial septal defects in adults. *N Engl J Med* 1999;**340**(11):839–846.

41. Chessa M, Carminati M, Butera G, et al. Early and late complications associated with transcatheter occlusion of secundum atrial septal defect. *J Am Coll Cardiol* 2002;**39**(6):1061–1065.

42. Beitzke A, Schuchlenz H, Gamillscheg A, et al. Catheter closure of the persistent foramen ovale: mid-term results in 162 patients. *J Interv Cardiol* 2001;**14**(2):223–229.

43. La Rosee K, Deutsch HJ, Schnabel P, et al. Thrombus formation after transcatheter closure of atrial septal defect. *Am J Cardiol* 1999;**84**(3):356–359, A9.

44. Acar P, Aggoun Y, Abdel-Massih T. Images in cardiology: Thrombus after transcatheter closure of ASD with an Amplatzer septal occluder assessed by three dimensional enchocardiographic reconstruction. *Heart* 2002;**88**(1):52.

45. Nkomo VT, Theuma P, Maniu CV, et al. Patent foramen ovale transcatheter closure device thrombosis. *Mayo Clin Proc* 2001;**76**(10):1057–61.

46. Vanderheyden M, Willaert W, Claessens P, et al. Thrombosis of a patent foramen ovale closure device: thrombolytic management. *Catheter Cardiovasc Interv* 2002;**56**(4):522–526.

47. Krumsdorf U, Ostermayer S, Billinger K, et al. Incidence and clinical course of thrombus formation on atrial septal defect and patent foramen ovale closure devices in 1,000 consecutive patients. *J Am Coll Cardiol* 2004;**43**(2):302–309.

48. Hung J, Landzberg MJ, Jenkins KJ, et al. Closure of patent foramen ovale for paradoxical emboli: intermediate-term risk of recurrent neurological events following transcatheter device placement. *J Am Coll Cardiol* 2000;**35**(5):1311–1316.

49. Chun DS, Turrentine MW, Moustapha A, et al. Development of aorta-to-right atrial fistula following closure of secundum atrial septal defect using the Amplatzer septal occluder. *Catheter Cardiovasc Interv* 2003;**58**(2):246–251.

50. Pinto FF, Sousa L, Fragata J. Late cardiac tamponade after transcatheter closure of atrial septal defect with Cardioseal device. *Cardiol Young* 2001;**11**(2):233–235.

51. Trepels T, Zeplin H, Sievert H, et al. Cardiac perforation following transcatheter PFO closure. *Catheter Cardiovasc Interv* 2003;**58**(1):111–113.

52. Hill SL, Berul CI, Patel HT, et al. Early ECG abnormalities associated with transcatheter closure of atrial septal defects using the Amplatzer septal occluder. *J Interv Card Electrophysiol* 2000;**4**(3):469–474.

53. Ries MW, Kampmann C, Rupprecht HJ, et al. Nickel release after implantation of the Amplatzer occluder. *Am Heart J* 2003;**145**(4):737–741.

54. Fukahara K, Minami K, Reiss N, et al. Systemic allergic reaction to the percutaneous patent foramen ovale occluder. *J Thorac Cardiovasc Surg* 2003;**125**(1):213–214.

55. Bullock AM, Menahem S, Wilkinson JL. Infective endocarditis on an occluder closing an atrial septal defect. *Cardiol Young* 1999;**9**(1):65–67.

56. Goldstein JA, Beardslee MA, Xu H, et al. Infective endocarditis resulting from CardioSEAL closure of a patent foramen ovale. *Catheter Cardiovasc Interv* 2002;**55**(2):217–220; discussion 221.

57. Casolo G, Gensini GF, Santoro G, et al. Anomalous origin of the circumflex artery and patent foramen ovale: a rare cause of myicardial ischaemia after percutaneous closure of the defect. *Heart* 2003;**89**(8):e23.

58. Ewert P, Berger F, Nagdyman N, et al. Masked left ventricular restriction in elderly patients with atrial septal defects: a contraindication for closure? *Catheter Cardiovasc Interv* 2001;**52**(2):177–180.

59. Latson LA. The CardioSEAL Device: History, Techniques, Results. *J Interven Cardiol* 1998;**11**:501–505.

60. Hausdorf G, Kaulitz R, Paul T, et al. Transcatheter closure of atrial septal defect with a new flexible, self-centering device (the STARFlex Occluder). *Am J Cardiol* 1999;**84**(9):1113–16, A10.

61. Zahn EM, Wilson N, Cutright W, et al. Development and testing of the Helex septal occluder, a new expanded polytetrafluoroethylene atrial septal defect occlusion system. *Circulation* 2001;**104**(6):711–716.

62. Rao PS, Berger F, Rey C, et al. Results of transvenous occlusion of secundum atrial septal defects with the fourth generation buttoned device: comparison with first, second and third generation devices. International Buttoned Device Trial Group. *J Am Coll Cardiol* 2000;**36**(2):583–592.

CHAPTER 18

Mesenteric Vascular Intervention

Fred Moeslein and Mark J. Sands

T he majority of vascular interventions that pertain to the mesenteric vessels are performed as a result of clinical manifestations of ischemia. The details of endovascular diagnosis and treatment of mesenteric ischemia will therefore constitute the major emphasis of this chapter. While other disease processes, such as gastrointestinal (GI) bleeding and GI tumors often necessitate endovascular diagnosis and treatment via the mesenteric vessels, they are outside the scope of this chapter.

ANATOMIC CONSIDERATIONS

The small (i.e., duodenum, jejunum and ileum) and large intestines (i.e., colon) are supplied by branches from three major arteries arising from the anterior surface of the lower thoracic and abdominal aortae: the celiac trunk, the superior, and inferior mesenteric arteries.

Arising at the level of the twelfth thoracic vertebra, the celiac trunk divides after 1 cm to 2 cm into the splenic, common hepatic, and left gastric branches (Fig. 18-1). The splenic branch has a tortuous leftward and posterior course toward the hilum of the spleen. The common hepatic branch courses rightward and anteriorly, dividing into the proper hepatic branch, which supplies the liver parenchyma and gallbladder, and the gastroduodenal artery, which provides branches to the stomach (i.e., right gastroepiploic) and proximal duodenum (i.e., superior pancreaticoduodenal).

The superior mesenteric artery (SMA) typically arises at the level of the first lumbar vertebra, just inferior to the celiac trunk (Fig. 18-2). It has a steep, inferior course as it courses toward the right, lower abdominal quadrant. To the left of the main vessel arise 10 to 15 jejunal and ilial branches supplying the respective portions of the small intestine (Fig. 18-3). To the right arise, in succession, the inferior pancreaticoduodenal artery that anastomoses with branches from the gastroduodenal artery, and the middle, right, and ileocolic branches, supplying the ascending and transverse colon (Fig. 18-3).

The inferior mesenteric artery (IMA) typically arises at the level of the third lumbar vertebra, and is usually much smaller than either the celiac trunk or SMA. It has a steep, inferior course in the midline, toward the pelvis (Fig. 18-4).

The left colic artery is the first and major branch of the IMA, supplying the descending colon. There are typically two to three small sigmoid branches of the IMA supplying the sigmoid colon. The IMA continues as the superior rectal artery supplying the proximal rectum, and anastomoses with the middle, and inferior rectal branches of the internal iliac artery.

Named Anastomoses between Mesenteric Vessels

The Marginal Artery of Drummond

This consists of a series of longitudinally anastomosing vessels along the mesenteric border of

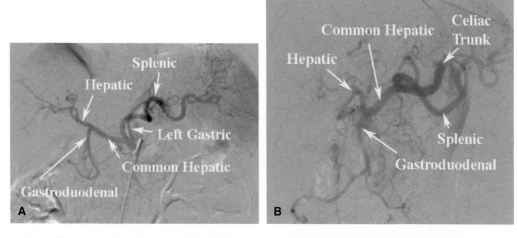

FIGURE 18-1 ● **Selective angiogram of the celiac trunk demonstrating its major branches.**
A: Posteroanterior (PA) angiogram. **B:** Lateral angiogram.

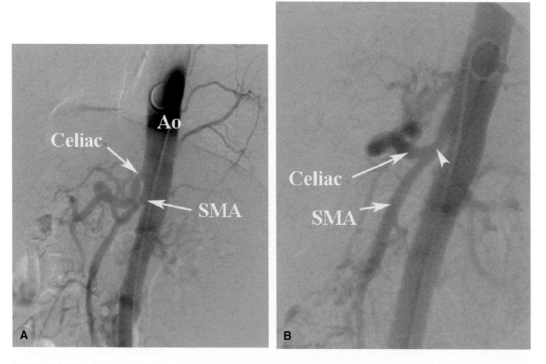

FIGURE 18-2 ● **Lateral aortogram demonstrating the relationship of the origins of the celiac trunk and superior mesenteric arteries (SMA). A:** Normal relationship showing the origin of the SMA, just inferior to the celiac trunk. **B:** Rare anomaly (<1%) in which the celiac trunk and SMA share a common origin (*arrowhead*). Ao, aorta.

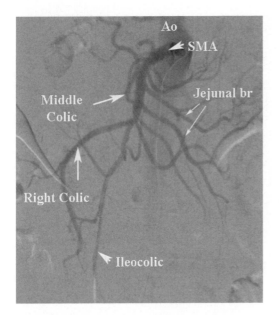

FIGURE 18-3 ● Selective angiogram of the superior mesenteric artery (SMA) demonstrating the jejunal and ileal branches, to the left, and the middle, right, and ileocolic branches to the right of the main vessel. Ao, aorta.

the large intestine, originating from arcades of the colic branches of the superior, and inferior mesenteric vessels.

Arc of Riolan

This refers to a direct communication between the superior, and inferior mesenteric arteries, via the left, and middle colic branches that anastomose at the splenic flexure (Fig. 18-5).

ACUTE MESENTERIC ISCHEMIA

Acute mesenteric ischemia (AMI) was first described by Antonio Beniviene in the fifteenth century. Over the last century, it has been increasingly recognized as a grave disease with an enigmatic presentation. In 1926, Cokkinis wrote:

> "occlusion of the mesenteric vessels is apt to be regarded as one of those conditions of which the diagnosis is impossible, the prognosis hopeless, and the treatment almost useless".

While some improvement in recognition and treatment of this disease has occurred since

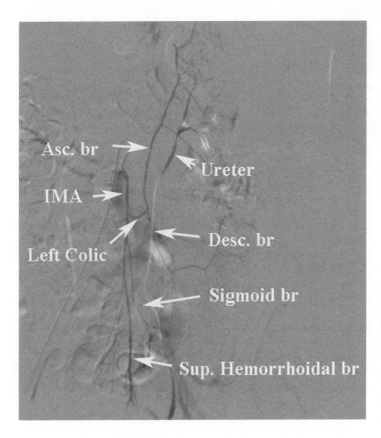

FIGURE 18-4 ● Selective angiogram of the inferior mesenteric artery (IMA) demonstrating its major branches. The left colic branch divides into ascending and descending branches, supplying the descending colon. Asc, ascending; Desc, descending; br, branch; Sup, superior.

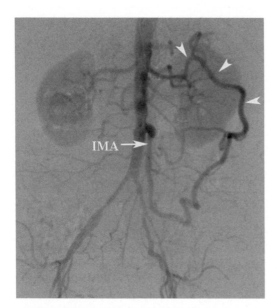

FIGURE 18-5 ● Abdominal aortogram demonstrating the Arc of Riolan (*white arrows*)—a direct connection of the superior mesenteric and inferior mesenteric arteries at the splenic flexure, provided by the left and middle colic branches.

TABLE 18-1

Etiology of a Acute Mesenteric Ischemia

Arterial occlusion (50%)
    Embolus—usually to the superior mesenteric artery
    Thrombotic occlusion
    Aortic aneurysm
    Vasculitis
    Fibromuscular dysplasia
    Trauma
Non-occlusive ischemia (25–35%)
    Systemic hypotension
    Cardiac failure
    Septic shock
    Mesenteric vasoconstriction
Venous occlusion (10–15%)
Extra-vascular etiologies (<5%)
    Incarcerated hernia
    Volvulus
    Intussusception
    Adhesive disease

Cokkinis penned these ominous words, nearly 80 years ago, it remains an entity with dire sequela. The reported average mortality rate of 71% is little changed over the last 50 years.

The great difficulty in treating AMI stems from the nebulous constellation of presenting signs and symptoms, and the lack of specific diagnostic tests. The classic presentation of AMI is abdominal pain that appears disproportionately expressed, relative to the patient's observed physical findings and persists beyond 2 to 3 hours. Other common presenting symptoms include fever, nausea, anorexia and diarrhea. In approximately 50% of cases, fecal occult blood is present, with melena or hematochezia occurring in up to 15% of cases. Clinical findings include leukocytosis (i.e., greater than 15,000) and metabolic acidosis in 75% and 50% of cases, respectively (1,2). However, as the initial diagnosis is often delayed, mostly owing to the non-specific nature of the earliest signs, it is not uncommon for a patient to present with an acute abdomen, including distension, rigidity and hypotension secondary to bowel infarction.

A diverse range of underlying etiologies cause AMI and are shown in Table 18-1. By far, the most common cause of AMI is embolic occlusion of the superior mesenteric artery (3). These emboli are usually cardiac in origin, and patients with valvular vegetations, arrhythmias, and mural thrombi from cardiac hypokinesia, are at increased risk. In 25% of AMI cases, occlusion of a pre-existing atherosclerotic lesion occurs. In this subset of patients, a history of intermittent episodes of abdominal pain, consistent with transient or chronic mesenteric ischemia, is often elicited, and for these patients the outcome may be particularly catastrophic, as a result of a generally reduced collateral reserve.

In up to one-third of AMI cases, ischemia results from under perfusion of the splanchnic bed, in the absence of actual occlusion. This hypoperfusion usually occurs secondary to decreased cardiac output or hepatorenal disease (4). The incidence of non-occlusive AMI is decreasing, possibly as a result of improved monitoring in the intensive care setting, with earlier correction of hemodynamic abnormalities.

AMI secondary to venous thrombosis, usually within the superior mesenteric vein, occurs in up

TABLE 18-2

Risk Factors for Acute Mesenteric Ischemia

Age >50 years
Cardiac disease
   Congestive heart failure
   Arrhythmias
   Recent or concurrent myocardial infarction
   Valvular disease
   Recent cardiac surgery
   Vasoconstrictor therapy
Hypovolemia
Hypotension
Sepsis
Hypercoagulable states
Prior arterial or venous emboli
Vasculitis
Trauma

to 15% of cases (5). In such cases, a search for underlying, hypercoagulable states is warranted. Lastly, extravascular etiologies, such as incarcerated hernia, volvulus, intussusception, and adhesive disease occur in a small percentage of cases.

As the presenting symptoms are largely nonspecific, the key to diagnosis is maintaining a high degree of clinical suspicion, coupled with recognition of at-risk individuals. The risk factors for AMI are listed in Table 18-2.

The utility of plain radiographs is limited, as the usual findings of ileus or mesenteric thickening are non-specific, and the more specific findings of intramural pneumatosis and portal venous gas are, relatively, late findings. Essentially, the key role for plain radiography is the rapid exclusion of perforation. Contrast-enhanced abdominal computed tomography (CECT) has revolutionized the detection of AMI. Important CECT findings include focal bowel wall thickening, submucosal edema or hemorrhage, pneumatosis, and portal venous gas with a sensitivity approaching 90% (6). Furthermore, CT angiography (CTA) may provide a non-invasive alternative

to conventional angiography, for the diagnosis and characterization of AMI (7). However, the gold standard for imaging of AMI remains digital subtraction angiography (DSA), which provides the most sensitive evaluation of the peripheral splanchnic circulation. Moreover, the procedure also allows for concurrent treatment, in selected patients.

Management of AMI is highly dependent on the underlying etiology and extent of disease. The cornerstone of management is adequate resuscitation, coupled with correction if possible, of the underlying pathophysiology (3). Without alleviation of the underlying hypotension, hypovolemia, or decreased cardiac output, any effort to increase splanchnic circulation would be ultimately, unsuccessful. Moreover, angiography is relatively contraindicated in the setting of hypotension or hypovolemia, as the splanchnic circulation is naturally vasoconstricted and as such, may mask any underlying ischemic mesenteric pathology. Furthermore, the administration of intra-arterial vasodilators, such as papaverine, is contraindicated in the setting of systemic hypotension or hypovolemia, because of the likelihood of causing a precipitous drop in systemic blood pressure by rapidly expanding the vascular bed volume. In individuals presenting with peritoneal signs, surgical exploration is universally accepted as the mainstay of therapy, as resection of infarcted bowel and embolectomy may be performed concomitantly, if needed.

Pre-operative angiographic evaluation of a patient with an acute abdomen and suspected AMI is controversial. Proponents argue that angiography provides essential information delineating the extent and location of splanchnic occlusions (Fig. 18-6), assessing mesenteric vasoconstriction and evaluation of the overall splanchnic circulation. Advocates also note that in selected patients, pre-operative infusion of vasodilators has been shown to limit the extent of the required resection, by reducing the amount of at-risk bowel that progresses to outright infarction (8). Critics argue that any unnecessary delay, prior to surgery, worsens the potential outcome.

The role of endovascular therapy in the management of AMI may be either adjunctive, or

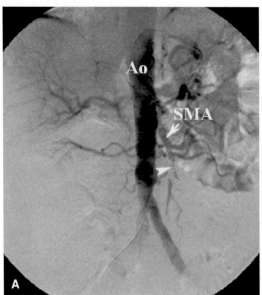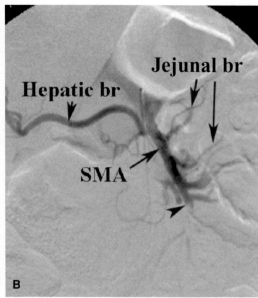

FIGURE 18-6 ● **Acute mesenteric ischemia.** This 83-year-old man presented with severe abdominal pain out of proportion to his clinical findings and with lactic acidosis. The patient gave a history of a recent Mallory-Weiss tear. Ao: aorta. **A:** Anteroposterior (AP) aortogram demonstrates cut-off of the superior mesenteric artery (SMA) (*arrowhead*). **B:** Selective angiography demonstrates abrupt occlusion of the SMA approximately 5 cm to 6 cm distal to the vessel origin (*arrowhead*). After consultation with the referring surgeon, the procedure was terminated and the patient went to the operating room for an SMA endarterectomy, with thrombectomy and small bowel resection, for treatment of the ischemic bowel.

in selected patients, the sole treatment modality. Intra-arterial papaverine administration has been used for the treatment of non-occlusive AMI (4). Several authors espouse the merits of surgery, coupled with adjunctive papaverine administration, for the management of mesenteric vasoconstriction in the setting of acute arterial occlusion (3,8). These groups have reported markedly lowered mortality rates (45 to 50%), and shorter bowel resections, with the coupled therapies. While surgery remains the mainstay of therapy for AMI, several recent reports have demonstrated the efficacy of stand-alone endovascular treatment. These therapies include intra-arterial administration of vasodilators, alone or in conjunction with intra-arterial thrombolytics (9,10). If endovascular thrombolytic therapy is to be pursued, appropriate patient selection is of vital importance. More obvious candidates are patients with comorbidities that present significant operative risk. Beyond this group, better candidates include individuals with less than 12 hours of symptoms, with partially occlusive superior mesenteric artery thrombus, or with occlusive

thrombus that lies distal to the ileocolic artery (11).

Endovascular Treatment of Non-occlusive AMI with Intra-Arterial Papaverine

Patient Selection and Preparation

Appropriate patients include individuals over the age of 50 years, with persistent abdominal pain lasting longer than 2 to 3 hours, with increased risk for AMI (Table 2), or individuals demonstrating findings consistent with AMI on abdominal CECT. Candidate patients need to undergo adequate resuscitation. In this setting, resuscitation must include restoring an adequate circulating blood volume, correcting cardiac arrhythmias, and relieving cardiac failure. This final point may be difficult, as cardiogenic shock and congestive heart failure may require systemic vasoconstrictor therapy for adequate management, but such treatment will likely aggravate, or precipitate, the underlying mesenteric ischemia. Close multidisciplinary coordination is

TABLE 18-3

Recommended Catheters and Wires for the Treatment of Acute Mesenteric Ischemia

Catheters
  Pigtail
  C2 Cobra
  SOS
  Simmons 1,2,3
Wires 0.035"
  Glidewire
  Bentson
  Rosen

essential for management of these clinically complex patients.

Access and Intervention

The recommended equipment for this procedure is shown in Table 18-3.

Femoral access is preferable for this procedure because this route allows the use of larger catheter sizes. After gaining arterial access, a 5 Fr sheath is used to maintain vascular access and facilitate catheter exchange. Unless otherwise stated, 0.035" guide-wire compatible systems are used for angiography and intervention. For the initial evaluation of the aorta and major branching vessels, a 5 Fr pigtail catheter is advanced past the mesenteric vessels (i.e., at level of T12). A routine aortogram in both the AP and the lateral projection is performed, in order to exclude proximal occlusions and other pathology.

Selective catheterization of the visceral arteries should then be performed, to assess the adequacy of splanchnic blood flow and the extent of mesenteric vasoconstriction. The authors favor engaging the mesenteric vessels with 5 Fr C2 Cobra catheters. In the setting of a tortuous aorta, or when the SMA has an unusually severe take-off angle, the authors use the 'Waltman loop technique' to aid engagement. With this technique, the Cobra catheter is engaged into the contralateral common iliac artery. Using a glidewire, the catheter is advanced into the distal, common iliac artery and the wire removed. At this point, for-

ward advancement of the Cobra catheter creates a large loop in the catheter, and eventually withdrawal of the tip of the catheter into the aorta. The catheter is then advanced to the site of origin of the vessel of interest.

Alternatively, catheters with preformed curves, such as the SoS or Simmons catheters, may be used. The Waltman loop technique is also effective for reshaping these preformed catheters in the common iliac artery. Reshaping these catheters in the thoracic aorta, proximal to the mesenteric vessels is less desirable, particularly if the aortic arch is used, owing to the increased risk of stroke.

If papaverine administration is warranted, the angiographic catheter should be sutured to the thigh, to prevent dislodgement over the course of therapy. Papaverine, diluted in saline to 1 mg/mL, may be administered at a rate of 30 mL to 60 mL per hour, intra-arterially. The concentration may be adjusted according to any fluid restrictions the patient may have. The duration of therapy varies but is usually administered for 12 to 24 hours. Prior to cessation of therapy, repeat angiography should be performed to assess for the presence of residual vasoconstriction. Approximately 30 minutes prior to repeat angiography, saline should be substituted for the papaverine. If vasoconstriction persists, continued papaverine administration is warranted. Intra-arterial administration of 5 days' duration has been reported (8).

Complications and Prognosis

As previously mentioned, AMI carries a high, associated mortality rate. However, with aggressive early intervention, survival rates approaching 50% have been reported (8). Potential complications include acute renal failure, secondary to contrast administration. There is a small chance of arterial thromboembolism, predominantly in the lower extremities. This risk increases in individuals with severe atherosclerotic disease of the aorta and iliac arteries. As this procedure is usually performed in conjunction with surgery, follow-up evaluation is usually tailored to the postoperative needs.

CHRONIC MESENTERIC ISCHEMIA

Chronic mesenteric ischemia (CMI) is an uncommon, but debilitating, disease. The first case reports are from the turn of the last century. Schnitzler described a patient, in 1901, with long-standing post-prandial pain that upon autopsy, was demonstrated to have an atherosclerotic occlusion of the SMA. Extension of this work by Conner and Mikkelson advanced the theory that chronic mesenteric ischemia was primarily caused by atherosclerotic occlusion or stenosis of the mesenteric vessels (12,13). The underlying etiology is atherosclerotic stenosis, or occlusion, in greater than 95% of CMI cases. While the mesenteric circulation is capable of supporting the metabolic demands of the resting gut, the diseased vasculature is unable to meet the increased metabolic needs of motility, secretion, and absorption, induced by digestion.

One of the great difficulties in the diagnosis of CMI is the insidious onset of symptoms. Classically, patients present with post-prandial, abdominal cramping, which may be quite severe. In the early disease process, symptoms predominantly occur after ingestion of large meals, but as the disease progresses, smaller prandial challenges are all that is required to evoke the painful response. As the disease progresses, other symptoms may arise, commonly including malabsorption and aberrant motility. Disease progression usually induces weight loss, which may be severe, and ultimately anorexia or sitophobia.

Patients normally present in the sixth and seventh decades of life (i.e., average age of onset is 60 years), and there is a slight female predominance. Importantly, there is a high prevalence of extravisceral atherosclerotic disease in patients with CMI. The most commonly effected extravisceral sites are the lower extremity, carotid, and coronary arteries. As with AMI, CMI is difficult to diagnose and is primarily a diagnosis of exclusion. Risk factors for CMI are given in Table 18-4.

As previously mentioned, the majority of CMI cases are caused by atherosclerotic disease of the proximal segments of the mesenteric arteries. These atheroma cause occlusion or stenosis of the proximal arterial segments but little, if any, distal pathology. Other rare etiologies include Takayasu arteritis, Buerger's Disease, fibromuscular dysplasia (Fig. 18-7), and post-radiation stenoses (14).

Conventional thinking holds that occlusion or stenosis of at least two mesenteric arteries is nec-

TABLE 18-4

Risk Factors for Chronic Mesenteric Ischemia

Age (older than 50)
Hypertension
Diabetes mellitus
Hyperlipidemia
Coronory artery disease
Renal disease
Smoking
Obesity
Sedentary lifestyle

essary to induce symptoms of CMI. However, this is an issue of great debate, as autopsy studies have demonstrated a high frequency of two- and three-vessel disease in asymptomatic individuals (15). The discrepancy between the observed frequency of CMI and the observed frequency of mesenteric stenoses is probably best explained by collateralization. The bowel has an immense potential for vascular collateralization. Celiac artery-to-SMA connection occurs primarily via the pancreatic-duodenal arteries. The marginal arteries of Drummond and Riolan's arch are the predominant SMA-to-IMA connections. In instances of three-vessel occlusion, recruitment of phrenic, lumbar and pelvic collaterals may occur.

Decreased collateral circulation may explain why certain individuals develop symptoms with occlusion of one vessel, while others may sustain atherosclerotic vascular disease of two or three vessels and remain asymptomatic. For example, patients with diabetes, or end-stage renal disease, may develop diffuse atherosclerotic disease of the mesentery and also appear to have a decreased ability to form collaterals. This may lead to the higher incidence of CMI observed in these populations. Furthermore, these observations support the practice of limited revascularization, as an effective therapy for CMI, because restoration of flow via any of the mesenteric arteries should allow adequate collateral flow into the territories of the other vessels.

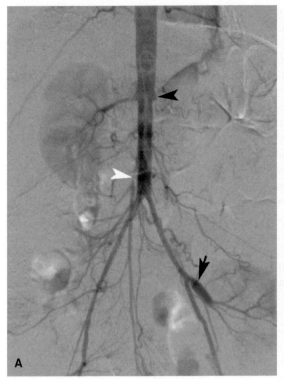
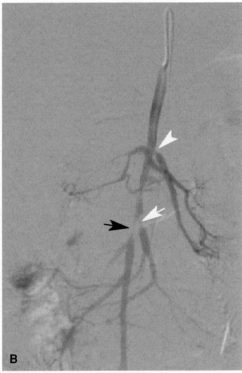

FIGURE 18-7 ● **Angiography from 40-year-old female with fibromuscular dysplasia and symptoms consistent with mesenteric ischemia. A:** Aortogram in posteroanterior (PA) projection demonstrates an absent celiac trunk, and evidence of disease in an atypical, non-ostial location in the superior mesenteric artery (SMA) (arrowhead). The inferior mesenteric artery is also occluded. Also note that the left renal artery is occluded (black arrow) and the left kidney has been reimplanted, off the common iliac artery (black arrow). **B:** Selective angiography of the SMA defining the extent of obstructive disease. Black arrowhead-stenosis in main SMA, white arrowheads-stenosis at origin of jejunal branches.

Diagnosis of CMI begins by exclusion of other etiologies, most specifically vascular, neoplastic, and inflammatory disease. In individuals complaining of worsening abdominal pain, in the setting of chronic pain, acute occlusive disease needs to be excluded. In the elderly population, abdominal pain and weight loss are particularly concerning for neoplasm, and more specifically pancreatic cancer. Retroperitoneal lymphoma also has a great propensity for causing epigastric pain, arising from compression of the celiac plexus. Gastroduodenal ulcers may cause chronic epigastric pain, and may be most easily assessed endoscopically.

Median arcuate ligament (i.e., of the diaphragm) syndrome, with resultant compromise of the proximal celiac artery, remains a controversial diagnosis. This entity usually occurs in young women and presents with abdominal bruits and abdominal pain that is alleviated by deep inspiration. Reliable detection of this entity by abdominal CECT has been reported (16).

Another rare entity that may cause abdominal pain is mesenteric artery aneurysm or dissection. These are readily detectable on CECT, MRA, or CT angiography (CTA).

In the setting of chronic abdominal pain, CECT has become the mainstay of initial imaging, owing to its sensitivity for a wide range of abdominal pathologies (17). Other imaging modalities may also play a role in the diagnostic workup. Duplex ultrasound (US) has been reported to be a sensitive screening test for proximal mesenteric artery stenosis. Peak systolic velocities greater than 275 cm per second, or end-diastolic velocities greater than 45 cm per second, have been shown to be highly specific for stenosis of greater than 75% (18). Both MR and CTA are quite sensitive for detection of proximal mesenteric arterial pathology (19,20). The role of conventional angiography in CMI is now mainly for pre-operative planning, or for endovascular treatment.

Owing to impaired mesenteric circulatory reserve, CMI patients are at markedly increased risk of suffering catastrophic bowel infarction, if an acute thrombus or embolus were to occlude one of the remaining vessels. Therefore, the impact of CMI treatment is two fold. First, it allows immediate resolution of symptoms and second, by increasing functional mesenteric circulatory reserve, it helps protect against potentially catastrophic acute insults.

The primary treatment for CMI has been surgical revascularization via bypass grafting or endarterectomy. However, successful endovascular treatment of both mesenteric stenosis and occlusion have been reported, and acceptance of this technique as a viable alternative therapy is growing. Endovascular therapies include percutaneous transluminal angioplasty (PTA) alone, or with stenting of stenosed SMA or celiac arteries (16,21). A small body of literature also supports the use of endovascular recanalization of occluded mesenteric arteries (Fig. 18-8) (22).

Percutaneous Transluminal Revascularization

Patient Selection

Patients presenting with post-prandial abdominal pain, weight loss, diarrhea, or gastroparesis should be evaluated to exclude more common non-CMI pathologies. In some institutions, abdominal CECT is usually the first diagnostic imaging study. In the patient with CMI, CT will often demonstrate one or more stenotic or occluded mesenteric arteries. In the event that CT fails to provide an etiology for the patient's symptoms, further evaluation with duplex ultrasound, MR or CTA is warranted if clinical suspicion is high. After one, or more, high-grade stenoses are detected, an angiogram is warranted.

Access and Intervention

While either a femoral or a brachial approach may be used, an initial attempt from the femoral approach is generally preferred. This is because of the reduced risk of ischemic complications, and that the femoral approach allows for larger caliber catheters, if needed. While initial reports favored the brachial approach, especially for celiac revascularization, modern, flexible catheters have alleviated most of the disadvantages of the femoral approach. Certainly, brachial access may be used if the femoral approach appears unsatisfactory or fails.

After gaining access, a 5 Fr sheath is placed, and 5000 U of heparin are administered, intravenously. Global aortic angiograms and selective angiography of the mesenteric vessels are performed as described above. At this point, a decision to proceed with revascularization should be based on an assessment of the severity of disease. In most reports, interventions were performed only when stenoses of greater than 70% were present in two or more vessels (Fig. 18-9).

If revascularization is to proceed, the SMA is the preferred vessel, based largely on technical considerations. This artery, in general, has fewer inherent turns than the celiac artery, which should allow a more technically simple procedure. If an occlusion is present, recanalization is more likely to succeed if a clearly defined stump may be detected on the lateral angiogram (Fig. 18-8).

The authors usually elect to cross stenotic lesions with an 0.035″ Glidewire, using the diagnostic catheter for support. After crossing the lesion, a guide catheter is telescoped over the diagnostic catheter, to the ostium of the mesenteric vessel, and the diagnostic catheter subsequently withdrawn. When using femoral access, a guide with an inferiorly directed primary curve should be chosen, such as a RES (renal standard), RDC (renal double curve) or IMA guide. Multipurpose guides are suitable when using brachial access. Selection of an appropriately sized angioplasty balloon is based on the diameter of the native vessel, and the length of the stenosis. As a reference, the average diameter of the celiac trunk is 5 mm to 7 mm, the SMA is 4 mm to 6 mm, and the IMA is 3 mm to 5 mm. The authors tend to dilate the balloon to a diameter that is 10 to 25% greater than the diameter of the vessel.

Following angioplasty, the authors routinely proceed to stent placement. In the typical ostial location of atherosclerotic lesions, the use of pre-mounted balloon-expandable stents (e.g., Genesis, Herculink) is strongly recommended. At this location, the superior radial force and precise placement of balloon-expandable stents

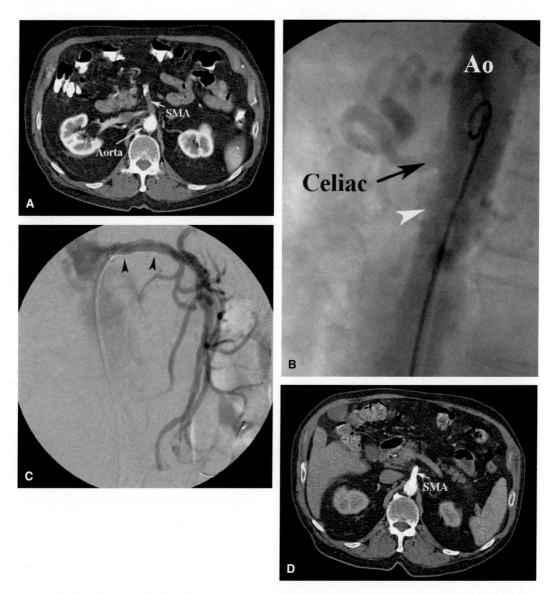

FIGURE 18-8 ● **Chronic superior mesenteric artery occlusion.** This 81-year-old man presented with progressive post-prandial pain, worsening food aversion, and weight loss. **A:** Contrast enhanced computed tomography (CECT) of the abdomen demonstrates a long segment of occlusion of the superior mesenteric artery (SMA) (indicated by the absence of contrast in the SMA). **B:** Lateral aortogram demonstrating a patent celiac artery and a stump just distal to the take off of the SMA, the typical location for atherosclerotic disease. Using a C2 Cobra catheter, and a Roadrunner guide wire, the obstruction was traversed, and two SMART control self-expanding stents were placed across the occlusion. **C:** Post-procedural lateral aortogram demonstrating patency of the stented SMA (*Location of stents indicated by black arrowheads*). **D:** Follow-up CECT, 3 days post-procedure, confirmed patency of the stented vessel.

offer significant advantages over self-expanding stents, which may be used in the non-ostial location. While angioplasty, alone, may be performed, most reports recommend adjunctive stenting, as the observed restenosis rate is markedly lower after stent placement. A post-stent angiogram in the AP and lateral projections is performed to assess residual stenosis. Postprocedure, patients should be placed on aspirin therapy (i.e., 100 mg to 325 mg per day).

If an occlusion is found during angiography, and if recanalization is to be attempted, then

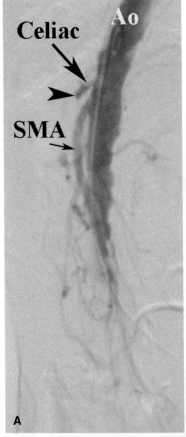

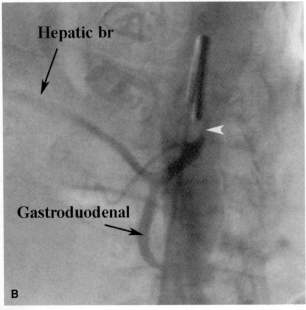

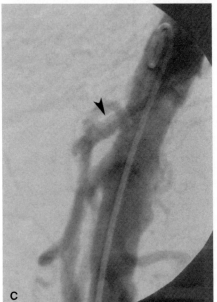

FIGURE 18-9 ● **Chronic celiac artery stenosis in an 86-year-old woman who presented with post-prandial pain.**
A: Aortography demonstrated a high-grade stenosis of the proximal celiac artery (*black arrowhead*). The inferior mesenteric artery was occluded at its origin. SMA: superior mesenteric artery. **B:** Selective celiac trunk angiography in oblique projection demonstrating high-grade stenosis in celiac trunk (white arrowhead). An initial attempt to cross the lesion from the femoral approach was unsuccessful. The patient was brought back 2 weeks later, for celiac intervention, using upper extremity arterial access. The celiac artery was engaged and the stenosis traversed using a 5 Fr SoS catheter and Bentson wire. Angioplasty of the stenosis was performed using a 4.5 mm × 2 cm Symmetry balloon. A post-dilation lateral aortogram demonstrated a reduction in stenosis, but because of a residual 17 mmHg arterial pressure gradient, a 5 mm × 5 cm Genesis stent was placed across the stenotic region. **C:** Lateral aortogram following stent placement demonstrating wide patency of the celiac artery.

modification of the above technique may be required. As before, the 5 Fr C2 Cobra catheter may be used. Alternatively a Simmons catheter may allow better purchase within the target vessel, by virtue of its reformed curve. In other instances, a guide catheter may be used to engage the vessel directly, in order to provide sufficient support for the wire to cross the lesion. Access from the brachial artery may provide a better orientation and angulation for crossing an occlusion, in some instances.

The catheter or guide should be placed in the arterial stump, and a directionally controlled guidewire (i.e., 0.035″ glidewire, moderate-support 0.014″ guidewire) should be advanced through the thrombus or occlusion. After the occlusion has been successfully traversed, and the true lumen reentered, an angiogram (i.e., though the lumen of an over-the-wire balloon passed distal to the occlusion) should be performed to assess the distal vasculature.

Subsequently, angioplasty and stenting across the lesion should be performed, as detailed above. Some authors have advocated the use of thrombolytics prior to recanalization (22). In general, this practice is not necessary unless there is clinical concern for an acute component to the occlusion.

Following angioplasty or stent deployment, angiography is performed to assess the adequacy of the procedure. The angiographic images are evaluated for the presence of residual stenosis, intimal dissection, and distal embolization. In some instances, intravascular ultrasound (IVUS) may be used to assess the degree of residual stenosis further, and determine the nature of any observed post-angioplasty dissection.

Follow-up Evaluation

Duplex US evaluation typically is performed prior to discharge, to evaluate flow in the mesenteric circulation. At the authors' institution, follow-up duplex US is performed, routinely, at 3 to 6 month follow-up. CTA or duplex US evaluation is performed yearly, thereafter, for surveillance to assess vessel patency.

Prognosis and Complications

Reported long-term success rates (i.e., 2 to 3 years) are approximately 90% for PTA with stenting, and rival those of surgical revascularization (14). Apart from vascular access issues, iatrogenic dissection during angioplasty has been reported. In most cases these have been successfully treated with stent deployment. There is also a small risk of distal embolization and subsequent infarction. Overall, the perioperative risks of endovascular revascularization are less than those of open surgical techniques (14).

CELIAC ARTERY AND INFERIOR MESENTERIC ARTERY DISEASE

The incidence of celiac arterial atherosclerotic disease was found in one study to be considerably less frequent than in the SMA (23). However, other angiographic studies demonstrate more stenoses of the celiac artery than of the SMA. This variance may be explained by the compression of the celiac artery by the crura of the diaphragm, or median arcuate ligament syndrome. Given the extensive collateral circulation between the celiac artery and the SMA, primarily through the pancreatic-duodenal arcade, compression of the celiac artery by the median arcuate ligament of the diaphragm, as a pathologic entity, is controversial. The role of angioplasty and stent placement is not established, as the source of compression is extraluminal.

Vascular compromise of the celiac artery and inferior mesenteric artery, from atherosclerotic disease, is certainly observed. While single-vessel disease is thought to be unlikely to result in mesenteric angina, such situations have been described. In such instances, endovascular intervention has resulted in symptomatic improvement.

There is one instance in which revascularization of an occluded splanchnic vessel should be considered, even in the absence of clinical symptoms; patients being considered for distal aortic surgery, or endograft placement, who possess a large, meandering artery being supplied by the IMA, due to the presence of an SMA stenosis or occlusion. Such patients are at considerable risk of mesenteric ischemia, should the IMA supply to the bowel be interrupted by the planned surgical or endovascular procedure, and revascularization of the SMA is indicated.

REFERENCES

1. Boley SJ, Sprayregen S, Veith FJ, et al. An aggressive roentgenologic and surgical approach to acute mesenteric ischemia. *Surg Annu*. 1973;5:355–378.
2. Kaleya RN, Boley SJ. Acute mesenteric ischemia: an aggressive diagnostic and therapeutic approach. 1991 Roussel Lecture. *Can J Surg*. 1992;35(6):613–623.
3. Brandt LJ, Boley SJ. AGA technical review on intestinal ischemia. American Gastrointestinal Association. *Gastroenterology*. 2000;118(5):954–968.
4. Trompeter M, Brazda T, Remy CT, et al. Non-occlusive mesenteric ischemia: etiology, diagnosis, and interventional therapy. *Eur Radiol*. 2002;12(5):1179–1187.
5. Kumar S, Sarr MG, Kamath PS. Mesenteric venous thrombosis. *N Engl J Med*. 2001;345(23):1683–1688.
6. Sheeran S. Acute mesenteric ischemia: recent advances in diagnosis and endovascular therapy. *Emergency Radiology*. 2000;7(4):231–236.
7. Kirkpatrick ID, Kroeker MA, Greenberg HM. Biphasic CT with mesenteric CT angiography in the evaluation of acute mesenteric ischemia: initial experience. *Radiology*. 2003;229(1):91–98.
8. Boley SJ, Feinstein FR, Sammartano R, et al. New concepts in the management of emboli of the superior mesenteric artery. *Surg Gynecol Obstet*. 1981;153(4):561–569.
9. Simo G, Echenagusia AJ, Camunez F, et al. Superior mesenteric arterial embolism: local fibrinolytic treatment with urokinase. *Radiology*. 1997;204(3):775–779.
10. Rivitz SM, Geller SC, Hahn C, et al. Treatment of acute mesenteric venous thrombosis with transjugular intramesenteric urokinase infusion. *J Vasc Interv Radiol*. 1995;6(2):219–223; discussion 224–228.
11. American Gastroenterological Association Medical Position Statement: guidelines on intestinal ischemia. *Gastroenterology*. 2000;118(5):951–953.
12. Mikkelsen WP. Intestinal angina: its surgical significance. *Am J Surg*. 1957;94:262.
13. Conner LA. A discussion of the role of arterial thrombosis in the visceral disease of middle life, based upon analogies form coronary thrombosis. *Am J Med Sci*. 1933;185:13.
14. Cognet F, Ben Salem D, Dranssart M, et al. Chronic mesenteric ischemia: imaging and percutaneous treatment. *Radiographics*. 2002;22(4):863–879; discussion 879–880.
15. Jarvinen O, Laurikka J, Sisto T, et al. Atherosclerosis of the visceral arteries. *Vasa*. 1995;24(1):9–14.
16. Nyman U, Ivancev K, Lindh M, et al. Endovascular treatment of chronic mesenteric ischemia: report of five cases. *Cardiovasc Intervent Radiol*. 1998;21(4):305–313.
17. Rha SE, Ha HK, Lee SH, et al. CT and MR imaging findings of bowel ischemia from various primary causes. *Radiographics*. 2000;20(1):29–42.
18. Perko MJ. Duplex ultrasound for assessment of superior mesenteric artery blood flow. *Eur J Vasc Endovasc Surg*. 2001;21(2):106–117.
19. Horton KM, Fishman EK. 3D CT angiography of the celiac and superior mesenteric arteries with multidetector CT data sets: preliminary observations. *Abdom Imaging*. 2000;25(5):523–525.
20. Meaney JF, Prince MR, Nostrant TT, et al. Gadolinium-enhanced MR angiography of visceral arteries in patients with suspected chronic mesenteric ischemia. *J Magn Reson Imaging*. 1997;7(1):171–176.
21. Steinmetz E, Tatou E, Favier-Blavoux C, et al. Endovascular treatment as first choice in chronic intestinal ischemia. *Ann Vasc Surg*. 2002;16(6):693–699.
22. Tytle TL, Prati RC, Jr. Percutaneous recanalization in chronic occlusion of the superior mesenteric artery. *J Vasc Interv Radiol*. 1995;6(1):133–136.
23. Goertler K, ed. *Das Gefassystem in Bauchraum aus der Sicht des Pathologen*. Stuttgart: Thieme; 1968. Bertelheimer H, Heisig N, eds. Aktuelle Gastroenterologie.

CHAPTER 19

Management of Complications: Surgical and Endovascular

Herbert D. Aronow and Kenneth Ouriel

Major complications of endovascular therapy include those that result in an unanticipated intensification in the level of care, prolongation of hospital stay, and occurrence of irreversible or prolonged morbidity, or death; all other complications are considered minor. Accepting the variation in specific outcomes captured and the manner in which they are defined, a number of operator-, patient-, procedure-, and lesion-related factors have been shown to predict an increased risk of complications (Table 19-1).

A number of large series, spanning the last 2 decades, indicate that major complications comprise nearly half of all endovascular therapeutic complications, and occur in approximately 5 to 6% of procedures; approximately 2 to 4% of these ultimately require surgical bail out (1–5). Vascular access site complications and distal embolization are the most common. Target site complications, such as perforation, severe dissection, and loss of intravascular foreign objects, occur much less frequently. The management, both endovascular and surgical, of these endovascular procedural complications will be reviewed herein.

VASCULAR ACCESS SITE COMPLICATIONS

Vascular access site complications are the most common adverse sequelae resulting from invasive catheter-based procedures. Among these, the most common include bleeding, formation of pseudoaneurysms and arteriovenous fistulae, dissection, and infection.

Bleeding

Localized bleeding at the access site is most commonly seen with femoral artery access use. In contrast, brachial and radial artery access are rarely associated with bleeding complications. Bleeding rates have declined with the widespread practice of cessation and occasionally, reversal, of heparin at the completion of the procedure, and a strategy of early sheath removal. Management of access site bleeding will depend upon the severity of the bleed and the hemodynamic impact on the patient. The first line of therapy should include compression (i.e., either manual or mechanical) at, and slightly above, the access site. For significant bleeds, prompt reversal of the effects of any anticoagulant, fibrinolytic, and some antiplatelet agents is indicated (Table 19-2).

When bleeding is accompanied by hemodynamic embarrassment, patients should be managed with aggressive fluid resuscitation (i.e., crystalloid and if necessary, colloid); pressors should be reserved for hemodynamic compromise refractory to volume resuscitation. In the event that these more conservative strategies fail, endovascular or surgical therapy should be considered.

Retroperitoneal bleeds complicate femoral artery access and occur in less than 0.5% of interventional procedures. The likelihood of a

TABLE 19-1

Factors Influencing Complications During Peripheral Vascular Intervention

Factor
Operator-related factors
Operator experience
Patient-related factors
Clinical presentation—e.g. claudication versus critical limb ischemia
Presence of co-morbidities
Lesion-related factors
Lesion stenosis versus occlusion
Severe lesion calcification
Vessel tortuosity
Presence of thrombus
Lesion location—e.g., aortoiliac versus superficial femoral artery
Procedure-related factors
Diagnostic versus interventional procedure

retroperitoneal bleed is increased with high femoral or back wall arterial punctures. The development of hypotension, with abdominal pain or distention during, or after, a procedure should raise suspicion for this complication. Ipsilateral lower quadrant fullness, tenderness, and guarding are particularly sensitive findings. It is important to emphasize that the diagnosis is primarily a clinical one, and therapy should never be delayed by attempts to obtain confirmation by diagnostic studies (i.e., computed tomography [CT] scan of abdomen and pelvis).

Initial stabilization should include compression over, and above, the femoral access site, volume resuscitation, reversal of anticoagulant/ fibrinolytic/antiplatelet effects, and pressors, used as described above. In the vast majority of cases, such therapies will be successful in stabilizing the patient. When these are unsuccessful, emergency angiography, from the contralateral-femoral artery or an upper extremity artery, should be performed to localize the source of bleeding. Balloon tamponade may be employed as an initial endovascular measure. Should this

measure fail, stent grafting (see below), or open surgical repair should be considered.

Pseudoaneurysm

In prospective ultrasonographic studies, the incidence of post-catheterization pseudoaneurysm ranges from about 1 to 8% (23–25), more commonly following interventional than diagnostic procedures. Most pseudoaneurysms occur in the femoral artery, as this is the most common site for vascular access; however these complications may occur at any arterial access site. In the groin, pseudoaneurysms are often associated with low arterial access. Clinical manifestations include pain, swelling, ecchymosis, an audible bruit or palpable thrill, and a pulsatile mass. Pseudoaneurysms may be complicated by rupture, prolonged pain and swelling adjacent to the vascular access site, neuropathy, skin necrosis, infection, and distal embolization (26).

Duplex ultrasound is the diagnostic modality of choice, typically revealing a poorly echogenic mass adjacent to the artery, and color Doppler revealing systolic flow in the neck of the aneurysm (Fig. 19-1).

Management options depend upon the pseudoaneurysm size and associated symptoms. Most small pseudoaneurysms (i.e., about 2 cm, or less) will spontaneously thrombose, over time; this may be documented by repeat ultrasound 2 to 4 weeks later, and they do not require treatment unless symptomatic. Nevertheless, many operators treat pseudoaneurysms, given that the alternative may entail a prolonged hospital stay, a delay in patient ambulation, and repeat ultrasound assessments. Treatment options for larger pseudoaneurysms include ultrasound-guided compression, thrombin or collagen injection, coil insertion, covered stenting, or surgical repair.

Ultrasound-Guided Compression

Ultrasound-guided compression was first described in 1991 (27), and quickly emerged as a first-line treatment for pseudoaneurysms, following endovascular procedures. The technique involves positioning the ultrasound probe immediately above the pseudoaneurysm neck (i.e., confirmed with color Doppler) and compressing it until flow is abolished. Repeat duplex ultrasound is performed 10 minutes later; if

TABLE 19-2

Summary of Agents Used to Reverse the Effects of Anticoagulant, Fibrinolytic, and Antiplatelet Agents Used During Peripheral Vascular Intervention

Drug	Reversal Agent	Dosage	Comment
Anticoagulant			
Unfractionated Heparin	Protamine	1 mg per 100 units of heparin IV (to max 50 mg)	Potential for allergic/anaphylactic reaction
Low molecular weight heparin	Protamine	1 mg per 100 anti—Xa units	Effect likely mediated by neutralizing higher molecular weight fractions of heparin. No effect on lower molecular weight fractions.
Direct antithrombins	N/A	—	No available reversal agents
Fibrinolytic	Fresh frozen plasma	15 ml/Kg	First-line therapy
	Cryoprecipitate	1 Bag per 10 Kg	First-line therapy
	Aminocaproic acid	Same dosing by oral or IV routes—5 g during first hour, followed by 1–1.25 g/hour for approximately 8 hours or until bleeding stops	Used as a last resort
Antiplatelet			
Glycoprotein IIb/IIIa agents			
Abciximab	Platelet transfusion	6 units, repeated if necessary	Produces partial reversal of effect
Tirofiban	N/A	—	Effect of drug wears off after ∼ 4 hours
Eptifibatide	N/A	—	Effect of drug wears off after ∼ 4 hours

thrombosis has occurred, it is considered a success. If flow persists, compression may be repeated several times but usually for no more than a total of 30 to 40 minute. The disadvantages of this approach include patient discomfort (i.e., conscious sedation is usually required), the large time commitment by the ultrasonographer, and limited efficacy (about 60 to 90% success) (26,28). The likelihood of success is further compromised in patients who are obese, have large pseudoaneurysms, and those who are anticoagulated.

Complications of ultrasound-guided compression are uncommon but include increased pain, pseudoaneurysm rupture, distal embolization, and deep vein thrombosis. Other methods may be employed for compression, including use of the heel of one's hand or a finger, with simultaneous ultrasound imaging, or the application of a mechanical-compression device, such as the Femostop or a C-clamp. In general, compression should be avoided in the presence of limb ischemia, infection, or with a tense hematoma. Although ultrasound-guided compression essentially replaced surgery as the primary mode of treatment for pseudoaneurysms, it too has now been replaced, largely, by thrombin injection as the procedure of choice.

Thrombin Injection

Injection of thrombin directly into the pseudoaneurysm sac to promote thrombosis was first

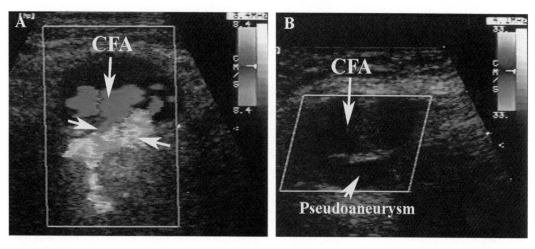

FIGURE 19-1 ● Common femoral artery pseudoaneurysm before **(A)** and after **(B)** percutaneous thrombin injection. From Mohler et al. Therapeutic thrombin injection of pseudoaneurysms: a multi-center experience. *Vasc Med.* 2001;6: 241–244. White arrows indicate neck of pseudoaneurysm. CFA, common femoral artery.

described in 1986 (29). Nevertheless, thrombin and other tissue adhesive injections were not commonly employed until more recently. Currently, pooled human thrombin preparations are used. Thrombin may also be harvested from patients' own blood, if they are not currently on anticoagulant therapy (30): thrombin is extracted from 30 to 60 mL of venous blood, in a procedure that requires approximately 30 to 60 minutes.

Regardless of its source, thrombin may be injected into the aneurysm sac through a number of techniques, including transarterial, percutaneous, and percutaneous with simultaneous balloon occlusion. Transarterial injection requires the introduction of a catheter into the arterial vasculature and its advancement into the pseudoaneurysm neck. Thrombin is then injected into the pseudoaneurysm sac (i.e., use of alternative agents such as collagen (31) and cyanoacrylate (32) have been described). As common femoral artery pseudoaneurysms usually require contralateral access, with aortoiliac crossover, this technique is relatively complicated, given the available alternatives, and should be reserved for those cases in which thrombin may not be injected percutaneously.

Percutaneous thrombin injection, without balloon protection, is the most commonly employed means used to treat pseudoaneurysm today. This technique may be performed in the outpatient setting, in a room equipped with an ultrasound machine and a 5 MHz to 7.5 MHz linear transducer.

The pseudoaneurysm, its neck, and adjacent vessels are identified on ultrasound, and a 19-gauge to 22-gauge needle is inserted under sterile conditions, through the skin into the sac, under ultrasound guidance. Thrombin is injected slowly, over approximately 10 seconds, until there is cessation of flow within the pseudoaneurysm. If flow in the neck persists, an additional dose is administered. Once the pseudoaneurysm sac thromboses, no additional thrombin should be injected, even when flow remains in the neck, as doing so might result in distal embolization.

There is significant variability in the amount of thrombin required to thrombose a pseudoaneurysm. On average, approximately 300 IU of thrombin are required, however multiloculated pseudoaneurysms may necessitate injections in multiple sites, and the use of more than 1000 IU of thrombin. In an attempt to prevent thrombin or thrombus from leaving the pseudoaneurysm sac and moving distally into the arterial tree, some operators have advocated simultaneous balloon inflation in the culprit artery, while injecting thrombin under ultrasound guidance. This technique requires reaccessing the arterial vasculature, and in the case of femoral artery pseudoaneurysms, using a contralateral approach. Since studies have shown no difference in complication rates after percutaneous thrombin injection, with or without balloon protection, and historically lower complication rates following the latter, balloon protection has, largely, been abandoned.

Some operators still use balloon protection (i.e., balloon sized 1:1 to the reference vessel diameter) for pseudoaneurysms with wide and short (i.e., less than 3 mm) necks.

Regardless of the thrombin injection method employed, a peripheral pulse examination should be performed at baseline, and again following the injection, to rule out significant distal embolization. Patients should remain on bed rest for 4 to 6 hours following thrombin injection. Some operators repeat an ultrasound exam the following day, others wait 7 to 10 days, and some do not repeat the ultrasound except when there are clinical findings to suggest persistence or recurrence of a pseudoaneurysm.

Overall, thrombin injection is successful in more than 93% of cases (26). While no randomized, head-to-head studies have compared ultrasound-guided compression with thrombin injection, historical success rates are much greater with the latter, and thrombin injection has therefore replaced compression, at most centers. The overall complication rate in most thrombin injection series is less than 4% (26). Distal embolization is the most common adverse outcome; aiming the needle away from the pseudoaneurysm neck during injection may reduce its incidence. Patients with minor symptoms of ischemia may be heparinized and carefully observed for clinical deterioration. If severe ischemia develops, patients should undergo emergency angiography, and distal embolization should be treated with mechanical or suction thrombectomy, or intra-arterial fibrinolysis. Surgical exploration and thrombectomy should be reserved for endovascular treatment failures.

Coil Embolization and Stent Grafting

If thrombin injection or ultrasound-guided compression fails, consideration should be given to an endovascular approach before proceeding to surgery. Surgery may be associated with significant morbidity and mortality in this cohort of patients with atherosclerotic vascular disease. Visualizing the pseudoaneurysm origin typically requires angiography from multiple projections, and often necessitates selective, superficial, and profunda femoral artery injections. The use of transarterial coil embolization, to treat pseudoaneurysms successfully, has been reported in a number of cases (32). For pseudoaneurysms with

smaller necks, 0.014″ coils may be delivered via a 3-Fr Tracker catheter; 0.035″ coils may be delivered through a 5-Fr angiographic catheter, for those with larger necks. Although coil embolization may be effective, it usually requires repeat arterial access; percutaneous coil embolization has been described) (33,34), is quite time consuming, may prevent shrinkage of the cavity after treatment, and may be associated with patient discomfort and pressure necrosis when placed superficially.

Stent grafting is another potential endovascular alternative (see below) (32,35). Despite its apparent efficacy in excluding pseudoaneurysm necks, a number of disadvantages preclude routine use. In particular, stent grafts may compromise important branch vessels, prohibit future vascular access at the same site, are associated with higher rates of subacute stent thrombosis and late stent failure, and are cost prohibitive for use as routine treatment of these complications.

Surgery

Given the spectrum of available non-surgical therapeutic options, surgical repair of a pseudoaneurysm should be reserved for uncontrolled hemorrhage at an incompressible site, rapid expansion, infection, local or distal limb ischemia, neuropathy, or failure of endovascular management (26).

Arteriovenous Fistulae

Arteriovenous fistulae (AVF) result from inadvertent punctures of the artery and adjacent vein during arterial access, and occur in about 0.4% of interventional procedures (Fig. 19-2) (36).

They are more common following low or high arterial punctures and in the setting of anticoagulation. Typically, AVF are clinically silent. When symptomatic, they manifest as extremity swelling and tenderness from venous distention, sometimes accompanied by arterial insufficiency, when severe. High-output heart failure may develop with significant arteriovenous shunting. On examination, a continuous murmur is pathognomonic. Most AVF are small in size and will close, spontaneously. Clinically relevant AVF require closure for relief of symptoms. Therapeutic options include ultrasound-guided compression, arterial stent graft placement (see

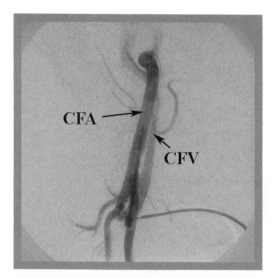

FIGURE 19-2 ● Asymptomatic right common femoral arteriovenous fistula discovered one year following a diagnostic left heart catheterization. CFA, common femoral artery; CFV, common femoral vein.

below), coil embolization, and surgical repair; the latter should be reserved for those patients who fail endovascular management.

Infection

Access site infection is an infrequent but potentially devastating complication of arterial access. It occurs in less than 1% of all cases, and may manifest as fever, a fluctuant mass, purulent wound drainage, or local pain. Typical culprit organisms include *Staphylococcus aureus* and *Staphylococcus epidermidis*. In addition to appropriate, empiric antibiotic coverage, surgical exploration and debridement is usually necessary.

DISTAL EMBOLIZATION

Distal embolization during endovascular procedures typically results from either atherothrombotic material dislodged during wiring, device manipulation, or device actuation.

Microembolization

Distal microembolization occurs frequently during endovascular procedures (37,38). It is detectable on real-time Doppler ultrasound examination, CT, magnetic resonance imaging (MRI),

organ-specific biochemical assays (e.g., creatine kinase), microscopic examination of debris retrieved from embolic protection devices, and occasionally on histologic examination of end-organ tissue specimens. The clinical manifestations of distal microembolization will depend on the burden of embolized material, the recipient vascular bed, and its tolerance to the microembolic insult.

In some vascular beds, microembolization is seldom clinically apparent (e.g., upper and lower extremity arterial vasculature) while in others, the result may be catastrophic (e.g., stroke in the cerebral bed, or worsening renal insufficiency in the renal vasculature), respectively. Because microemboli culminate in a more down-stream insult, collateral circulation is less well able to ameliorate its impact than in the case of macroemboli; ultimately, microemboli reside in capillaries subtended by these collateral vessels.

The management of distal microembolization should be directed both at prevention and treatment, although the former is clearly more effective. Embolic protection devices may be used to minimize microembolization during endovascular procedures (see Chapter 6). When microembolization during an endovascular procedure may not be prevented, the available therapeutic options are limited. Pharmacologic management, in this situation, is based upon data extrapolated from the treatment of slow flow, and no reflow, in the coronary vasculature, and includes the use of intra-arterial verapamil (100 mcg to 200 mcg boluses) or adenosine (24 mcg to 96 mcg boluses) (39,40). Likewise, while the platelet glycoprotein (GP) IIb/IIIa inhibitors—abciximab, integrelin, and tirofiban—confer clinical benefit by reducing platelet aggregation and preventing distal embolization in the coronary bed, their clinical benefits are less well established in the peripheral vasculature. Data to support the routine, prophylactic or therapeutic use of these agents, in the setting of peripheral arterial intervention, are preliminary (41–43).

Macroembolization

Macroembolization (i.e., embolization of large particulate atherothrombotic material) is one of the most common complications of endovascular intervention. Macroembolization is defined

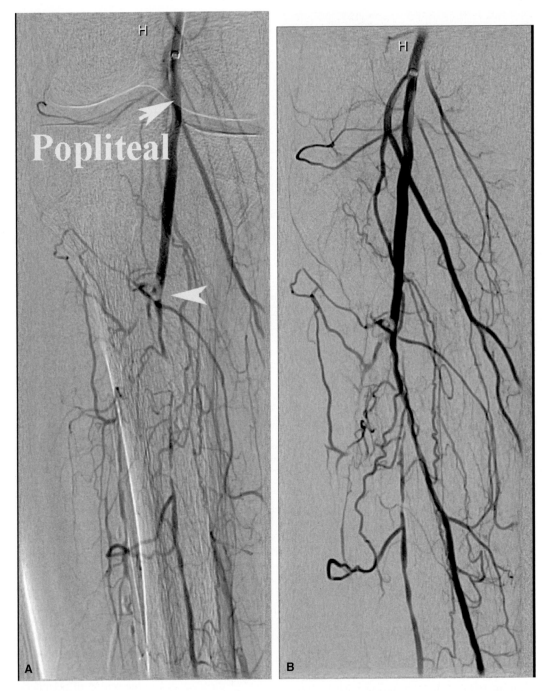

FIGURE 19-3 ● **A:** Distal atheromatous embolization to the right tibioperoneal trunk (*indicated by arrowhead*) during an intervention performed for limb salvage. **B:** angiogram following angioplasty performed at the anterior tibial-tibioperoneal trunk bifurcation.

angiographically as a new occlusion of the distal parent vessel, or any of its branches, post-intervention (Fig. 19-3).

In the lower extremities, it occurs in approximately 2 to 5% of procedures and is more com-

mon following recanalization of total occlusions than in treatment of stenoses (1,5,44). A number of therapeutic maneuvers are available for the treatment of distal macroembolization, including aspiration (45–47), mechanical thrombectomy

(48), angioplasty (49), thrombolysis and surgery (50).

Appropriate management will depend on the size and composition of the embolus, and the location of the embolized fragment. Smaller emboli may sometimes be aspirated through a low-profile aspiration catheter (e.g., Export Catheter, Pronto Extraction Catheter), advanced beyond the angioplasty site to the area of occlusion. Larger emboli may be managed in a number of ways. Negative pressure (i.e., through use of a Luer-lock syringe) may be applied to a diagnostic- or guide catheter in order to affix the embolus to the distal tip; the catheter and embolus may then be removed as a single unit, via the vascular sheath. If this method fails (e.g., when the embolus is too large, nondeformable or irregular in shape), emboli may be captured using a similar method, but advanced into a less important distal branch where redundant circulation exists, and released (i.e., the "push and park" method) (44); this method should be reserved for cases when no other viable alternatives exist.

Snares or baskets may also be of use in securing and removing an embolus (i.e., see intravascular foreign object retrieval, later in this chapter), especially when primarily atheromatous in composition. In cases where the embolus is predominately thrombotic, angioplasty to mold the embolus against the vessel wall, mechanical thrombectomy (e.g., Angiojet), coil retrieval (Merci Retrieval System), or local fibrinolysis may be employed. If the above measures fail to relieve on-going, end-organ, or limb ischemia, surgical embolectomy with a Fogarty catheter should be considered.

PERFORATIONS

Perforations were once among the most dreaded complications of endovascular therapy. While their incidence has remained relatively constant over time, evolution in equipment and techniques have led to a paradigm shift, from surgical to endovascular management (6). In the face of a vascular perforation, the most critical issue is location. Bleeding into the thoracic, abdominal, or pelvic cavities represents a life-threatening emergency. Hence, perforations of the innominate artery, proximal left common carotid artery, proximal subclavian artery, aorta, and iliac vessels, are the most serious. Perforations into

compartmentalized spaces are likely to be self-limited. The elevated pressure in the space is responsible for compartment syndromes, but also limits further hemorrhage, making the complication less life-threatening. Exceptions to the rule exist; for example, perforation of the internal carotid may produce a hematoma that compromises the airway, and therefore poses a significant risk.

Wire perforations tend to occur distally in the vascular tree and are usually minor. Stiffer, straight-tipped, and hydrophilic wires are more likely to produce this complication. Major perforations are most commonly associated with vessel angioplasty and stenting, which produce frank vessel tearing and perforation. This often results from oversizing of balloons or stents. Since heavy lesion calcification provides resistance to full balloon or stent expansion, higher inflation pressures are often used in this circumstance, which increases the risk of perforation. Heavy vessel calcification, in itself, is also likely to increase the predisposition to vessel tearing at normal inflation pressures.

Prompt recognition of vascular perforation is essential, as hematoma formation or hemodynamic compromise may occur, rapidly. In general, one should manage vessel perforation with simultaneous pharmacologic and mechanical interventions. Prompt reversal of anticoagulation is indicated. Intravenous fluids and pressor agents should be administered as necessary for hemodynamic stabilization. Mechanical approaches include prolonged balloon inflation, stent grafting, and coil embolization; when these fail, open surgery (i.e., repair or bypass) is indicated.

Prolonged Balloon Inflation

Multiple, prolonged (i.e., several minutes each) balloon inflations (i.e., 1.2:1 balloon: artery ratio), at lower than nominal pressure, may allow time for a perforation to seal; this strategy may be more effective for wire, rather than device perforations but may be attempted in either situation (Fig. 19-4). Angiography between balloon inflations will confirm whether this maneuver has achieved hemostasis.

Stent Grafting

Stent grafts are composite devices comprising a metallic skeleton in association with

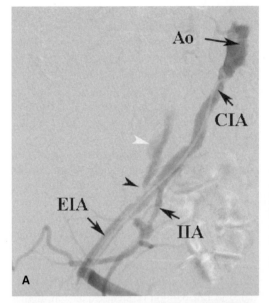

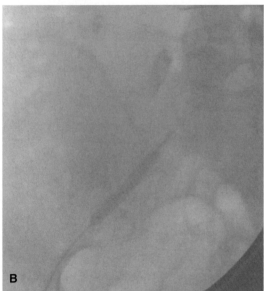

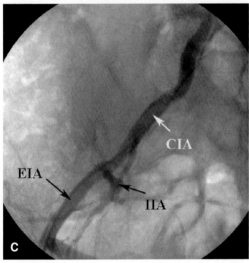

FIGURE 19-4 ● **Endovascular repair of right external iliac artery perforation. A:** Perforation (*indicated by black arrowhead*) of the right external iliac artery into the pelvic space (*indicated by white arrowhead*) following advancement of a wire and catheter. **B:** A Wholey wire was quickly advanced across the site of the perforation into the distal aorta and a 6.0 × 40-mm Opta-Pro balloon was inflated for several minutes. **C:** Final angiography showing complete cessation of flow through perforation achieved using prolonged balloon inflation alone. Ao, aorta; CIA, common iliac artery; EIA, external iliac artery; IIA, internal iliac artery.

FIGURE 19-5 ● **Management of complicated left common iliac artery (CIA) perforation. A:** Baseline pelvic aortogram demonstrating proximal occlusion of the left CIA. The occlusion was approached in an antegrade manner, using left brachial artery access. The wire exited through the vessel wall and an angioplasty balloon was advanced over the wire before this complication was recognized. This resulted in perforation of the left CIA, which did not resolve with reversal of anticoagulation and prolonged inflation of a 6.0 × 20 mm Opta-Pro balloon inflated at the origin of the left CIA. **B:** Subsequent angiogram from the right common femoral artery (CFA) demonstrating perforation of the left CIA at the site of occlusion (*indicated by black arrowheads*). **C:** Prolonged inflation of 18 mm (diameter) × 2.0 cm (length) XXL balloon (introduced from the right CFA) in the distal aorta was performed to achieve hemostasis. **D:** A 6-Fr shuttle sheath was introduced from the right brachial artery and a 4.0 × 20 mm Opta-Pro balloon was passed into the origin of the left CIA. Two tornado coils (10-mm diameter) were deployed in the stump of the left CIA. **E:** Final angiography demonstrating sealing of the perforation. Black arrowhead indicates the position of the coils.

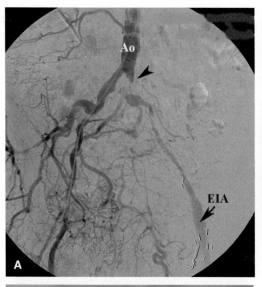

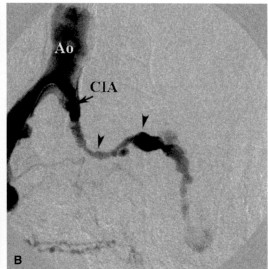

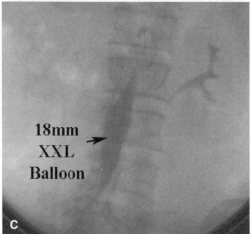

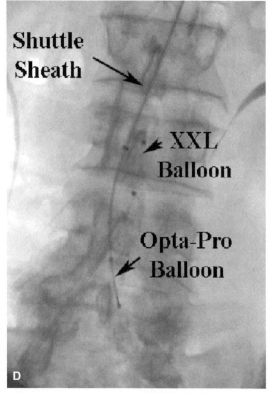

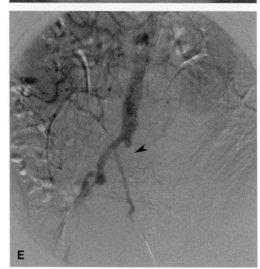

synthetic graft material. The graft material either may be attached to the external or internal surface of the stent, or may be sandwiched between two stents. Most stent grafts are self-expanding (e.g., aSpire, Cragg Endopro System I [not available in the United States], Hemobahn/Viabahn, and Wallgraft), and are available in sizes ranging from 6 mm to 14 mm, in diameter. The Jostent is the only available, balloon-expandable, covered stent; its availability in the United States is limited to 3-mm, 4-mm, and 5-mm diameter sizes, and hence is useful for treating perforations in smaller vessels.

The advantage of using a stent graft is the efficiency with which it may be deployed. For this reason, when conservative measures and balloon tamponade fail, stent grafting should be considered, particular in hemodynamically unstable patients. Nevertheless, there are a number of noteworthy disadvantages to stent grafting. Blood flow to important side branches may be compromised by the graft (e.g., internal iliac artery). Vascular access sites (e.g., common femoral artery) may no longer be accessible subsequent to their deployment, an issue that may be particularly germane in patients with vascular disease who are likely to need repeat intervention. Finally, the use of graft material results in a bulkier device profile than uncovered stents, necessitating the use of larger delivery systems (7 Fr to 14 Fr). As a result, these devices may be associated with a greater frequency of vascular access site complications.

Coil Embolization

Coil embolization is generally reserved for situations where conservative measures or balloon tamponade have failed (Fig. 19-5). Pushable or detachable bare, coated, or biologically active coils may be successfully deployed within the perforated vessel (if its occlusion is expected to occur without clinical sequelae) or into the perforation tract itself. Unlike pushable coils, their detachable counterparts may be withdrawn, if improperly positioned.

In addition to the general approach to managing vascular perforations outlined above, a few caveats regarding particular vascular territories are noteworthy, and are defined below.

Aortic

During peripheral arterial intervention, the situations in which aortic perforation is likely to occur include stenting of the aortic bifurcation, recanalization of occlusions of the iliac or origins of the great vessels of the aortic arch, when approaching from the periphery toward the aorta, and during aneurysm exclusion procedures (12). Low-pressure balloon inflation may be attempted for very small, and hemodynamically insignificant, perforations. It is important to have a small supply of larger diameter balloons for use in the aorta, in such emergency situations (e.g., XXL, with diameters ranging between 12 mm and 18 mm; MAXI LD, with diameters ranging between 14 mm and 25 mm). When this fails, an attempt at stent grafting, using an appropriately sized aortic stent graft, may be worthwhile provided there are no important aortic branches that may be covered by the stent (13). Otherwise, the patient will need to proceed to emergency surgery.

Renal

Renal artery perforation may occur in the setting of diagnostic or therapeutic catheterization, and may occur in as many as 3.6% of renal artery interventions. Back pain at the time of stent deployment or angioplasty is a sign of overexpansion of the renal artery and ostium, and should serve as a caution against further dilation.

Iliac

If a covered stent is required to treat an iliac artery perforation, coverage of the internal iliac artery with the stent graft should be avoided whenever possible, as it may cause buttock claudication, impotence, and rarely, bowel necrosis.

Infrainguinal

The infrainguinal territory includes the common femoral, superficial femoral, popliteal, and infrapopliteal arteries. Lower extremity arterial perforations are a relatively uncommon complication of peripheral angioplasty procedures. Estimates from large series range from 0.2 to 4% of cases (3,8). Hemorrhage in these vessels is usually not life-threatening, but may be limb threatening (Fig. 19-6) (8). Unabated, the accumulation of blood in the thigh or calf may culminate

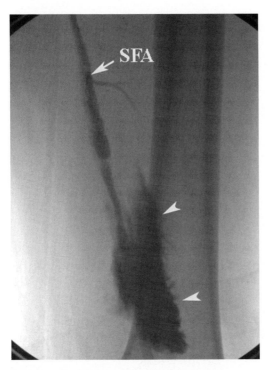

FIGURE 19-6 ● **Complicated superficial femoral artery (SFA) perforation.** Angiogram of the distal left SFA demonstrating significant perforation and extravasation of contrast into the thigh (*indicated by white arrowheads*). Failure to seal this perforation would place the patient at high risk for a compartment syndrome.

in a compartment syndrome, necessitating fasciotomy for decompression and limb salvage.

In the superficial femoral artery (SFA), perforations may occur in which a connection between the SFA and the adjacent deep vein is created (Fig. 19-7). This is a relatively benign form of perforation, since there is little risk of hemorrhage or compartment syndrome. In the authors' experience, this form of perforation usually responds to prolonged balloon inflation or placement of nitinol self-expanding stents.

Subclavian

If covered stents are used to treat a subclavian-artery occlusion, care must be taken not to 'jail' (i.e., cover) the vertebral or internal mammary artery (IMA) branches. Occlusion of the vertebral artery may culminate in cerebral embolization or ischemia, when contralateral vertebral artery disease is present. Occlusion of the IMA may sacrifice a potential, or real, coronary-artery bypass graft conduit.

FLOW-LIMITING DISSECTIONS

During peripheral vascular intervention, two major forms of dissection, retrograde and antegrade (Figs. 19-8 and 19-9), may occur.

Retrograde dissections typically occur when obtaining vascular access as a result of the wire uplifting plaque, as it passes retrograde, toward the aorta. Because antegrade flow typically 'tacks' up these dissections, a conservative approach is generally adopted, provided antegrade flow may be shown to be normal. In the case of an iliac dissection during femoral artery access, this will necessitate obtaining access from an arm artery or the contralateral femoral artery, and performing antegrade angiography of the iliac artery.

In contrast, antegrade dissections are propagated by antegrade flow, increasing the risk of limiting, or abolishing, flow to vital structures, and warrant a more aggressive management strategy. Treatment of an antegrade dissection requires that the guidewire be passed distal to the site of dissection. If a dissection occurs during attempts to wire a stenosis (i.e., no guidewire in the distal vessel lumen), all efforts to traverse the stenosis (i.e., even if subintimal), and re-enter the true vessel lumen, should be made. If the dissection occurs following guide-catheter or sheath manipulation, balloon angioplasty or stenting (i.e., proximal or distal edge dissection), it is critical to preserve guidewire position. The approach to a flow-limiting dissection depends upon the location of the dissection. At important flexion points, where repeated vascular access is likely (e.g., common femoral or popliteal arteries), or where stent deployment is generally contraindicated, prolonged low-pressure balloon inflation may be performed in an effort to 'tack up' the intima. In all other situations, and when prolonged balloon angioplasty fails, stenting is the treatment of choice for flow-limiting dissections.

INTRAVASCULAR RETRIEVAL

With the rapid evolution of endovascular therapeutic procedures, the need to retrieve intravascular foreign objects and embolized atheromatous debris has become more common. The spectrum of foreign objects to be captured and removed has expanded beyond catheter and wire

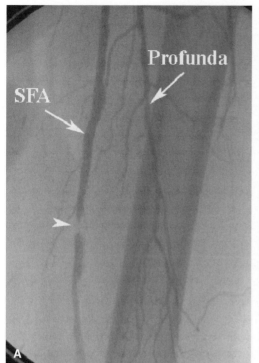

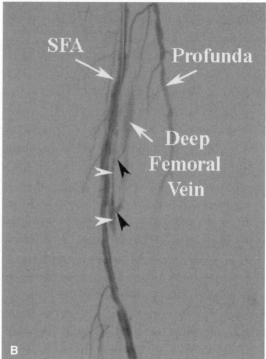

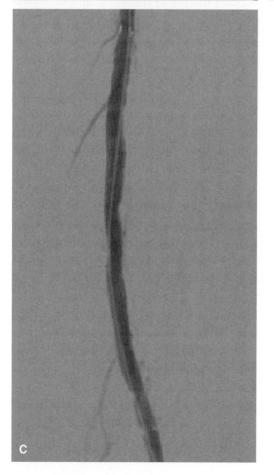

FIGURE 19-7 ● **Benign form of superficial femoral artery (SFA) perforation. A:** Baseline angiogram demonstrating severe stenosis in the left mid-SFA. **B:** Angiogram following angioplasty demonstrating a tear in the wall of the SFA, evidenced by staining of the adventitia (*white arrowheads*), and flow from the SFA (*indicated by black arrowheads*) into the adjacent deep femoral vein. **C:** Final angiography following deployment of self-expanding stent in the SFA.

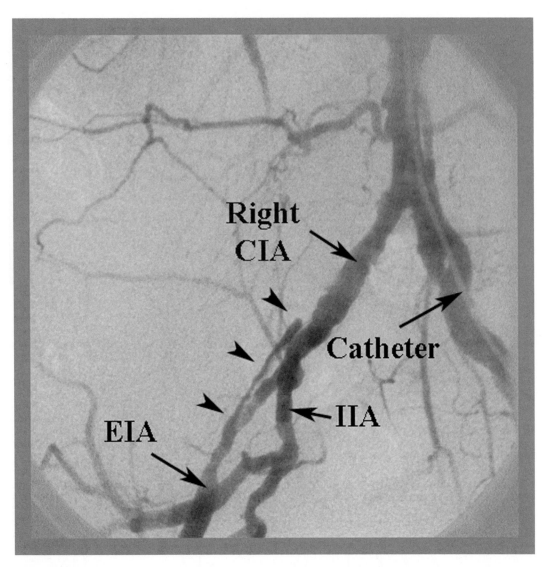

FIGURE 19-8 ● Example of retrograde dissection created by wire during retrograde common femoral artery access. Black arrowheads demonstrate extent of dissection. CIA, common iliac artery; EIA, external iliac artery; IIA, internal iliac artery.

fragments to include stents, balloons, embolization coils, and vena caval filters, among others. Successful retrieval occurs more than 90% of the time, in some series (51). Femoral arterial or venous access is used most frequently, both because this is usually the primary access site for the index procedure, and because these larger diameter vessels will typically accommodate the larger sheaths and guide catheters required for object removal. The ultimate goal in addressing misplaced or lost foreign objects depends upon the nature of the object itself. Most often the aim is to remove or at least relocate the object into a more favorable peripheral vascular segment.

As the spectrum of objects in need of retrieval has grown, so has the armamentarium available for their removal; it now includes snares, baskets, tip-deflecting wires, balloon catheters, forceps, and others (Fig. 19-10).

Early self-made snares opened in a parallel fashion. While it was possible to adjust the loop diameter, it was difficult to direct the snares toward intravascular objects for retrieval. The

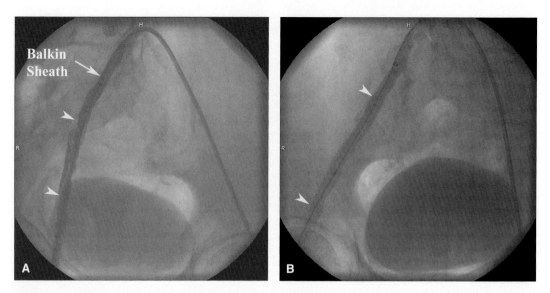

FIGURE 19-9 ● Example of antegrade dissection created during advancement of a Balkin sheath from the left common femoral artery into the contralateral common iliac artery. **A:** Angiogram demonstrating antegrade dissection in right external iliac artery (*extent of dissection indicated by white arrowheads*). **B:** Angiogram following placement of nitinol self-expanding stent (*ends of stent indicated by white arrowheads*) to cover the dissection.

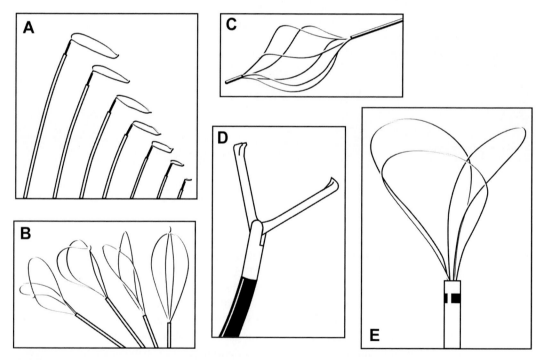

FIGURE 19-10 ● Examples of snares, baskets, and forceps used to retrieve foreign bodies during peripheral vascular intervention. **A:** Goose-neck snare, **B:** Dimension articulating stone baskets, **C:** EPflex grasping basket, **D:** Olympus grasping forceps, **E:** En-snare device.

nitinol gooseneck snare and microsnare (Amplatz) have overcome this disadvantage. The snare and its delivery catheter are advanced through a 5-Fr multipurpose guide catheter but may be used with a variety of catheter shapes and diameters. The snare loop is at a 90° to the snare shaft, and the loop diameter is chosen to match or approximate the diameter of the vessel of interest. When this device fails, a variety of other devices are available.

Snares and baskets are the safest devices since there is little risk of vessel perforation. Forceps should only be used as a last resort, since vessel perforation becomes a significant risk with their use. Before introducing a snare or other retrieval device into the vasculature, it is important to upsize the sheath or guide catheter as necessary, so that the captured object and its retrieval device may be removed as a single unit.

CONCLUSION

An absolute increase in the number of attendant procedural complications is likely to accompany the steady growth in endovascular procedural volume. It should be remembered that "an ounce of prevention is worth a pound of cure." The best way to get out of trouble is to avoid getting there in the first place. To this end, operators should recognize the limits of their experience and skill during case selection, review each successive procedural step, and ensure that all necessary equipment is available before initiating the procedure. Despite these preventive measures, complications will still occur. Having established comfortable working relationships with other operators experienced within one's own specialty or related specialties will be essential in these circumstances.

REFERENCES

1. Gardiner GA, Jr., Meyerovitz MF, Stokes KR, et al. Complications of transluminal angioplasty. *Radiology.* 1986;159:201–208.
2. Becker GJ, Katzen BT, Dake MD. Noncoronary angioplasty. *Radiology.* 1989;170:92–94.
3. Belli AM, Cumberland DC, Knox AM, et al. The complication rate of percutaneous peripheral balloon angioplasty. *Clin Radiol.* 1990;41:380–383.
4. Morse MH, Jeans WD, Cole SE, et al. Complications in percutaneous transluminal angioplasty: relationships with patient age. *Br J Radiol.* 1991;64:5–9.
5. Matsi PJ, Manninen HI. Complications of lower-limb percutaneous transluminal angioplasty: a prospective analysis of 410 procedures on 295 consecutive patients. *Cardiovasc Intervent Radiol.* 1998;21:361–366.
6. Lewis DR, Bullbulia RA, Murphy P, et al. Vascular surgical intervention for complications of cardiovascular radiology: 13 years' experience in a single centre. *Ann R Coll Surg Engl.* 1999;81:23–26.
7. van Lankeren W, Gussenhoven EJ, Pieterman H, et al. Comparison of angiography and intravascular ultrasound before and after balloon angioplasty of the femoropopliteal artery. *Cardiovasc Intervent Radiol.* 1998;21:367–374.
8. Hayes PD, Chokkalingam A, Jones R, et al. Arterial perforation during infrainguinal lower limb angioplasty does not worsen outcome: results from 1409 patients. *J Endovasc Ther.* 2002;9:422–427.
9. Dabbagh A, Chakfe N, Kretz JG, et al. Late complication of a Greenfield filter associating caudal migration and perforation of the abdominal aorta by a ruptured strut. *J Vasc Surg.* 1995;22:182–187.
10. Arafa OE, Pedersen TH, Svennevig JL, et al. Vascular complications of the intraaortic balloon pump in patients undergoing open heart operations: 15-year experience. *Ann Thorac Surg.* 1999;67:645–651.
11. Okabayashi H, Shimada I, Soga Y, et al. [Emergent operation after percutaneous transluminal coronary rotational atherectomy (ROTABLATOR)]. *Kyobu Geka.* 1997;50:1077–1080; discussion 1080–1082.
12. Malina M, Brunkwall J, Ivancev K, et al. Late aortic arch perforation by graft-anchoring stent: complication of endovascular thoracic aneurysm exclusion. *J Endovasc Surg.* 1998;5:274–277.
13. Bautista-Hernandez V, Moya J, Martinell J, et al. Successful stent-grafting for perforation of the thoracic aorta by an intraaortic balloon pump. *Ann Thorac Surg.* 2002;73:956–958.
14. Allaire E, Melliere D, Poussier B, et al. Iliac artery rupture during balloon dilatation: what treatment? *Ann Vasc Surg.* 2003;17:306–314.
15. Baltacioglu F, Cimsit NC, Cil B, et al. Endovascular stent-graft applications in iatrogenic vascular injuries. *Cardiovasc Intervent Radiol.* 2003;26:434–439.
16. Lin PH, Bush RL, Weiss VJ, et al. Subclavian artery disruption resulting from endovascular intervention: treatment options. *J Vasc Surg.* 2000;32:607–611.
17. Bartorelli AL, Trabattoni D, Agrifoglio M, et al. Endovascular repair of iatrogenic subclavian artery perforations using the Hemobahn stent-graft. *J Endovasc Ther.* 2001;8:417–421.
18. Becker GJ, Benenati JF, Zemel G, et al. Percutaneous placement of a balloon-expandable intraluminal graft for life-threatening subclavian arterial hemorrhage. *J Vasc Interv Radiol.* 1991;2:225–229.
19. Xenos ES, Freeman M, Stevens S, et al. Covered stents for injuries of subclavian and axillary arteries. *J Vasc Surg.* 2003;38:451–454.
20. Kato N, Sze DY, Semba CP, et al. Custom-made stent-graft of polytetrafluoroethylene-covered Wallstents: technique and applications. *J Vasc Interv Radiol.* 1999;10:9–16.
21. Schoder M, Cejna M, Holzenbein T, et al. Elective and emergent endovascular treatment of subclavian artery aneurysms and injuries. *J Endovasc Ther.* 2003;10:58–65.
22. Kiemeneij F, Laarman GJ, Odekerken D, et al. A randomized comparison of percutaneous transluminal

coronary angioplasty by the radial, brachial and femoral approaches: the access study. *J Am Coll Cardiol.* 1997; 29:1269–1275.

23. Eichlisberger R, Frauchiger B, Schmitt H, et al. [Aneurysma spurium following arterial catheterization: diagnosis and follow-up]. *Ultraschall Med.* 1992;13: 54–68.
24. Moote DJ, Hilborn MD, Harris KA, et al. Postarteriographic femoral pseudoaneurysms: treatment with ultrasound-guided compression. *Ann Vasc Surg.* 1994;8:325–331.
25. Katzenschlager R, Ugurluoglu A, Ahmadi A, et al. Incidence of pseudoaneurysm after diagnostic and therapeutic angiography. *Radiology.* 1995;195:463–466.
26. Morgan R, Belli AM. Current treatment methods for postcatheterization pseudoaneurysms. *J Vasc Interv Radiol.* 2003;14:697–710.
27. Fellmeth BD, Roberts AC, Bookstein JJ, et al. Postangiographic femoral artery injuries: nonsurgical repair with US-guided compression. *Radiology.* 1991;178:671–675.
28. Wiley JM, White CJ, Uretsky BF. Noncoronary complications of coronary intervention. *Catheter Cardiovasc Interv.* 2002;57:257–265.
29. Cope C, Zeit R. Coagulation of aneurysms by direct percutaneous thrombin injection. *AJR Am J Roentgenol.* 1986;147:383–387.
30. Quarmby JW, Engelke C, Chitolie A, et al. Autologous thrombin for treatment of pseudoaneurysms. *Lancet.* 2002;359:946–947.
31. Hamraoui K, Ernst SM, van Dessel PF, et al. Efficacy and safety of percutaneous treatment of iatrogenic femoral artery pseudoaneurysm by biodegradable collagen injection. *J Am Coll Cardiol.* 2002;39:1297–1304.
32. Waigand J, Uhlich F, Gross CM, et al. Percutaneous treatment of pseudoaneurysms and arteriovenous fistulas after invasive vascular procedures. *Catheter Cardiovasc Interv.* 1999;47:157–164.
33. Lemaire JM, Dondelinger RF. Percutaneous coil embolization of iatrogenic femoral arteriovenous fistula or pseudo-aneurysm. *Eur J Radiol.* 1994;18:96–100.
34. Jain SP, Roubin GS, Iyer SS, et al. Closure of an iatrogenic femoral artery pseudoaneurysm by transcutaneous coil embolization. *Cathet Cardiovasc Diagn.* 1996;39:317–319.
35. Thalhammer C, Kirchherr AS, Uhlich F, et al. Postcatheterization pseudoaneurysms and arteriovenous fistulas: repair with percutaneous implantation of endovascular covered stents. *Radiology.* 2000;214:127–131.
36. Johnson LW, Esente P, Giambartolomei A, et al. Peripheral vascular complications of coronary angioplasty by the femoral and brachial techniques. *Cathet Cardiovasc Diagn.* 1994;31:165–172.
37. Al-Hamali S, Baskerville P, Fraser S, et al. Detection of distal emboli in patients with peripheral arterial stenosis

before and after iliac angioplasty: a prospective study. *J Vasc Surg.* 1999;29:345–351.
38. Topol EJ, Yadav JS. Recognition of the importance of embolization in atherosclerotic vascular disease. *Circulation.* 2000;101:570–580.
39. Piana RN, Paik GY, Moscucci M, et al. Incidence and treatment of 'no-reflow' after percutaneous coronary intervention. *Circulation.* 1994;89:2514–2518.
40. Rosales OR, Eades B, Assali AR. Cardiovascular drugs: adenosine role in coronary syndromes and percutaneous coronary interventions. *Catheter Cardiovasc Interv.* 2004;62:358–363.
41. Shlansky-Goldberg R. Platelet aggregation inhibitors for use in peripheral vascular interventions: what can we learn from the experience in the coronary arteries? *J Vasc Interv Radiol.* 2002;13:229–246.
42. Ouriel K, Castaneda F, McNamara T, et al. Reteplase monotherapy and reteplase/abciximab combination therapy in peripheral arterial occlusive disease: results from the RELAX trial. *J Vasc Interv Radiol.* 2004;15: 229–238.
43. Almeda FQ, Schaer GL. Noncardiac applications of glycoprotein IIb/IIIa inhibitors. *Catheter Cardiovasc Interv.* 2004;62:530–538.
44. Higginson A, Alaeddin F, Fishwick G, et al. "Push and park": an alternative strategy for management of embolic complication during balloon angioplasty. *Eur J Vasc Endovasc Surg.* 2001;21:279–282.
45. Murray JG, Brown AL, Wilkins RA. Percutaneous aspiration thromboembolectomy: a preliminary experience. *Clin Radiol.* 1994;49:553–558.
46. Cleveland TJ, Cumberland DC, Gaines PA. Percutaneous aspiration thromboembolectomy to manage the embolic complications of angioplasty and as an adjunct to thrombolysis. *Clin Radiol.* 1994;49:549–552.
47. Wagner HJ, Starck EE, Reuter P. Long-term results of percutaneous aspiration embolectomy. *Cardiovasc Intervent Radiol.* 1994;17:241–246.
48. Kasirajan K, Haskal ZJ, Ouriel K. The use of mechanical thrombectomy devices in the management of acute peripheral arterial occlusive disease. *J Vasc Interv Radiol.* 2001;12:405–411.
49. Papavassiliou VG, Walker SR, Bolia A, et al. Techniques for the endovascular management of complications following lower limb percutaneous transluminal angioplasty. *Eur J Vasc Endovasc Surg.* 2003;25:125–130.
50. Hoch JR, Tullis MJ, Acher CW, et al. Thrombolysis versus surgery as the initial management for native artery occlusion: efficacy, safety, and cost. *Surgery.* 1994;116:649–656; discussion 656–657.
51. Gabelmann A, Kramer S, Gorich J. Percutaneous retrieval of lost or misplaced intravascular objects. *AJR Am J Roentgenol.* 2001;176:1509–1513.

Index

Note: Page numbers followed by t indicate tables; page numbers followed by f indicate figures.